Diseases of the Spinal Cord

Elke Hattingen • Stefan Weidauer
Matthias Setzer • Johannes C. Klein
Frank Vrionis
Editors

Diseases of the Spinal Cord

Novel Imaging, Diagnosis and Treatment

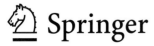

Editors
Elke Hattingen
Institute for Neuroradiology
Goethe-University
Frankfurt
Germany

Stefan Weidauer
Department of Neurology
Sankt Katharinen Hospital
Frankfurt
Germany

Matthias Setzer
Department of Neurosurgery
Goethe-University
Frankfurt
Germany

Johannes C. Klein
Brain Imaging Center (BIC)
Department of Neurology
Goethe-University
Frankfurt
Germany

Frank Vrionis
University of South Florida
H. Lee Moffitt Cancer Center
Tampa
USA

ISBN 978-3-642-54208-4   ISBN 978-3-642-54209-1 (eBook)
DOI 10.1007/978-3-642-54209-1
Springer Heidelberg New York Dordrecht London

Library of Congress Control Number: 2014949350

© Springer-Verlag Berlin Heidelberg 2015
This work is subject to copyright. All rights are reserved by the Publisher, whether the whole or part of the material is concerned, specifically the rights of translation, reprinting, reuse of illustrations, recitation, broadcasting, reproduction on microfilms or in any other physical way, and transmission or information storage and retrieval, electronic adaptation, computer software, or by similar or dissimilar methodology now known or hereafter developed. Exempted from this legal reservation are brief excerpts in connection with reviews or scholarly analysis or material supplied specifically for the purpose of being entered and executed on a computer system, for exclusive use by the purchaser of the work. Duplication of this publication or parts thereof is permitted only under the provisions of the Copyright Law of the Publisher's location, in its current version, and permission for use must always be obtained from Springer. Permissions for use may be obtained through RightsLink at the Copyright Clearance Center. Violations are liable to prosecution under the respective Copyright Law.
The use of general descriptive names, registered names, trademarks, service marks, etc. in this publication does not imply, even in the absence of a specific statement, that such names are exempt from the relevant protective laws and regulations and therefore free for general use.
While the advice and information in this book are believed to be true and accurate at the date of publication, neither the authors nor the editors nor the publisher can accept any legal responsibility for any errors or omissions that may be made. The publisher makes no warranty, express or implied, with respect to the material contained herein.

Printed on acid-free paper

Springer is part of Springer Science+Business Media (www.springer.com)

Contents

1	**Introduction**...	1
	Friedhelm E. Zanella, Helmuth Steinmetz, and Volker Seifert	

Part I Anatomy of the Spine and Spinal Cord

2	**Anatomy of the Spine and Spinal Cord**	5
	Se-Jong You and Elke Hattingen	
3	**Structures of the Spinal Canal**..............................	29
	Se-Jong You and Elke Hattingen	

Part II Imaging Methods

4	**Magnetic Resonance Imaging (MRI) Methods**	39
	Thomas W. Okell, Elke Hattingen, Johannes C. Klein, and Karla L. Miller	
5	**Advanced MRI Methods**	85
	Thomas W. Okell, Elke Hattingen, Johannes C. Klein, and Karla L. Miller	
6	**CSF Dynamics**...	93
	Andreas Gottschalk	
7	**Contrast-Enhanced MR Myelography**	101
	Elke Hattingen and Jürgen Beck	
8	**Myelography and Post-myelographic CT**......................	107
	Elke Hattingen and Stefan Weidauer	

Part III Malformations of the Spine

9	**Malformations of the Spine**	117
	Luciana Porto	

Part IV Diseases of Extramedullary Origin

10 Diseases of Extramedullary Origin: Degenerative Diseases 159
Stefan Weidauer, Michael Nichtweiß, Werner Wichmann,
and Elke Hattingen

**11 Extramedullary Space-Occupying Pathologies:
Epidural and Intradural Extramedullary Disorders** 201
Stefan Dützmann and Matthias Setzer

12 Spinal Trauma... 243
Matthias Setzer

13 Meningeal Disorders....................................... 271
Marlies Wagner and Johannes C. Klein

Part V Diseases of the Spinal Cord

14 Pathophysiological Regards................................ 303
Michael Nichtweiß

15 Inflammation of the Spinal Cord............................ 315
Michael Nichtweiß, Elke Hattingen, and Stefan Weidauer

**16 Metabolic-Toxic Diseases and Atrophic Changes of the
Spinal Cord**.. 369
Michael Nichtweiß, Elke Hattingen, and Stefan Weidauer

17 Gray Matter Diseases of the Spinal Cord.................... 389
Johannes C. Klein

18 Intramedullary Spinal Cord Tumors 395
Kamran Aghayev and Frank Vrionis

**19 Vascular Diseases of the Spine and Spinal Cord and Basics
of Spinal Angiography and Vascular Interventions**.............. 411
Joachim Berkefeld, Stefan Weidauer, and Elke Hattingen

20 Spinal Cord Infarction..................................... 435
Stefan Weidauer, Michael Nichtweiß, and Joachim Berkefeld

Index 453

Introduction

Friedhelm E. Zanella, Helmuth Steinmetz, and Volker Seifert

Spinal diseases constitute a big significant and constantly increasing of the daily practice of neuroradiologists, neurologists and neurosurgeons. Once considered as a stepchild of the neuro-specialities, spinal diseases have also moved into the focus of many practitioners and general radiologists spending much of their clinical and research efforts in this area.

This book is primarily written for last-year residents and fellows in neuroradiology, radiology, neurosurgery and neurology, but it should also be useful for orthopaedic surgeons and advanced spine practitioners.

The editors give an overview of imaging findings in spine and spinal cord diseases with special regard to the anatomical structures of the spinal canal and the spinal cord. This approach should give support to differentiate the pathologies affecting the structures of the spinal canal. It was an utmost concern to illustrate the different pathologies with educative radiological images. However, this book should not replace current neuroradiological picture books. The description of pathophysiological aspects and of clinical findings together with characteristic lesion patterns might enable the reader to interpret diagnostic radiological images in daily clinical practice and to decide sometimes very urgent therapeutic consequences. Instructive

---

F.E. Zanella
Institute for Neuroradiology, Goethe-University,
Schleusenweg 2-16, D-60528 Frankfurt, Germany
e-mail: zanella@em.uni-frankfurt.de

H. Steinmetz
Department of Neurology, Goethe-Universität,
Schleusenweg 2-16, D-60528 Frankfurt, Germany
e-mail: h.steinmetz@em.uni-frankfurt.de

V. Seifert
Department of Neurosurgery, Goethe-Universität,
Schleusenweg 2-16, D-60528 Frankfurt, Germany
e-mail: v.seifert@em.uni-frankfurt.de

tables as well as boxes containing key imaging features were added for differential diagnostic considerations.

The book chapters have been organized in an intuitive and logical sequence. After a thorough overview on the spine and spinal cord anatomy in Sect. II (Chaps. 2 and 3), Sect. III (Chaps. 4, 5, 6, 7, 8) especially MR imaging techniques for the spine, spinal canal and spinal cord including MR angiography, diffusion tensor imaging, CSF dynamics and MR myelography. However, the Chap. 8 of this section addresses traditional myelography and post-myelographic CT investigations, since these techniques have especially to be proven especially valuable in patients who undergo instrumentation techniques in which high-quality MR images are difficult to obtain and also in patients with contraindications for MRI. Section IV (Chap. 9) provides an overview on malformations of the spine and spinal cord, which occur most often in children.

In Sect. V (Chaps. 10, 11, 12, 13) tumorous, degenerative and inflammatory diseases of extramedullary origin are described in detail, and characteristics as well as therapeutic managements of the most important spinal fractures and traumatic spinal cord injuries are reviewed. Chapter 13 of this section deals with disorders of meningeal origin and illustrates relevant neoplastic and inflammatory leptomeningeal diseases. The Sect. VI (Chaps. 14, 15, 16, 17, 18, 19, 20) deals with diseases of the spinal cord with special regard to intramedullary imaging finding on MRI. Pathophysiology, characteristic lesion patterns and also some hints regarding therapeutic options of neoplastic, inflammatory, metabolic-toxic and vascular diseases of the spinal cord are displayed. Chapter 17 addresses especially grey matter diseases.

With the help of additional 13 experts in different fields of clinical neurosciences with special regard to neuroradiology, we have tried to concentrate a broad expertise in this book project. This textbook is comprehensive and yet readable. We hope that the book will enhance the field of spine and spinal cord diseases in clinical practice and ultimately will improve the care for our patients.

Part I
Anatomy of the Spine and Spinal Cord

Anatomy of the Spine and Spinal Cord

2

Se-Jong You and Elke Hattingen

Contents

2.1	Introduction	5
2.2	Vertebral Column and Vertebral Segments	6
	2.2.1 Vertebral Column	6
	2.2.2 Vertebrae	6
	2.2.3 Intervertebral Discs	17
	2.2.4 Joints	20
	2.2.5 Ligaments	24
	2.2.6 Intervertebral Foramina	26

2.1 Introduction

This chapter refers to the structures which surround the spinal cord, giving descriptions of their MR imaging features. These depictions take special regard to the MR imaging characteristics of the developing spine, which may be confounding for an inexperienced viewer. Structures of the spine include the bony and soft tissues forming the spinal canal as well as soft structures which cover the subarachnoid space. Pathologies from all these structures may affect the spinal cord, either due to compression (see Chap. 4) or as consequence of an inflammatory or tumorous disease (Chap. 5).

S.-J. You (✉) • E. Hattingen
Institute for Neuroradiology, Goethe-University,
Schleusenweg 2-16, D-60528 Frankfurt, Germany
e-mail: se-jong.you@kgu.de; elke.hattingen@kgu.de

2.2 Vertebral Column and Vertebral Segments

2.2.1 Vertebral Column

The vertebral column normally consists of 33 spinal vertebrae. There are 7 cervical, 12 thoracic and 5 lumbar articulating vertebrae, while the 5 sacral elements fuse to the os sacrum and the 4–5 coccygeal elements form the coccyx. The number of the coccygeal elements is variable, whereas the number of cervical vertebrae is normally constant. The number of spinal vertebrae varies from 32 to 35.

Imaging: In the lateral view, the vertebral column presents several curves. In the thoracic spine and the pelvis, a kyphotic curve is formed already during foetal development. The lordotic curve develops in the cervical spine when the child is able to hold up its head and to sit upright during the first year of life, while in the lumbar spine the lordotic curve develops at around 12 months when the child begins to stand and walk.

The remainder of this chapter focuses on the non-fused presacral part of the vertebral column.

Figure 2.1 shows a lateral plain film of the cervical spinal canal.

2.2.2 Vertebrae

The common vertebra consists of the body and the arch, which enclose the vertebral foramen. The body consists of a loose trabecular bone, the spongiosa, which contains the bone marrow and is encased by the corticalis. The vertebral bodies increase in width from C2 to L3 and then decrease again in the lower lumbar spine towards the coccyx. The superior and inferior surfaces of the vertebral body are called endplates and consist of a ringlike cortical bone that surrounds the hyaline cartilage plates, which are remnants of the epiphysis of the vertebral body.

The epiphysis of the vertebral body undergoes a ring-like ossification at the age of 8 years and fuses with the vertebral body by the age of 18–21 years.

Imaging: The non-ossified epiphysis and the adjacent intervertebral disc account for the wide intervertebral distance between the ossified centres in children on CT and plain films (Fig. 2.2).

At the posterior surface, an irregular-shaped aperture can be found for the exit of the basivertebral veins from the body of the vertebra. The perivenous fat leads to a bright signal in MRI on T1w. Typically, a strong enhancement can be detected after administration of intravenous contrast agent.

> The non-ossified epiphysis and the adjacent intervertebral disc account for the wide intervertebral distance between the ossified centres in children on CT and plain films.

2 Anatomy of the Spine and Spinal Cord

Fig. 2.1 Alignment of the cervical spine. The following three lines normally show smooth curves: Anterior vertebral line along the anterior margins of the vertebral bodies. Posterior vertebral line which follows the posterior margins of the vertebral bodies. Spinolaminar line at the junction of the spinous processes with laminae. Note, in adults the width of the prevertebral soft tissue should be less than 7 mm at the level of C2 (*star*) and 22 mm at C6 (*arrow*)

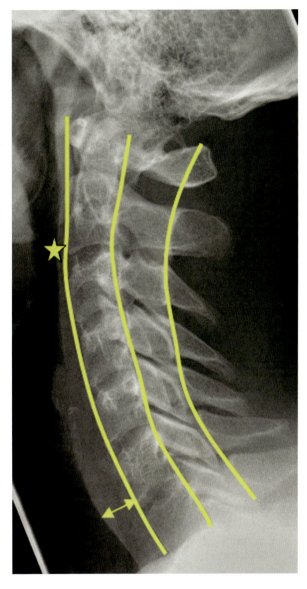

During the first months of life, the appearance of the vertebral bodies on MRI occurs through three subsequent stages:

First month (Fig. 2.3):

The enchondral ossification centres of the vertebral bodies show a lower signal in T1w compared to muscles (Fig. 2.3a). The basivertebral veins appear as a horizontal band of high signal intensity in the centre of the osseous part. The adjacent cartilaginous endplates are markedly hyperintense on T1w

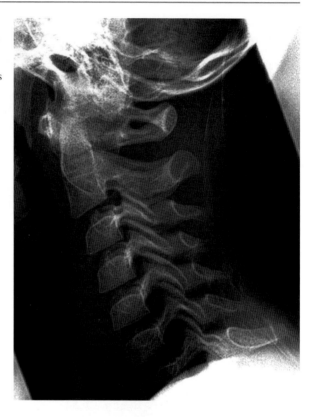

Fig. 2.2 Lateral view of the cervical spine in a 4-year-old male. Image shows wide intervertebral distance due to mainly non-ossified epiphysis of the vertebral bodies and intervertebral discs. Lateral view radiograph

compared to the osseous portion and are each about half the size of the central vertebral component (Fig. 2.3b). In T2w imaging, the osseous part of the vertebral body appears hypointense, while the endplates appear mildly hyperintense compared to muscles (Fig. 2.3c). The administration of contrast agent enhances the cartilaginous endplates and the central osseous portion.

One to six months (Fig. 2.4): The osseous portion of the vertebral body increases in signal intensity on T1w, starting at the superior and inferior portions of the body until the entire vertebral body is involved. Increasing signal intensity can also be detected on T2w until the body becomes isointense with the endplates at the age of 3 months.

From the age of about 7 months (Fig. 2.5): The vertebral bodies become hyperintense on T1w imaging compared to the cartilaginous endplates and surrounding muscles, while the cartilaginous endplates undergo ossification and therefore decrease in signal and incorporate into the vertebral body. On T2w imaging, the whole vertebral body now shows a homogenous and mildly hyperintense signal compared to muscles.

In children and adults the signal intensity of the vertebral body depends on its marrow contents.

Imaging: For children, haematopoietic marrow is dominant resulting in a relatively low signal intensity on T1w in MRI (Figs. 2.3, 2.4 and 2.5). The red marrow

2 Anatomy of the Spine and Spinal Cord

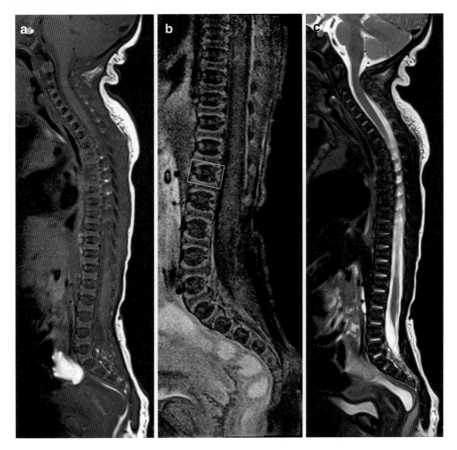

Fig. 2.3 Spine in a 2-day-old newborn. The rectangle in (**b**) marks the contour of the first lumbar vertebral body. Note the hyperintense and prominent cartilaginous endplates on T1w and less obvious on T2w. Sagittal T1w (**a**), sagittal T1with spectral fat saturation (**b**) and sagittal T2w (**c**)

contains intermixed fat so that its signal intensity in T1w is higher compared to muscles and also compared to the intervertebral disc. The haematopoietic marrow markedly enhances after administration of contrast agent.

Fatty conversion of the marrow starts at the age of 8–12 years around the central venous plexus, yielding increasing signal of the vertebral body on T1w. With increasing age, the replacement of the red marrow by fatty marrow continues.

- In older patients the vertebral bodies can show inhomogeneous signal due to focal fatty deposits and fibrous components, which may be misdiagnosed as pathology (Fig. 2.6).
- The contrast enhancement of the vertebral body decreases with fatty conversion and is normally absent in older children and adults.

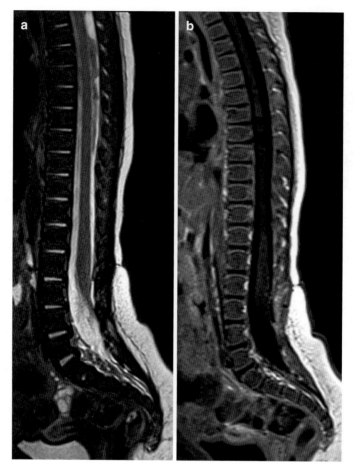

Fig. 2.4 Spine in a 7-week-old infant. The cartilaginous endplates are less prominent and hyperintense on T1w. Contrast-enhanced sagittal T1w (**a**) and sagittal T2w (**b**)

The anterior part of the arch, which on both sides extends from the dorsolateral part of the body, is the pedicle. The dorsal part of the arch is formed by the paired lamina, which join at midline to the spinous process.

Ossification of the dorsal parts of the arch occurs at the age of 2–3 years, while fusion of the anterior part of the arch with the vertebral body takes place at the age of 3–6.

At each side, the transverse processes arise from the lateral parts of the arch. Moreover, a total of four articular processes can be found at the junction of pedicles and lamina which are called zygapophyses. Each side has a superior and inferior process, which articulates with zygapophyses of the adjacent vertebrae to the facet joint. The area between the superior and inferior articular processes is called the interarticular portion (Fig. 2.7).

Around the beginning of puberty, secondary apophyseal ossification centres can be seen at the edges of the spinous and the transverse processes. Synostosis occurs by completion of growth and can be mistakenly diagnosed as a traumatic bone fragment.

2 Anatomy of the Spine and Spinal Cord

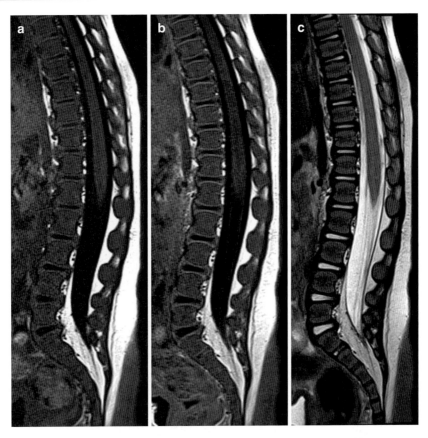

Fig. 2.5 Spine in an 8-month-old infant. Incorporation of the endplates into the vertebral body continues. On T2w the whole vertebral body now shows a homogenous signal. Note the high signal of the nucleus pulposus of the intervertebral disc on T2w. Sagittal T1w (**a**), contrast-enhanced sagittal T1w (**b**) and sagittal T2w (**c**)

Intervertebral (neural) foramen
- Bounded by the pedicles, the facet joints, ligamentum flavum, the posterior surface of the vertebral body and the intervertebral disc
- Contains nerve roots, dorsal root ganglion, arteries, veins and fat

Vertebral canal
- Formed by the vertebral body and arch along with the adjacent vertebrae
- Extends from the foramen magnum to the sacrum
- Contains the spinal cord with its meninges, the cerebrospinal fluid, spinal nerve roots and small vessels

Lateral recess
- The anterolateral portion of the spinal canal
- Bounded anteriorly by the intervertebral disc and the vertebral body, posteriorly by the superior articular process, and laterally by the pedicle
- Merging into the intervertebral foramen
- Contains the spinal nerve roots (Fig. 2.8)

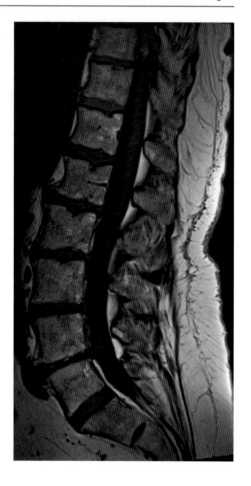

Fig. 2.6 Spine in a 69-year-old male. Sagittal T1w MRI of the lumbar spine shows inhomogeneous signal of the vertebral bodies in this older male due to focal fat deposits

2.2.2.1 Specific Characteristics of the Spine
Cervical Spine (Fig. 2.9)

The first cervical vertebra, the atlas, does not have a vertebral body; instead, paired lateral masses are connected through anterior and posterior arches (Fig. 2.9a). On the inner side of the anterior arch, a facet articulates with the dens axis, which represents a part of the original body of the atlas from phylogenetical point of view. The lateral masses carry the articular facets which articulate with the axis (yellow arrow in Fig. 2.9b) and the occipital condyles. Moreover, there is no spinous process (Fig. 2.9c). The second cervical vertebra, the axis, has a large corpus that is fused to the cranially projecting odontoid process (dens) (Fig. 2.9b, c). A fusion defect may result in an os odontoideum. The os odontoideum may result in craniocervical instability and cord compression (Fig. 2.10).

The relatively small cervical vertebral bodies C3–C7 are broader in the transversal dimension compared to the sagittal dimension (Fig. 2.11a). The lateral edges of the superior surface of the vertebral body turn superiorly and form the uncinate

2 Anatomy of the Spine and Spinal Cord

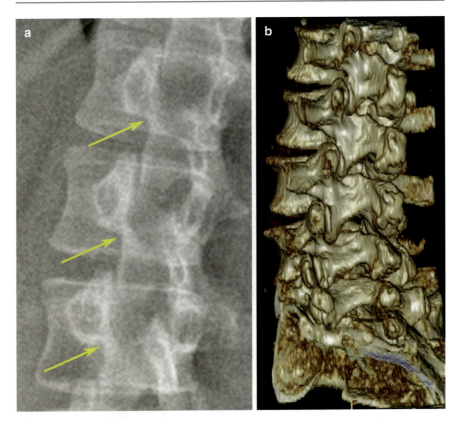

Fig. 2.7 The interarticular portion. On plain film the interarticular portion can be seen best on oblique views. The posterior part of the vertebra forms the "scotty dog". The neck of the dog represents the interarticular portion which appears as a collar if spondylosis is existent (*yellow arrows*). Oblique view radiograph (**a**) and oblique VRT-CT (**b**)

processes (Fig. 2.11b) which also can be found at the first thoracic vertebral body. The transverse process contains an anterior portion ending in a tubercle which is the homologue of the rib in the thoracic spine.

- Cervical ribs arising from C7 are found in 0.5 % of the population.
- Cervical rip syndrome: The presence of a cervical rib can cause thoracic outlet syndrome due to compression of the lower trunk of the brachial plexus or of the subclavian artery.

The posterior part of the transverse process, which also ends in a tubercle, is the true transverse process.

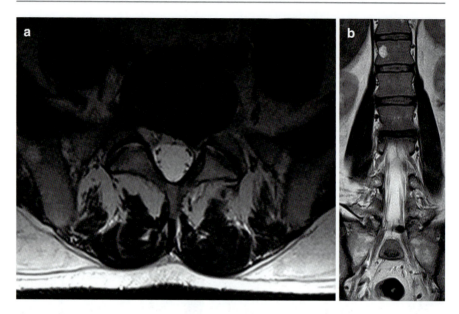

Fig. 2.8 The lateral recess with disc herniation and nerve root compression. The lateral recess is the lateral extension of the spinal canal and contains the spinal roots which can be affected, e.g. due to disc herniation at the segment L 4/5 as in this patient with a left L5 syndrome. Axial (**a**) and coronal (**b**) T2w

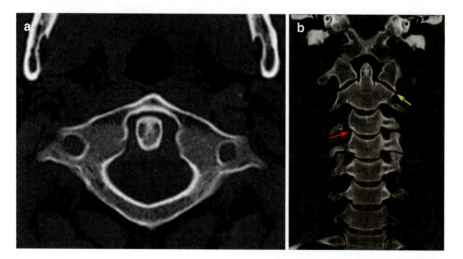

Fig. 2.9 Cervical spine, multislice-CT with axial (**a**), coronal (**b**) and sagittal (**c**) reformations. In the frontal view of the cervical spine, the lateral masses of C1 and C2 normally align (*yellow arrow* in **b**). Note the uncinate processes (*red arrow* in **b**). The atlanto-dental width is normally under 3 mm in adults (**a, c**)

Fig. 2.9 (continued)

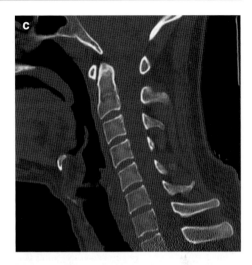

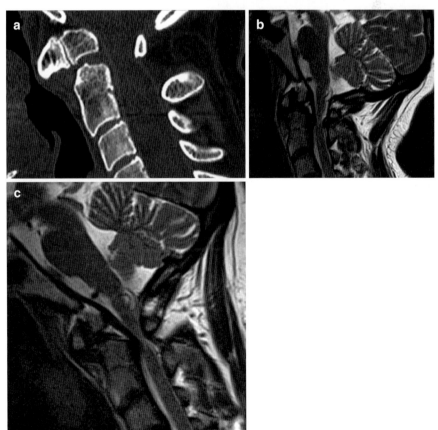

Fig. 2.10 Os odontoideum. The os odontoideum (**a**) may result in craniocervical instability and spinal cord compression (**b**) due to narrowing of the spinal canal which may aggravate under flexion (**c**). Note that the atlas and os odontoideum of the axis are a functional union which move anteriorly during anteflexion of the head

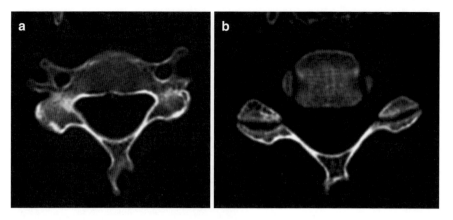

Fig. 2.11 Cervical spine, axial multislice CT. The transverse foramen can be found in each cervical vertebra and contains the vertebral artery with the exception of C7 (**a**). The intervertebral foramen is bounded by the uncovertebral and facet joints (**b**)

Transverse foramen (Fig. 2.11a):
- Located between both portions of the transverse process
- Can be found in each cervical vertebra
- Contains vertebral veins and plexus of sympathetic nerves
- Contains the vertebral artery with the exception of C7

The spinous processes of C3–C5 are relatively short and bifid, whereas the spinous process of C7 is the longest in the cervical spine.

Vertebra prominens (Fig. 2.1):
- C7 bearing the longest spinous process of the cervical spine
- Helps to identify C7 on lateral view of plain films and MRI

The articular surfaces are orientated approximately 45° superiorly from the transverse plane. Superior facets are directed posteriorly, cranially and slightly medially, while the inferior facet is directed to the opposite.

Function: In cervical spine lateral flexion, ventral flexion, dorsal extension and, to a lesser degree, rotation are possible. The vertebral canal is large and triangular in shape.

Thoracic Spine

The thoracic bodies are roughly heart shaped and in the sagittal view slightly wedge shaped. There are costal articular facets on both lateral parts of all thoracic vertebral bodies, which articulate with the heads of the ribs, while facets on transverse processes that articulate with the costal tubercles can only be found on vertebrae T1–T10. Spinous processes are relatively long and are directed caudally.

Function: The facet joints are orientated coronally, which, also because of the rib cage, limits flexion and extension. Rotation and lateral flexion between the thoracic vertebrae are possible to a certain extent.

The vertebral canal is round in shape and relatively small compared to the posterior element size.

Lumbar Spine

Lumbar vertebral bodies are large and oval with strong pedicles and lamina, while the lumbar lateral processes are long and are in fact homologous with the ribs. Therefore, they are called costal processes. The original transverse processes only exist as small tubercles at the dorsal part of the base of the costal processes and are called accessory process. Adjacent to the superior articular processes, an additional tubercle, the mamillary process, can be seen.

Superior articular processes face dorsomedial; inferior articular processes face anterolateral, while at the level of L5–S1, the configuration of the facets is nearly coronal.

Function: Lumbar articulations allow flexion and extension, moderate lateral flexion and rotation to a small degree, due to the configuration of the facets.

The largest diameter of the vertebral canal can be found at the thoracolumbar junction (Fig. 2.12).

Imaging

Cervical spine: Intervertebral foramina are orientated anterolaterally below the pedicles at approximately 45° to the sagittal plane (Fig. 2.13a); oblique views of radiographs and MR images give the optimal access to the intervertebral foramina and its contents (Fig. 2.13b, c).

Lumbar spine: Intervertebral foramina are orientated laterally below the pedicles at approximately 90° to the sagittal plane, best seen in lateral view (Fig. 2.13d).

2.2.3 Intervertebral Discs

The intervertebral discs are located between the cartilage endplates on the superior and the inferior surfaces of vertebrae C2/3 to L5/S1. They are connected especially to the posterior longitudinal ligament. They account for approximately ¼ of spinal column height, while their thickness varies; the thinnest are in the upper thoracic spine, while the thickest can be found in the lower lumbar spine. Intervertebral discs are wedge shaped and therefore account for the characteristic curves of the spine.

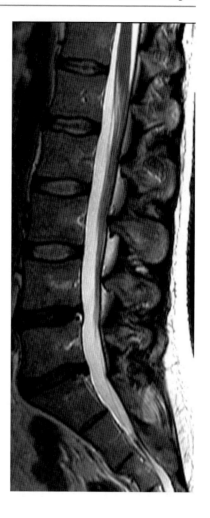

Fig. 2.12 Lumbar spine. The largest diameter of the vertebral canal is the thoracolumbar junction. Intervertebral discs show different amounts of water loss due to disc degeneration which leads to a decreased signal intensity of the nucleus pulposus on T2w

The discs comprise of the central nucleus pulposus and the peripheral annulus fibrosus. The annulus fibrosus consists of 15–25 fibrous lamellae, which surround and constrain the nucleus pulposus. The outer annulus attaches to both the longitudinal ligaments and the epiphyseal ring of vertebral bodies as well as to the hyaline cartilage plates, forming a strong connection to the vertebral body.

Imaging: The annulus shows a low signal on T2w and is sensory innervated by branches of the ventral primary ramus of the spinal nerve. Nucleus pulposus represents a remnant of the notochord. The major macromolecular components are proteoglycans. The nucleus has a high water content, accounting for the high signal in T2w especially in children and young adults (Figs. 2.3, 2.4 and 2.5). Until the age of 2, the disc is vascularised. In older children, nutrients to the disc diffuse via the endplates.

2 Anatomy of the Spine and Spinal Cord

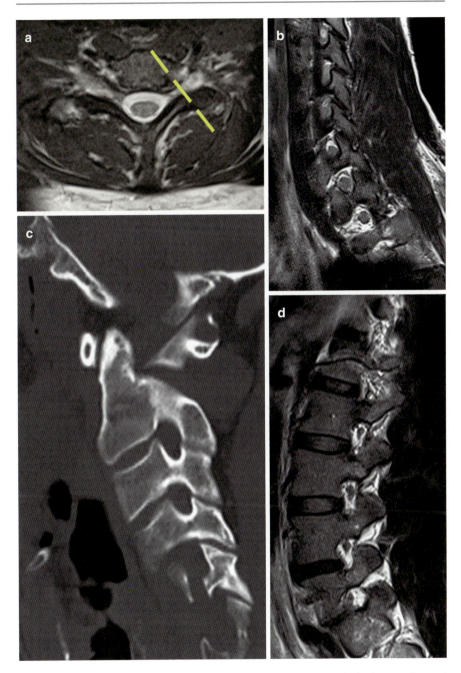

Fig. 2.13 Intervertebral foramina. The intervertebral foramina in the cervical spine are orientated anterolaterally; thus, oblique angulations 45° to the sagittal plane (**a**) allow optimal access to the neural foramina and its contents (**b**, **c**). In contrast intervertebral foramina in lumbar spine are orientated laterally and therefore best seen in lateral view (**d**). Oblique angled T2w of the cervical spine (**b**) and oblique angled CT reformations (**c**)

On T2w, a horizontal linear area of reduced signal can be detected which is called the intranuclear cleft and represents a fibrous transformation of the nucleus pulposus (Fig. 2.12).

- Up to age 2 intervertebral discs enhance mildly after administration of contrast agent.
- From the second decade, signal of the discs decreases in T2w due to disc degeneration and water loss (Fig. 2.12).

2.2.4 Joints

From segment C2/3 to L5/S1, the vertebrae articulate in three joint complexes: two synovial joints between articular processes, called facet joints, and a secondary cartilaginous joint between vertebral bodies, which are symphyses.

Other non-synovial articulations comprise fibrous articulations between lamina, transverse and spinous processes as well as uncinate processes of the cervical spine (C3–C7). The uncinate processes are best depicted in the anterior-posterior view of the spine (Fig. 2.14, red arrow).

2.2.4.1 Facet Joint

The facet joints are true synovial joints covered by hyaline cartilage consisting of articular processes, the zygapophyses. The superior facet surface is directed dorsally, the inferior facet surface ventrally.

Imaging: On axial images the anterior facet is the superior facet of the lower vertebra, while the posterior facet belongs to the inferior facet of the upper vertebra (Fig. 2.11b).

Locked facet: The inferior articular facet of the superior vertebral body is locked in front of the superior facet of the inferior vertebral body.

Function: The orientation of the joints is obliquely sagittal in the lumbar spine to protect the discs from axial rotation and coronal in cervical and thoracic spine to protect against shear. The capsule of the facet joint is a continuation of the ligamentum flavum.

2.2.4.2 Craniocervical Junction

The craniocervical junction comprises the occiput, atlas and axis, their articulations and ligaments (Fig. 2.15).

The atlanto-occipital joints consist of the paired convexly formed inferior articular facet of the occipital condyle and the concavely formed superior articular facet of the atlas.

2 Anatomy of the Spine and Spinal Cord

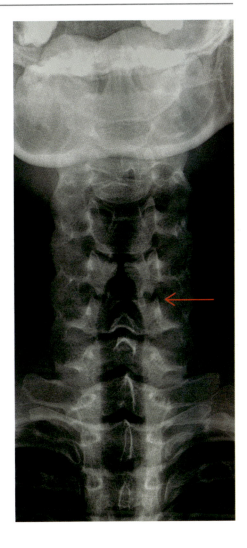

Fig. 2.14 Uncinate processes and uncovertebral joints are best seen in frontal view as on this AP view radiograph of the cervical spine (*red arrow*)

The median atlanto-axial joint is a pivot-type synovial joint between the dens axis and the anterior arch of C1 and transverse ligament, which takes course behind the dens. The paired lateral atlanto-axial joints comprise the inferior articular facet of the atlas and the superior articular facet of the axis.

Function

- Atlanto-occipital joints: Mainly extension and flexion
- Median antlanto-axial joint: Mainly rotational movement
- Paired lateral atlanto-axial joints: Allow the upper neck to move laterally

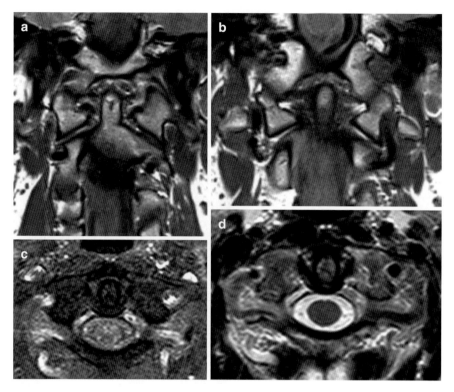

Fig. 2.15 The craniocervical junction. Paired atlanto-occipital joints and paired lateral atlanto-axial joints (**a**, **b**). The ligamentum transversum appears as a dark band on MRI. It connects both lateral masses of the atlas and takes course dorsally of the dens. Axial contrast-enhanced T1w with spectral fat saturation (**c**) and axial T2w (**d**). Lig. transversum (**b**) and Ligg. alaria (**a**) appear as horizontal dark bands on these coronal T1w images

Imaging: The width of the atlanto-dental interval (red line in Fig. 2.16) is normally less than 3 mm in adults and under 5 mm in children and flexion. In children (to age 8), a physiologic anterior displacement up to 4 mm can be seen at level C2–C3 and less frequently at level C3–C4.

> Wackenheim line (yellow line in Fig. 2.16): The posterior surface of clivus normally points to posterior odontoid tip which should be located directly inferior to the clivus. This relationship does not change in flexion or extension (see also Fig. 9.1).

Normally, the odontoid tip is less than 5 mm above the Chamberlain line, which extends from the hard palate to the opisthion.

2 Anatomy of the Spine and Spinal Cord

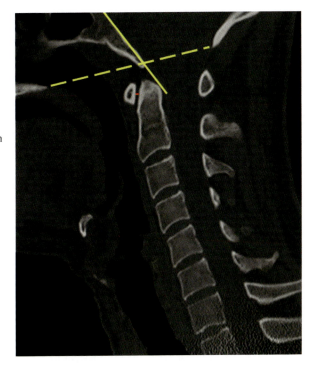

Fig. 2.16 Chamberlain line (*dashed line*) extends from the hard palate to the opisthion. Wackenheim line (*continuous line*) follows the posterior surface of clivus and points to the posterior part of the odontoid tip. The width of the atlanto-dental intervall is normally less than 3 mm in adults (*red line*). Sagittal CT reformation

- Chamberlain line (dotted yellow line in Fig. 2.16): Extends from the hard palate to the opisthion.
- Basilar impression: An odontoid tip at least 5 mm or more above the Chamberlain line defines a basilar impression.

In the frontal view of the craniocervical junction, it should be noted that lateral masses of C1 and C2 normally align, whereas overlapping lateral masses can be a normal variant in children.

2.2.4.3 Uncovertebral Joint
Uncovertebral joints, also called joints of Luschka, are exclusively found in the cervical spine with the exception of the segment C1–C2. The uncovertebral joints are oblique, cleft-like cavities between the superior surfaces of the uncinate processes and the lateral parts of the inferior surface of the adjacent vertebral body (red arrows in Figs. 2.9b and 2.14).

2.2.5 Ligaments

2.2.5.1 Anterior and Posterior Longitudinal Ligament

The anterior longitudinal ligament follows the ventral surface of the vertebral bodies and extends from skull to sacrum. It is mainly attached to the ends of each vertebral body and only loosely attached to the intervertebral discs. The posterior longitudinal ligament extends on the posterior surface of the vertebral bodies and adheres tightly to the posterior surface of the annulus fibrosus, the adjacent margins of the vertebral bodies and also to the periost of the pedicles.

Imaging: The posterior longitudinal ligament is not adhered to the midportion of the vertebral bodies where a fat-filled space can be detected on MRI, containing epidural veins. At the level of the intervertebral discs, those ligaments usually cannot be distinguished from the annulus fibrous as they appear dark on T1w and T2w as all ligaments and show no contrast enhancement.

Function: The longitudinal ligaments are involved in maintaining the spinal curvatures.

2.2.5.2 Ligaments of the Craniocervical Junction

Cruciate Ligament and Tectorial Membrane

The cruciate ligament is formed by the transverse ligament and longitudinal bands. The transverse ligament connects both lateral masses of the atlas and takes course dorsally to the dens to which it has an articular connection as part of the median atlanto-axial joint (Fig. 2.15). The longitudinal component extends to the ventral part of the foramen magnum and the dorsal surface of the corpus axis, where it is in direct continuation with the deep part of the posterior longitudinal ligament. Usually it cannot be separated from the adjacent tectorial membrane on MR imaging.

The tectorial membrane is a strong band that covers the cruciate ligament and the dens dorsally. It is a prolongation of the superficial part of the posterior longitudinal ligament which ends at the basilar part of the occipital bone slightly above the foramen magnum where it is covered by the dura mater (Fig. 2.17). The tectorial membrane is mainly inseparable from the adjacent dura on MR imaging.

Odontoid Ligaments

The odontoid ligaments comprise of the alar and apical ligament. The alar ligaments are paired ligaments that arise at the posterolateral apex of the dens and extend to the lateral margins of the foramen magnum (Fig. 2.15a). The apical ligament is located between the alar ligaments and connects the apical end of the dens with the ventral margin of the foramen magnum. It represents the fibrous remnant of the notochord (Fig. 2.17).

Anterior and Posterior Atlanto-occipital Membrane

Skull and atlas are connected through the atlanto-occipital membrane. The anterior part of the membrane is a cranial prolongation of the anterior longitudinal ligament and extends from the anterior arch of the atlas to the basilar part of the occipital bone and consists of dense fibres. The posterior atlanto-occipital membrane extends from

2 Anatomy of the Spine and Spinal Cord

Fig. 2.17 Ligaments of the craniocervical junction. This midsagittal view shows (from anterior to posterior): The anterior atlanto-occipital membrane is a continuation of the anterior longitudinal ligament, the apical ligament, the tectorial membrane and the posterior atlanto-occipital membrane with adjacent dura mater

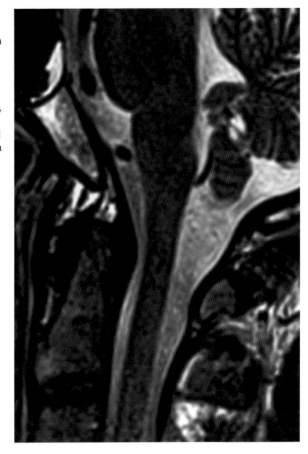

the dorsal arch of the atlas to the dorsal margin of the foramen magnum. It consists of elastic fibres and is adherent to the dura mater. The lateral part of the membrane is perforated on both sides by the vertebral arteries which enter the vertebral canal.

Functions

Tectorial membrane and longitudinal part of the cruciate ligament:
- Limits the ventral flexion of the head

Transverse ligament (part of cruciate ligament):
- Prevents the dens from moving dorsally to the spinal canal and injuring the medulla oblongata or from anterior dislocation of the atlas on axis during flexion, respectively

Odontoid ligaments:
- Inhibit the rotation and the lateral flexion of the head

Anterior part of the atlanto-occipital membrane:
- Inhibits the dorsal extension of the head (dense fibres)

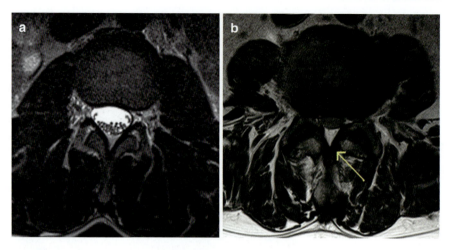

Fig. 2.18 Ligamentum flavum. The ligamentum flavum appears normally as a dark thin band on T1w and T2w (**a**). In degenerative spine diseases, this ligament is often thickened which can contribute to stenosis of the vertebral canal (*yellow arrow* in **b**)

2.2.5.3 Ligamentum Flavum

Ligamentum flavum is a fibroelastic ligament, which extends between the laminae of two adjacent vertebrae from C2 to the lumbosacral junction. It extends from the capsule of the facet joint to the junction of the lamina with the spinous process in the dorsal part of the vertebral canal. In the lumbar spine, this ligament encompasses the ventral part of the facet joints and forms parts of the dorsal border of the lateral recess and the intervertebral foramen.

Imaging: The ligaments are thin in the cervical spine and most thick in the lumbar region and appear as hypointense structures on both T1w and T2w (Fig. 2.18).
Function: They extend the vertebral column dorsally and therefore assist the back muscles in resuming an upright posture after flexion.

2.2.6 Intervertebral Foramina

The intervertebral foramen (Fig. 2.19), also known as the neural foramen, is bounded above and below by the pedicles, posteriorly by the interarticular part of the vertebral arch, the capsule of the facet joint and the ligamentum flavum and anteriorly by the posterior surface of the vertebral body and the intervertebral disc. The intervertebral foramen is the continuation of the lateral recess of the vertebral canal.

The foramen contains nerve roots, dorsal root ganglion, arteries and veins. The remainder of the intervertebral foramen is filled with fat.

2 Anatomy of the Spine and Spinal Cord

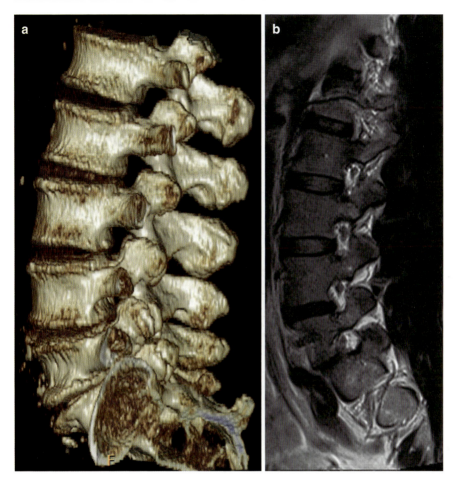

Fig. 2.19 Intervertebral foramina contain spinal nerves and vessels and are surrounded by fat, thus allowing a good discrimination of the structures especially on T1w. 3D volume-rendering CT (**a**) and sagittal T2w (**b**)

> Intervertebral foramen and nerve root
> *Cervical spine*:
> - The nerve root is named for the lower segment that it runs between, e.g. at C5–C6 segment passes the C6 nerve root.
>
> *Thoracic and lumbar spine*:
> - The nerve root is named for the upper segment that it runs between, e.g. at L4–L5 segment passes the L4 nerve root.

The spinal nerves pass through the cervical neural foramen in its lower part at the level of the intervertebral discs.

The spinal nerves pass through the thoracic and especially through the lumbar intervertebral foramen in the superior part of the foramen. These oval-shaped foramina are relatively small in the cervical spine and gradually increase in size towards the lumbar spine. In the cervical spine, the foramina are orientated in a 45° oblique plane (see also Sect. 2.2).

- Cervical intraforaminal disc herniation usually affects the nerve root, whereas the lumbar nerve roots often leave the intervertebral foramen above the herniated disc.
- Perform oblique angulated slices perpendicular to the axis of cervical intervertebral foramina to see the extent of disc herniation!

Structures of the Spinal Canal

Se-Jong You and Elke Hattingen

Contents

3.1 Meninges 29
3.2 Spaces 31
3.3 Nerve Roots: Cauda Equina 33

3.1 Meninges

The meninges of the spine comprise the following three layers:

The dura (pachymeninx) forms the outermost layer of the meninges and consists of dense, tough, connective tissue. It forms the dural sac, which continues from the dura of the brain where it is connected to the periost of the skull. Caudally, the dural sac extends normally at the level of the second sacral vertebra but may occasionally terminate already at the level L4 or L5. Ventrally, fibrous bands attach the dura to the posterior longitudinal ligament.

Tubular prolongations of the dura extend around the roots of each nerve (Fig. 3.1). These *dural sleeves* cover the ventral and the dorsal roots and extend anteriorly, laterally and caudally into the lateral recess and through the epidural space to the intervertebral foramina where the dura fuses with the capsule of the ganglion and the epineurium of the spinal nerve. Also consider Fig. 3.1 which shows the initial lateralisation of the nerve root passing the dural sleeve before entering in the lateral recess.

S.-J. You (✉) • E. Hattingen
Institute for Neuroradiology, Goethe-University,
Schleusenweg 2-16, D-60528 Frankfurt, Germany
e-mail: se-jong.you@kgu.de; elke.hattingen@kgu.de

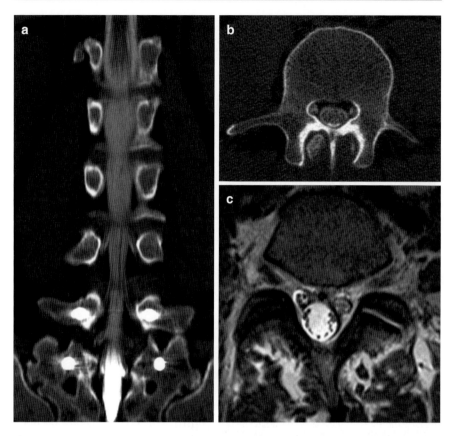

Fig. 3.1 Lateral extensions of the dura, myelography with coronal and axial reformats (**a**, **b**) and axial T2w (**c**). The lateral extensions of the dura are the dural sleeves containing the nerve roots as well as CSF thus allowing assessment of the root sleeves on MRI (**c**) and myelography (**a**, **b**)

Imaging: The dura can be detected on MRI as a thin black line on T2w. After the application of contrast agent, an enhancement can be seen due to a lack of endothelial tight junctions of the vessels.

The arachnoid is attached to the dura, follows its contours and also extends within the dural sleeves. It forms a fine network of connective tissue fibres that extend to the innermost layer of the meninges. An incomplete longitudinal midline membrane, which connects the pia and the cord dorsally to the dura, is called septum posticum and can be found in the cervical and the upper thoracic spine. It partially divides the subarachnoid space.

The pia is the innermost and thinnest layer of the meninges and is adherent to the surface of the cord and spinal nerve roots. It also enters the dural sleeves where it fuses with the arachnoid. Caudally it covers the filum terminale. Pia and arachnoid are also called leptomeninges.

The denticulate ligament exists between level C1 and L1 and consists of flat fibrous perforated sheets that support the spinal cord. It extends laterally from the pia between ventral and dorsal roots, inserts into the dura mater and therefore

3 Structures of the Spinal Canal 31

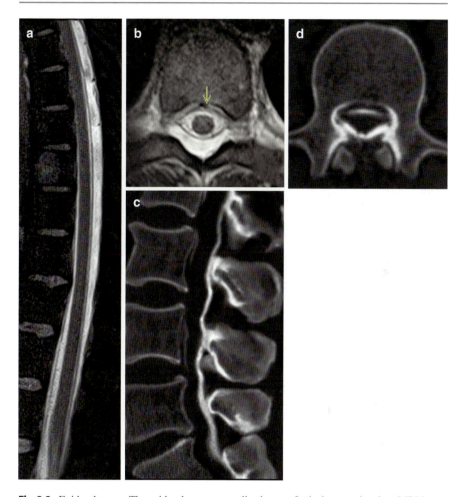

Fig. 3.2 Epidural space. The epidural space normally shows a fat-isointense signal on MRI imaging. In this case, the epidural space shows a water-isointense signal on fat-saturated T2w due to CSF leakage which caused intracranial hypotension (*arrow*) (**a, b**). An epidural blood patch was performed to seal the leakage (**c, d**). CT shows the epidural distribution of the applied hyperdense mixture of blood and contrast media. The undulating appearance of the epidural space on the sagittal reformations (**d**) is due to respiratory motion artifacts. Axial CT (**c**) and sagittal reformations (**d**)

partially separates the subarachnoid space in an anterior and a posterior part. There are 20–22 pairs of denticulate ligaments.

3.2 Spaces

The real and potential spaces of the vertebral canal are located between the meningeal layers or adjacent structures. A potential space is only present postmortem or due to pathologic conditions, such as haemorrhage.

The epidural space (Fig. 3.2) is located between the dura and surrounding margins of the vertebral canal and extends from the foramen magnum to the posterior

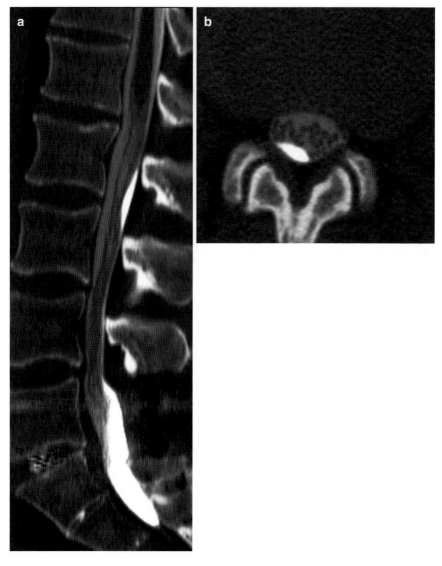

Fig. 3.3 Subdural space. The subdural space is only a potential space. Myelography was performed with accidental application of parts of the contrast agent in the subdural space at level L2-L3. Post-myelographic CT scan with sagittal (**a**) and axial (**b**) reformations

sacrococcygeal ligament. It contains mainly fat, small arteries, the internal vertebral venous plexus, lymphatics and dural sleeves. The anterior epidural fat progressively increases in thickness from L1 to L5, especially in individuals where the dural sac terminates already at the lower lumbar spine.

Between the dura and the outer surface of the arachnoid, there is a potential subdural space (Fig. 3.3). Cerebrospinal fluid pressure presses the arachnoid against the dura, thus closing this space.

3 Structures of the Spinal Canal

The subarachnoid space is located between the inner surface of the arachnoid and pia. It contains cerebrospinal fluid, vessels, spinal cord ligaments, nerves and the filum terminale (see also Chap. 8). The subpial space is another potential space.

> The subarachnoid space of the spine is incompletely separated by the denticulate ligament and the septum posticum.

Imaging

> Contents of spinal compartments:
> Extradural compartment:
> Includes the epidural space, the vertebral bodies, the neural arches, the intervertebral discs and the paraspinal muscles
> Intradural extramedullary compartment:
> Includes subarachnoidal space, spinal cord ligaments, nerve roots, cauda equina and filum terminale
> Intramedullary compartment:
> Comprises the spinal cord and the pia

3.3 Nerve Roots: Cauda Equina

There are normally 31 pairs of spinal nerves: eight cervical, 12 thoracic, 5 lumbar, 5 sacral and 1 coccygeal pair, which emerge from the vertebral canal through their respective intervertebral foramen with the exception for the first spinal nerve pair, which emerges between the atlas and the occipital bone. The cervical nerves are numbered by the vertebra below. Because of the existence of an 8th cervical nerve pair, which exits between vertebrae C7 and T1, the thoracic, the lumbar and the sacral nerves are numbered by the vertebra above.

Each spinal nerve is formed by the union of a ventral and a dorsal nerve root, which exit from their respective hemichords. The ventral root consists of 4–7 filaments, which exit the chord at the anterolateral sulcus. It contains mainly efferent somatic fibres. The dorsal root enters the chord at the posterolateral sulcus and consists of 4–10 filaments. It contains afferent fibres, whereas both ventral and dorsal roots contain also visceral autonomic axons. The roots are surrounded by pia and cross the subarachnoid space until they reach their respective dural sleeve, which emerges from the anterolateral surface of the dural sac.

Within the dural sleeve, the nerve roots cross the lateral recess and the epidural space and finally reach the intervertebral foramen. Both roots unite in or adjacent to

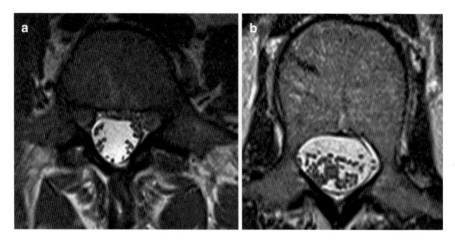

Fig. 3.4 Cauda equina. Characteristic distribution of the nerve roots at the level of lower spine (**a**) and conus medullaris (**b**). Axial T2-weighted images

the intervertebral foramina to the main trunk of the spinal nerve which extends for only a short distance until it divides into the dorsal and ventral rami. The dorsal root itself forms the spinal ganglion, which is located in the intervertebral foramen.

Because of the differing growth of the vertebral column and the spinal cord, the caudal termination of the cord, conus medullaris, ends most commonly between T12 and L1 (Fig. 3.4), in newborns at the level of the third lumbar vertebra. Therefore, the remaining lumbar, sacral and coccygeal roots, which form the cauda equina, have a descending and relatively long course through the subarachnoid space until they exit the vertebral canal at their appropriate intervertebral foramina.

> Cauda equina: lumbar, sacral and coccygeal roots coursing craniocaudally through the subarachnoid space until they exit the vertebral canal at their appropriate intervertebral foramina

In the supine position, the roots in the lower lumbar spine lie in a U-shaped configuration within the posterior portion of the dural sac (Fig. 3.4). The sacral roots are located dorsally and medially, the lumbar roots lie more laterally and anteriorly; and in the upper lumbar spine, the ventral roots remain anteriorly. The roots at the cervical and upper thoracic spine have a relatively short horizontal or even ascending course.

3 Structures of the Spinal Canal

The intrathecal nerve roots normally do not enhance after admission of intravenous contrast agents due to the intact blood-nerve barrier.

In contrast, the dorsal root ganglion shows strong enhancement due to the lack of the barrier.

> Contrast enhancement of the dorsal root ganglion should not be mistaken as inflammation or metastatic disease.

The filum terminale internum extends inferiorly from the conus medullaris and consists mainly of connective tissue, glia and leptomeninges. Normally, it measures 2 mm or less in diameter. It has a branch of the anterior spinal artery, which causes enhancement after admission of a contrast agent. It perforates the caudal end of the dural sac. The extradural continuation is called filum terminale externum, which attaches on the dorsum of the first or second coccygeal segment.

Part II
Imaging Methods

Magnetic Resonance Imaging (MRI) Methods

4

Thomas W. Okell, Elke Hattingen, Johannes C. Klein, and Karla L. Miller

Contents

4.1 Introduction 40
4.2 Why Use MRI for Spinal Imaging? 40
    4.2.1 Advantages of MRI 40
    4.2.2 Challenges of MRI 41
4.3 Where Does the MRI Signal Come From? 42
    4.3.1 Components of an MRI Scanner 42
    4.3.2 Processes Underlying MRI 42
    4.3.3 What Is a Pulse Sequence? 46
4.4 Basic Image Contrasts: T1, T2, T2* and Proton Density 47
    4.4.1 What Influences Image Contrast? 47
    4.4.2 T1 Weighting 48
    4.4.3 T2 Weighting 48
    4.4.4 Proton Density Weighting 50
    4.4.5 T2* Weighting 51
    4.4.6 Measures of Image Quality: Signal and Contrast-to-Noise Ratios 53
4.5 Image Formation and Artefacts 57
    4.5.1 From Signals to Images 58
    4.5.2 Image Artefacts 70

T.W. Okell (✉) • K.L. Miller
FMRIB Centre, Nuffield Department of Clinical Neurosciences,
University of Oxford, Oxford, UK
e-mail: tokell@fmrib.ox.ac.uk

E. Hattingen
Institute for Neuroradiology, Goethe-University,
Schleusenweg 2-16, D-60528 Frankfurt, Germany
e-mail: elke.hattingen@kgu.de

J.C. Klein
Brain Imaging Center (BIC), Department of Neurology, Goethe-University,
Schleusenweg 2-16, D-60528 Frankfurt, Germany
e-mail: klein@med.uni-frankfurt.de

4.6	Tricks to Improve Image Quality	76
	4.6.1 Reducing Physiological Fluctuations	76
	4.6.2 Suppression of Adjacent Tissues	77
	4.6.3 Inversion Recovery	78
	4.6.4 Fat Suppression	78
	4.6.5 Contrast Agents	80
4.7	Suggested Imaging Protocols	82
Further Reading		84

4.1 Introduction

Magnetic resonance imaging (MRI) has become increasingly important for the evaluation of spinal cord disease. In this chapter we discuss why MRI is so well suited for this purpose, along with some of its potential problems. In order to help interpret MR images, we then give an intuitive overview of the origin of the MR signal, how contrast can be generated between different tissue types or lesions, the image formation process and some common image artefacts. Finally, we discuss tricks to improve image quality and reduce artefacts before providing some suggested spinal imaging protocols.

4.2 Why Use MRI for Spinal Imaging?

There are an ever-increasing range of methods for generating images of the human body, so why chose magnetic resonance imaging for looking at the spine? In this section we examine some of the benefits as well as the drawbacks of using MRI for spinal imaging (Table 4.1).

4.2.1 Advantages of MRI

Perhaps the most striking feature of the images produced by a well-optimised MRI protocol is the superb contrast between different types of soft tissue. This sets MRI apart from other standard imaging methods, such as X-ray-based computed tomography (CT). Moreover, tissue contrast in MRI is very flexible and can be modified using a wide variety of techniques to help highlight certain characteristics of the

Table 4.1 The main benefits and drawbacks of using MRI for spinal imaging

Advantages	Disadvantages
Excellent soft tissue contrast	Some contraindications
Flexible "contrast" (information)	Relatively slow and expensive
Good spatial resolution	Limited availability
No ionising radiation	Unintuitive artefacts
Allows multi-planar imaging	Lacks specificity

tissues. Combining information from a set of such images can aid differentiation between various types of lesion, such as a cyst or a tumour.

Unlike most other imaging methods, MRI is capable of acquiring images in any desired orientation. This is particularly advantageous for spinal imaging where a sagittal view of the spinal column is often more informative than a series of axial slices produced by most other imaging modalities. In addition, there is no intrinsic limit on the spatial resolution that can be achieved in any given direction, unlike CT where the minimum slice thickness is fixed by the size of the X-ray detectors. As we will see, however, image quality and timing considerations limit what can be achieved in practice.

Another major advantage of MRI is the absence of ionising radiation used with other methods, such as X-rays and nuclear medicine. This is of particular importance in children and in patients who require regular imaging investigations. However, there are a number of drawbacks to using MRI, as we shall see in the next section.

4.2.2 Challenges of MRI

As with any imaging technique, MRI also has its disadvantages. There are a number of patient groups who are prohibited from being scanned due to the interaction of various medical implants or other contraindications with the magnetic fields necessary for MR imaging. These include most cardiac pacemakers and certain types of aneurysm clips and stents. In addition, the most common "tube-like" scanners are unsuitable for patients with severe claustrophobia, although wider diameter or "open" designs are becoming available, helping alleviate this to some extent.

MRI scanners are also relatively expensive. As a result the majority of imaging examinations tend to be performed with modalities such as CT or ultrasound where possible. This situation is not aided by the relatively long time required for a typical MRI exam, meaning that patient throughput is quite low. However, recent technical advances are allowing much more rapid imaging, some of which we will discuss later in this chapter.

There are a range of confounds that affect the unique image formation process and lead to a variety of errors or "artefacts" in the images, which are often unintuitive to those not familiar with MRI. In addition to compromising diagnostic image quality, these artefacts can masquerade as anatomical structure (or pathology), making artefact recognition an important part of the diagnostic process. Later in this chapter we will describe artefacts commonly found in spinal MR images along with a variety of methods for their reduction.

Although soft tissue contrast in MRI is excellent, it is less well suited to looking at tissues with low water density, such as bone, which is better visualised with X-ray methods. In addition, MRI generally lacks the specificity of nuclear medicine investigations where the radiotracer targets the tissues of interest, although this is an active research area in MRI. Despite these problems, MRI is often the modality of choice for examining the spine. We will spend the remainder of this chapter discussing how MR images are generated along with common artefacts.

4.3 Where Does the MRI Signal Come From?

In order to understand how different types of MR images are formed, it is first important to have an appreciation of where the MR signal originates. In this section we give an overview of the main components that an MRI scanner requires and how these relate to the various processes that are crucial for detecting an MR signal.

4.3.1 Components of an MRI Scanner

The main components that make up a MRI scanner (see Fig. 4.1) are:
- A *strong magnet (usually superconducting)*: this creates a large uniform magnetic field (B_0). For standard cylindrical MRI scanners, B_0 points along the axis of the cylinder. By convention this is labelled the "z" direction. For clinical MRI scanners, B_0 is typically 1.5 or 3 tesla (abbreviated to T), which is tens of thousands of times stronger than the earth's magnetic field.
- A *transmit radio-frequency (RF) coil*: this allows radio waves to be transmitted into the subject, creating a time-varying magnetic field (B_1). A large "body" transmit coil is built into the main body of most scanners.
- A *receive radio-frequency (RF) coil*: this measures the MR signal from the subject and is often composed of a series of individual elements (a "multichannel" coil). Modern scanners provide a broad selection of receive coils that are tailored to the anatomy of interest.
- *Gradient coils*: these three coils create variations in the main magnetic field in three different directions, which are necessary for signal localisation (described in Sect. 4.5.1). Gradients are built into the main body of the scanner.

As the reader will see, these components of the MRI scanner hardware relate closely to the processes that underlie different aspects of MRI image formation (outlined in Sect. 4.3.2).

For spinal imaging a specific spine RF receive coil is often used (Fig. 4.1). This coil is sometimes built into the subject table of the scanner to allow imaging of the spine whilst the subject lies in a supine position. This coil generally consists of an ensemble of small elements, each of which provides high sensitivity to a small region and which in combination allow a large region of the spine to be imaged. Because the received signal is much stronger in regions of the body close to the coil, clear visualisation of anterior tissues often requires an additional coil array on top of the patient to obtain high signal in both anterior and posterior regions.

4.3.2 Processes Underlying MRI

There are a number of basic processes that occur to allow the measurement of the MR signal. These processes are summarised here and shown graphically in Fig. 4.2.
- *Polarisation* – The main magnetic field (B_0) "magnetises" the hydrogen nuclei of water molecules within the subject. Each hydrogen nucleus is magnetic, like a

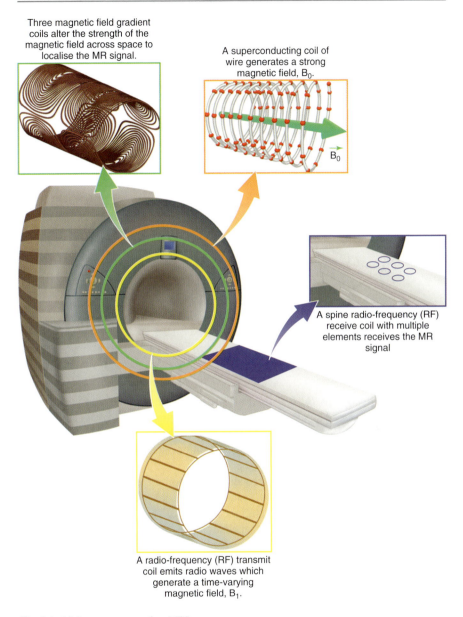

Fig. 4.1 Main components of an MRI scanner

tiny bar magnet or compass needle. In the absence of an external magnetic field, these nuclei are randomly oriented (pointing in random directions) so their effects average out to result in no net magnetic field. However, just like a compass needle, when the hydrogen nuclei are brought into the strong B_0 field, they tend to line up with it, creating a net magnetisation, which we call M, pointing in

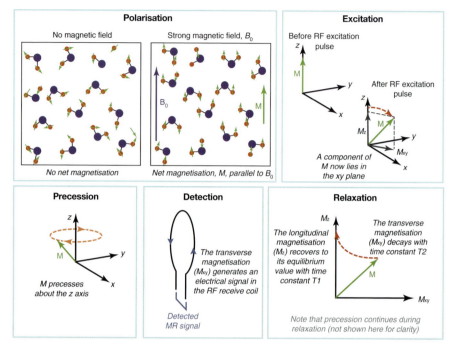

Fig. 4.2 Processes involved in MRI

the same direction as B_0. It is this magnetisation, M, that we measure in MRI. Note that hydrogen nuclei present in non-water sources are also magnetised, but they tend to produce very little MR signal, so we shall focus largely on the water signal in this chapter. One important exception is fat, which is discussed in Sects. 4.5.2.2 and 4.6.4.

- *Excitation* – The transmit radio-frequency (RF) coil creates a time-varying magnetic field (B_1) which "excites" the magnetisation. This means that M is rotated away from its normal orientation (aligned with B_0). The result is that M now has some component within the plane at right angles to B_0: the "transverse" plane. Excitation is crucial, because only components of M within the transverse plane are measureable (see "Detection").
- *Precession* – Once the magnetisation, M, has been excited it begins to "precess" or rotate about B_0, in the same manner that a gyroscope precesses when knocked off its axis. The rate of this precession is proportional to the strength of B_0.
- *Detection* – The precessing magnetisation is detected by the radio-frequency (RF) receive coil, which has been tuned to the precession frequency. Magnetisation precessing near the RF coil induces an electrical signal that can be recorded. The strength of this signal is proportional to the size of the M within the transverse plane.
- *Relaxation* – After the magnetisation has been excited, there is a strong force driving the magnetisation to reorient itself to its preferred position aligned with

4 Magnetic Resonance Imaging (MRI) Methods

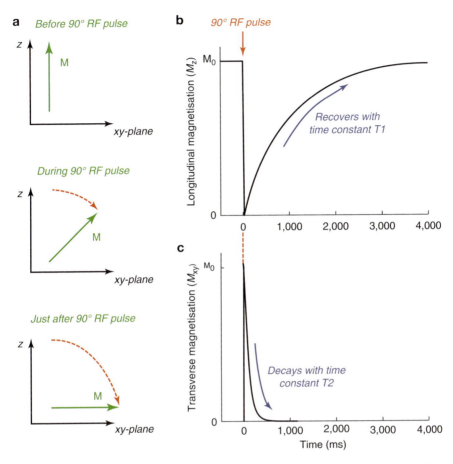

Fig. 4.3 Relaxation processes following a 90° RF excitation pulse: (**a**) The magnetisation, *M*, is initially aligned with B_0 (along *z*) before being rotated through 90° into the transverse (*xy*) plane by the RF pulse; (**b**) After the RF pulse (at time 0), the longitudinal (*z*) component of the magnetisation is zero, but recovers back towards its equilibrium value (M_0) with time constant T1; (**c**) The transverse (*xy*) magnetisation created by the RF pulse decays to zero with time constant T2. For this simulation we assumed T1 = 1 s and T2 = 100 ms

B_0. However, this process is not simply a reversal of excitation in which the magnetisation rotates back into alignment with B_0. Instead, relaxation is composed of two (somewhat) independent processes: the component of the magnetisation in the transverse plane disappears faster than the component aligned with B_0 (the "longitudinal" magnetisation) regrows. This leads to a temporary loss of magnetisation that recovers over time in a process called "relaxation". The loss of transverse magnetisation is characterised by time T2, whilst regrowth of longitudinal magnetisation takes characteristic time T1, with T2<<T1. An example of relaxation following a 90° RF excitation pulse is given in Fig. 4.3.

> *Some important terminology*
>
> *x, y and z*: The main magnetic field, B_0, creates a coordinate system for our MR experiments. B_0 points along the longitudinal axis, which is labelled "z" by convention. The plane at right angles to B_0 is the transverse, or "xy", plane. MRI involves manipulating the magnetisation in this 3D coordinate frame. Depending on the direction of the magnetisation, it will have some longitudinal component (M_z) and some transverse component (M_{xy}), and only M_{xy} generates the MR signal. In general *x, y* and *z* are the left-right, anterior-posterior and inferior-superior directions, respectively.
>
> *Flip angle*: This is the angle between the *z* axis and the magnetisation at the end of the RF excitation pulse. It is determined by the strength of the B_1 field and its duration.
>
> *Resonance frequency*: The precession frequency of the magnetisation is also referred to as the "resonance" frequency. At common field strengths (e.g. 1.5–3 T), this is in the radio-frequency (RF) range. A RF pulse must be tuned to this frequency in order to excite the magnetisation. The received MR signal produced by the precessing magnetisation is also at this frequency, which is why we need both RF transmit and RF receive coils in MRI.

4.3.3 What Is a Pulse Sequence?

Whilst the main magnetic field (B_0) is static (i.e. remains on at all times), the RF transmit and gradient magnetic fields are manipulated during an MRI scan with precise control on the order of microseconds. This prescription of carefully timed RF transmit, gradient and signal detection events constitute a "pulse sequence" that is designed to generate the desired MRI signal.

As we will see, the precise gradient waveforms determine the spatial extent and resolution of the image. Image contrast is largely determined by the excitation flip angle and timing parameters. Two of the most important timing parameters (shown in Fig. 4.4) are:

- *The repetition time, TR*: the time between one excitation RF pulse and the next
- *The echo time, TE*: the time between the RF excitation pulse and the point at which the signal is recorded

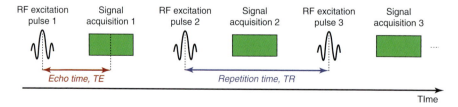

Fig. 4.4 A schematic of a simple pulse sequence showing the repetition time, TR, and the echo time, TE

4 Magnetic Resonance Imaging (MRI) Methods

In the next section we shall explore how these pulse sequence timing parameters and tissue relaxation properties can be utilised to generate contrast between different types of tissue with MRI.

4.4 Basic Image Contrasts: T1, T2, T2* and Proton Density

4.4.1 What Influences Image Contrast?

The ability to distinguish between different tissue types within an image is dependent on there being large signal differences, or high contrast, between them. One of the keys to the excellent soft tissue contrast in MRI is that different tissues have different relaxation properties (i.e. T1 and T2 differ between tissues). In addition, some tissues have a greater concentration of water than others, leading to a higher density of hydrogen nuclei (protons), resulting in higher signal. These properties form the basis of the basic image contrasts in MRI. Examples of T1-weighted, T2-weighted and proton density (PD)-weighted images are shown in Fig. 4.5.

The weighting between these three factors can be adjusted relatively simply by modifying the timing of the image acquisition. In this section we discuss how contrast due to T1, T2 or proton density can be isolated and maximised. We will also describe T2* weighting, which is closely related to T2 weighting.

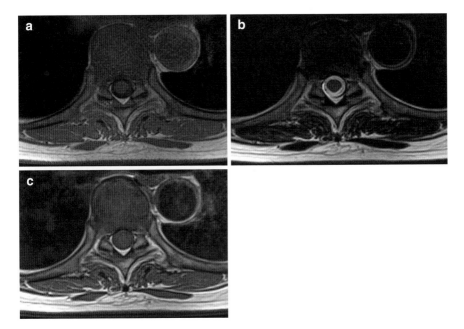

Fig. 4.5 Typical spinal images with (**a**) T1 weighting, (**b**) T2 weighting and (**c**) proton density weighting

4.4.2 T1 Weighting

As discussed above, after excitation the longitudinal magnetisation, M_z, recovers back to its equilibrium position with characteristic "time constant" T1. Tissues with a short T1 recover back to equilibrium quickly, whilst those with a long T1 recover more slowly. Regions with a liquid composition, such as those containing cerebrospinal fluid (CSF), tend to have longer T1 values than areas that are more solid or fatty, such as white matter.

Achieving contrast between tissues based on T1 poses a challenge, given that T1 is a property of the z magnetisation, but only the x-y component of the magnetisation can be directly observed. However, let us consider what happens if we do not allow the magnetisation to fully recover back to its equilibrium location before applying another RF excitation pulse (i.e. if the repetition time, TR, is short relative to T1). Tissues with a short T1 recover more quickly and will therefore have a greater longitudinal magnetisation just before the next RF excitation pulse. This means that when the longitudinal magnetisation is rotated into the transverse plane, tissues with a short T1 will produce a greater amount of transverse magnetisation and therefore a greater signal than tissues with a long T1. By modifying the TR, we have generated contrast between two tissues with different T1 values, resulting in a "T1-weighted" image. This is illustrated in Fig. 4.6. It is worth noting that these images will also be influenced by proton density, although in most situations T1 weighting will dominate.

> *Aside: spoiling*
> Any transverse magnetisation remaining just prior to the next RF excitation pulse can interfere with signals in subsequent TR periods. Therefore, most pulse sequences using a short TR utilise a technique called spoiling. This process attempts to destroy any residual transverse magnetisation just before the next RF pulse is played out, preventing this interference from occurring.

4.4.3 T2 Weighting

Just as the TR changes the T1 weighting, the T2 weighting is controlled by the time between the excitation and signal acquisition: the echo time (TE). Figure 4.7 shows that the transverse magnetisation, and therefore the signal, decays from the tissue with a short T2 more rapidly than the signal from the tissue with a long T2. Therefore, using a longer TE introduces contrast based on differences in T2. This contrast can be optimised by picking a TE that maximises the signal difference between the two tissue types.

Again, introducing a relatively simple change in the pulse sequence timing allows us to generate contrast between different tissue types based on their relaxation properties. However, as for T1-weighted images, the proton density will also influence the signal strength in T2-weighted images.

4 Magnetic Resonance Imaging (MRI) Methods

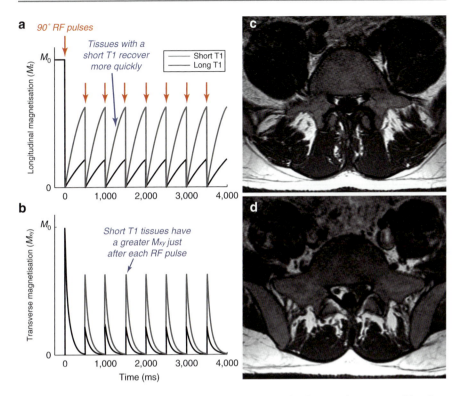

Fig. 4.6 Producing T1 weighting using a short TR: Here we simulate two tissues, one with a short T1 (0.5 s, *grey*) and one with a long T1 (2 s, *black*), during a pulse sequence with a relatively short TR period (0.5 s) so that the magnetisation cannot fully recover to its equilibrium position; (**a**) the longitudinal magnetisation of the tissue with a short T1 recovers more fully just prior to the next RF pulse (shown with *red arrows*); (**b**) As a result the transverse magnetisation produced by the excitation RF pulse is greater for the tissue with a short T1, resulting in a higher signal from that tissue. Note that this is not the case for the first RF pulse but the first few pulses are often ignored to allow the signal to reach a stable "steady state". Here we have used a RF excitation flip angle of 90° for simplicity, but in practice lower flip angles are commonly used to optimise the signal strength produced from this kind of pulse sequence; (**c**) An axial T1-weighted image of the lumbar spine, where the hyperintense fat signal allows us to discriminate between the lumbar dural sac and the nerval roots in the lumbar recesses; (**d**) Left-sided disc herniation, clearly visible in this T1-weighted image, compresses the left nerve root in the lateral recess

It is worth noting that a T2-weighted image often appears to have inverted contrast compared to a T1-weighted image (i.e. a region with a high intensity on a T2-weighted image often has a low intensity on a T1-weighted image). This is because tissues with a long T1 often have a long T2 as well. This gives high signal in a T2-weighted image since the signal decays more slowly, but in T1-weighted images the longitudinal magnetisation does not recover quickly during the short TR period and therefore produces a low signal.

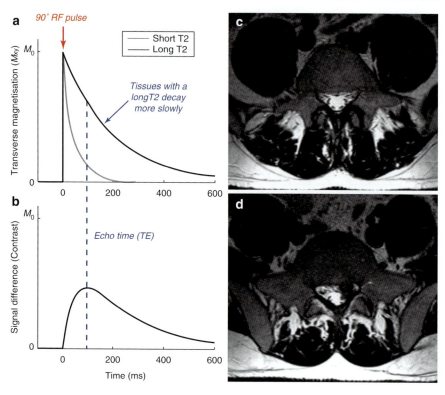

Fig. 4.7 Producing T2 weighting using a long TE: (**a**) Again, we simulate two tissues, one with a short T2 (50 ms, *grey*) and one with a long T2 (200 ms, *black*), during a pulse sequence with a relatively long TE (100 ms). During the long echo time, the transverse magnetisation of the tissue with a short T2 decays rapidly, giving only a small signal. The transverse magnetisation of the tissue with a long T2 decays much more slowly, yielding a higher signal. (**b**) The signal difference, or contrast, between the two tissues varies over time. By picking the correct echo time we have maximised the contrast between these two tissues. Note that we assume here that the TR period is long relative to the T1 values of these tissues so the longitudinal magnetisation has fully recovered before the next RF excitation pulse. (**c**) Axial T2-weighted images corresponding to the T1-weighted images in Fig. 4.6. The nerve roots within the dural sac and in the lateral recesses are well delineated as dark spots. The disc herniation in (**d**) shows low signal intensity due to reduced water content

4.4.4 Proton Density Weighting

In some cases it is advantageous to generate images that isolate proton density as contrast, rather than being weighted by T1 or T2. We already know from the discussions above that using a long TR allows the longitudinal magnetisation to recover fully, irrespective of the T1, and therefore minimises T1 weighting. In addition, using a short TE prevents the signal from decaying significantly before it is measured, thereby minimising T2 weighting. Therefore, images acquired with a long TR and short TE are only weighted by water content or proton density.

Proton density (PD)-weighted images of the spine are used differently to those in cerebral imaging: PD is not used to differentiate the grey and white matter structures

	>>> *More T2 weighting* >>>	
	Short TE	**Long TE**
Short TR	T1 weighting	T1 and T2 weighting (useless!)
Long TR	PD weighting	T2 weighting

>>> More T1 weighting >>>

Table 4.2 Relationships between TR, TE and the resulting image contrast

Note that using a short TR and a long TE results in combined T1 and T2 weighting which tend to cancel each other out. For example, a tissue with a long T1 often has a long T2, giving a low signal due to the T1 weighting but a high signal from the T2 weighting. Conversely a tissue with a short T1 often has a short T2, giving a high signal from T1 weighting but a low signal from T2 weighting. Therefore, the resulting images have low signal and very little contrast

of the spinal cord due to the insufficient contrast of these very small structures, but it is advantageous for depicting soft tissue structures like ligaments and intervertebral discs.

The relationships between TR, TE and the type of image contrast obtained are summarised in Table 4.2.

4.4.5 T2* Weighting

We have seen above that after excitation, the transverse magnetisation decays with time constant T2. However, this is not the whole story. If there is any unevenness (inhomogeneity) in the main magnetic field (B_0), then this causes the magnetisation at different positions to precess at slightly different frequencies. As a result, the transverse magnetisation at different positions no longer adds together to give a strong, coherent signal, but begins to partially cancel out or "dephase" (Fig. 4.8). The result is that the signal decays more quickly than would be expected from T2 alone. This faster decay occurs with a time constant T2*, which is always less than T2.

Why isn't the magnetic field uniform?
Unevenness, or inhomogeneity, in the magnetic field can come from a number of sources. When the subject is placed in the scanner, this distorts the main magnetic field, leading to large-scale inhomogeneity. Most scanners attempt to correct for this using a process known as "shimming", but the results are never perfect. In addition, such inhomogeneity can be present at the microscopic level due to the presence of certain substances that distort the magnetic field, such as deoxyhaemoglobin in blood vessels.

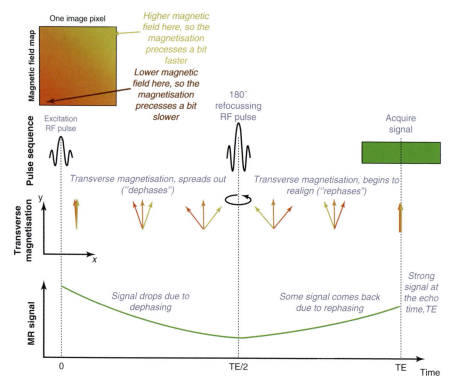

Fig. 4.8 Dephasing due to an inhomogeneous magnetic field and rephasing with a spin-echo refocusing pulse: Within one pixel of an image there is some variation in the magnetic field strength, causing the magnetisation at different locations to precess at slightly different frequencies. After excitation the transverse magnetisation begins to spread out (dephase). Some of the transverse magnetisation partially cancels out, leading to loss of signal. Note that we do not show precession due to B_0 here for clarity. A 180° refocusing pulse flips (mirrors) the magnetisation, so that it then begins to realign, leading to a strong coherent signal at the echo time, TE (a spin echo). Note that there is still some inherent T2 decay that cannot be recovered using a spin echo

This signal loss or dephasing can be reversed by the addition of a 180° RF pulse between the excitation RF pulse and the signal acquisition. This refocuses the dephased magnetisation and forms what is known as a "spin echo". In spin-echo pulse sequences the signal is therefore observed to decay with time constant T2, whereas in gradient echo sequences, where no 180° refocusing pulse is used, the signal decays more quickly, with time constant T2* (Fig. 4.9). Gradient echo sequences with a long TE are therefore said to have T2* weighting.

In some cases this additional signal loss can give useful contrast between otherwise similar tissues. For example, the build-up of blood products in the tissue reduces the T2*, making images with T2* weighting ideally suited to identifying haemorrhage. T2*-weighted sequences also better differentiate bony structures from disc materials compared to T2-weighted sequences, as the low signal of bone

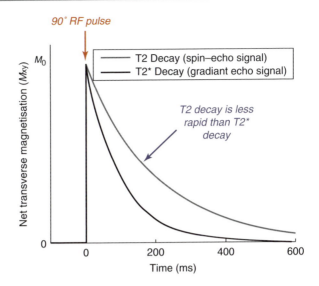

Fig. 4.9 T2* decay: The signal decays more rapidly than would be expected due to T2 alone because of inhomogeneities in the magnetic field, giving a shorter apparent time constant T2*. In this simulation we assume T2 = 200 ms and T2* = 100 ms

contrasts well with the hyperintense discs. Some previous reports reveal that T2*-weighted images are superior to T2-weighted images for detecting spinal cord lesions, even at 3 T, and provide good contrast between grey and white matter. However, T2*-weighted sequences suffer from artefacts in regions of strong magnetic field inhomogeneity, as discussed in Sect. 4.5.2.1. These artefacts can simulate lesions and result in overestimation of osteophytes.

One method for reducing these artefacts involves acquiring signals at multiple echo times after each excitation RF pulse. Combining the images obtained from each echo results in relatively high SNR images with reduced artefacts whilst retaining good tissue contrast (Fig. 4.10). These sequences are sometimes referred to as Multi-Echo Data Image Combination (MEDIC) or Multiple Echo Recombined Gradient Echo (MERGE).

4.4.6 Measures of Image Quality: Signal and Contrast-to-Noise Ratios

Given the variety of different methods for generating images with MRI, it is useful to have measures of image quality to allow an objective comparison to be made. One important feature of medical images is the "noise level". Noise is the random error in an image, which reflects how robust the underlying signal is and is generally reflected in how grainy or speckled an image appears. Noise in images can obscure important features, rendering them non-diagnostic. Measurement of noise is therefore useful in judging image quality.

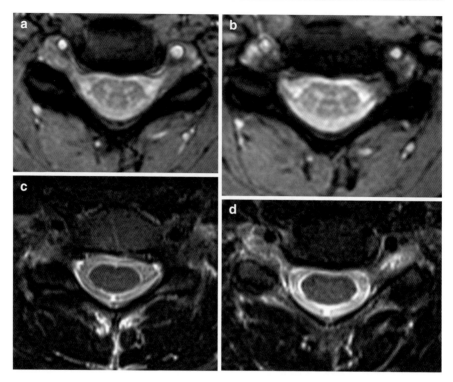

Fig. 4.10 Axial images (**a**, **b**) of the cervical spine showing high grey-white matter contrast produced by a multi-echo (MEDIC) sequence, which is not present in the T2-weighted images (**c**, **d**). Note the signal loss of bony structures in the MEDIC sequence

Where does "noise" in MR images come from?
Noise or random fluctuations in the signal arise from two main sources in MR images. Thermal noise arises from the actual heat (i.e. resistance) of the patient's body and/or electronics, which adds to the currents detected by the RF coil. Physiological processes such as cardiac or respiratory pulsation also lead to pseudorandom fluctuations referred to as "physiological noise".

One common metric of image quality is signal-to-noise ratio (SNR). SNR is defined as the mean signal strength within a defined region of interest divided by the standard deviation of the noise. High SNR is desirable since it implies that the signal dominates over the noise, resulting in clear images.

Signal-to-noise ratio definition

$$\text{SNR} = \frac{\text{Mean Signal}}{\text{Standard Deviation of the Noise}}$$

4 Magnetic Resonance Imaging (MRI) Methods

The main factors that affect the SNR are:

- *Main magnetic field strength (B_0)*: As discussed in Sect. 4.3.2, the main magnetic field causes the water molecules to "polarise" or line up in the same direction, resulting in the net magnetisation that we measure with MRI. The stronger the main magnetic field, the greater this polarising effect is, resulting in a higher net magnetisation and therefore an increased SNR.
- *RF receive coil*: RF receive coils are more sensitive to regions of the body which are close to them. Therefore, placing the receive coil as close to the region of interest as possible will increase the signal and therefore improve the SNR. In addition, coils that cover a large volume tend to pick up more noise, reducing the SNR. Using a series of smaller coil elements together can provide the SNR benefit of using a smaller coil with the better coverage of a larger coil. Note that these "multichannel" or "phased-array" coils can be hard to distinguish from single-channel coils since the individual elements are often concealed within casing.
- *Pulse sequence timing*: As discussed above, the timing of the pulse sequence can alter the measured signal strength and therefore the SNR. For example, using a long TE to generate T2 weighting means that the signal decays to a greater degree, resulting in lower signal strength and thus a lower SNR.
- *Voxel volume*: A voxel is a three-dimensional (3D) pixel, which is typically visualised as a single point in an image. As its name suggests, however, voxels are characterised by a 3D volume. For example, if the in-plane resolution is 2×2 mm with slice thickness 5 mm, the voxel volume is $2 \times 2 \times 5 = 20$ mm^3. The higher the voxel volume, the more water molecules contribute to the signal in that voxel, giving a stronger signal and therefore higher SNR. This is one of the factors that limits the maximum achievable spatial resolution in MRI.
- *Bandwidth*: When magnetic field gradients are used in MRI to localise the signals (see Sect. 4.5.1), they cause the magnetisation at different locations to precess at different frequencies. The measured MR signal is a combination of these different frequencies, and the range of frequencies is known as the bandwidth. Because there is approximately an equal amount of noise at each frequency, using a higher bandwidth allows more noise to enter into the measurement, reducing the SNR.
- *Signal averaging*: If the same image is acquired multiple times and then averaged, this tends to boost the SNR. This is because the noise in each image is random and so tends to be reduced by averaging, whereas the true signal is constant, so is reinforced by the averaging process. However, averaging only increases SNR with the square root of the number of averages (so averaging two repeats only increases SNR by $\sqrt{2} = 1.414$).

Images with different SNR values but constant contrast are shown in Fig. 4.11. Very low SNR values mean that the anatomy and detail in the image are very difficult to discern. However, beyond a certain point, the information required from the image is clear, so increasing the SNR further may not provide any further advantage.

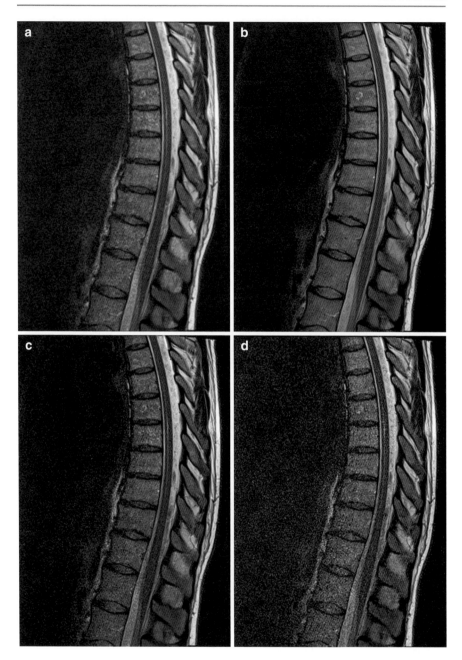

Fig. 4.11 Images with varying SNR but constant contrast. Here we define the relative SNR of the image in (**a**) as relative SNR = 1; (**b**) relative SNR = 1.22; (**c**) relative SNR = 0.7; (**d**) relative SNR = 0.5

Another measure of image quality is contrast-to-noise ratio (CNR). This is a closely related measure that specifically considers the contrast, or signal difference, between two specific tissue types (or sometimes, between two images taken under different conditions). CNR is then calculated by taking the difference between the mean signals of the two tissues (conditions) and dividing by the standard deviation of the noise.

> *Contrast-to-noise ratio definition*
>
> $$CNR = \frac{\text{Mean Signal}(\text{tissue 1}) - \text{Mean Signal}(\text{tissue 2})}{\text{Standard Deviation of the Noise}}$$

CNR therefore provides a measure of whether two tissues (conditions) can be distinguished from each other. For example, CNR = 1 indicates that the signal difference between two tissues types is of the same size as the noise in the image, making it very difficult to see any difference between them. This kind of measure can be useful, for example, when optimising the signal to distinguish a particular type of lesion from healthy tissue.

It is worth noting that images with a high SNR do not necessarily have a high CNR. For example, if the contrast of interest is between two tissues with the same proton density but different T2 values, then a short echo time will give a high signal and therefore high SNR. However, there will be almost no contrast between the two tissues since no time has been allowed for T2 decay to occur, resulting in a low CNR.

SNR and CNR provide useful objective measures for comparing different MR images but they do not completely encapsulate image quality. For example, these measures do not account for differences in spatial resolution, the level of spurious signals (artefacts), how long it takes to acquire the images, etc. They are therefore most useful when comparing images that are otherwise matched.

4.5   Image Formation and Artefacts

We have seen in the previous sections how the MRI pulse sequence can be modified to generate different signal strengths from each tissue type. However, the signal that is measured by the RF receive coil comes from the entire subject. How then do we generate images? In other words, how do we localise where the measured signal is coming from? The trick to this rather magical process lies in the use of magnetic field gradients and some clever mathematics. In this section we will discuss how the MR signals are localised and how this process influences errors, or artefacts, in the resulting images.

4.5.1 From Signals to Images

4.5.1.1 Magnetic Field Gradients

All MRI scanners contain a set of three gradients (see Fig. 4.1). When one of these is switched on, it causes the magnetic field strength to vary with position along a specific direction. For example, if the "z" gradient is turned on, then the magnetic field strength towards the subject's feet is reduced, but near the head it is increased, as shown in Fig. 4.12a. Similarly, application of the "x" or "y" gradient causes variation in the magnetic field strength across the left-right or anterior-posterior direction, respectively. Note that the magnetic field gradients do not change the *direction* of the magnetic field, which always points along the z axis, they only change its *strength*.

As we discussed in Sect. 4.3.2, the precession frequency of the magnetisation is proportional to the magnetic field strength it experiences. Therefore, using a gradient to cause a variation in the magnetic field strength across a given direction also causes the precession frequency of the magnetisation to vary in that same direction, as shown in Fig. 4.12. It is this difference in the precession frequency that allows us to localise the MR signal, as we shall see below.

4.5.1.2 Slice Selection

The first step in localising where the measured signal is coming from often involves selecting a single plane, or "slice", for imaging within the subject. The necessary insight lies in the fact that in order to excite the magnetisation (i.e. rotate it into the transverse plane to generate a signal), the transmit RF pulse must be played out at the exact precession frequency of the magnetisation. If the frequency is too high or too low, it will not affect the magnetisation and therefore not generate any MR signal. The trick here is to apply the transmit RF pulse in the presence of a magnetic field gradient which causes the precession frequency of the magnetisation to vary with position. As a result, the frequency of the RF pulse will only match the precession frequency of the magnetisation at one location along the gradient direction (i.e. a single plane) within the subject, and therefore, only a single slice is excited (see Fig. 4.13). Because we only detect signal that has been excited, the rest of the imaging process can proceed with confidence that all signal originates from this slice alone.

The position of the excited slice can be shifted by simply modifying the frequency of the transmitted RF pulse to match the frequency of the desired slice. Furthermore, the orientation of the slice is determined by the direction of the applied magnetic field gradient. For example, transmitting the RF pulse in the presence of a gradient in the z (inferior-superior) direction excites an axial slice, whereas using a gradient in the x (left-right) direction yields a sagittal slice.

Note that in practice the transmitted RF pulse can contain multiple frequencies. By transmitting simultaneously at all frequencies within a given range, we excite a corresponding range of locations (i.e. a slice with a certain thickness). The range of transmitted frequencies and the size of the applied gradient control the thickness of the excited slice.

Fig. 4.12 Magnetic field gradients: (**a**) Applying the gradient in the z direction causes a linear variation in the magnetic field strength across this direction; (**b**) This results in a linear variation in the precession frequency of the magnetisation in the z direction

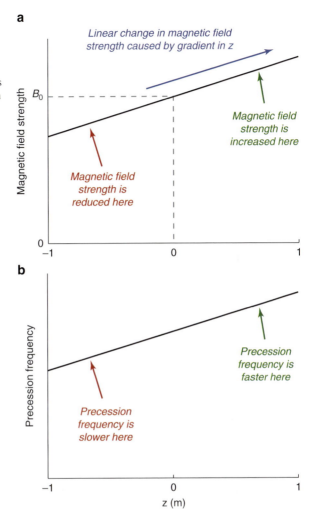

4.5.1.3 Spatial Localisation

Once a slice of magnetisation has been excited, the signal that we measure will only come from this slice, but how do we now generate a two-dimensional image? This is one of the trickiest concepts to grasp in MRI, but is directly relevant to image quality, speed and understanding artefacts.

Frequency Encoding

The key to spatial localisation is that when a magnetic field gradient is applied, the precession frequency of the magnetisation varies across space. If such a gradient is applied after the magnetisation has been excited, the frequency of the signals produced by the water molecules will depend on their location along the direction of the applied gradient. Therefore, by measuring the frequency of the MR signal in the

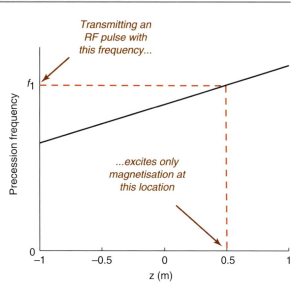

Fig. 4.13 Slice selection: If a magnetic field gradient is applied in the z direction the precession frequency varies linearly across z. Playing out an RF pulse with frequency f_1 only excites magnetisation with precession frequency equal to f_1. This occurs at a specific location along the z axis (0.5 m in this case), exciting a single axial slice within the subject

presence of a gradient, we can work backwards to determine the location at which that signal was generated. The process of recording the MR signal in the presence of a gradient is often referred to as "frequency encoding", since spatial location is encoded in the frequency of the MR signal.

In practice there will be signals generated from a whole range of locations across the slice. The RF receive coil picks up all of these signals simultaneously, so the total signal measured is the sum of the signals from all the water molecules in the excited slice. To map out the distribution of the water molecules, we use a mathematical procedure known as the "Fourier transform", which tells us how much signal is present at each frequency. Since the relationship between frequency and location is determined purely by the applied gradient, we can deduce how much signal originates from each location. A simple example of this process is described in Fig. 4.14 and an analogy, which some may find useful, is given in the textbox.

Phase Encoding

Using the techniques discussed thus far, we can excite the magnetisation in a single slice and determine the distribution of this magnetisation along a single direction. However, we have not yet obtained a two-dimensional image of this slice. In order to do this, it turns out that the concept of frequency encoding can be generalised into two dimensions in a process known as "phase encoding". This involves turning on a magnetic field gradient at right angles to the frequency encoding direction for a brief period before the frequency encoding gradient is turned on and the signal is recorded. This causes the magnetisation at different locations to add together or cancel out in a way that is dependent on their position. This step is repeated a number of times with different amounts of phase encoding. Image formation in MRI involves pooling measurements made with both phase and frequency encoding to determine the spatial distribution of magnetisation across the excited slice.

4 Magnetic Resonance Imaging (MRI) Methods 61

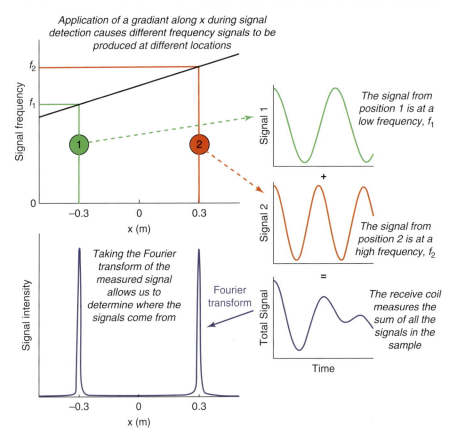

Fig. 4.14 Frequency Encoding: Here we consider a simple imaging experiment where there are only two sources of MR signal, located at $x=\pm 0.3$ m from the centre of the scanner. After the RF excitation pulse, the x gradient is switched on. This causes a variation in the precession frequency across the x direction, so source 1 produces a signal at a lower frequency than source 2. The RF receive coil measures the sum of signals from all the sources. However, taking the Fourier Transform of this total signal tells us how much signal intensity there is at each frequency. With knowledge of the applied gradient strength, this allows us to determine how much of the signal originates from each location along the x-axis. In other words, the spatial position along x was "encoded" in the frequency of the MR signal

k-Space

Hopefully it has become clear by this point that MRI is quite different from most other imaging methods, in that the measured signal at any point in time does not come from a single region within the subject, but from the entire subject. The reconstruction of images relies on a mathematical procedure, the Fourier transform, which translates the raw measured signals into maps of the spatial distribution of that signal. This process involves an intermediate step that allocates signals acquired over time to corresponding points within a conceptual domain called "*k*-space". Each point in *k*-space represents a different "spatial frequency" within the image,

Frequency encoding and gremlins

Spatial localisation is a tricky concept, so we explore it here using a slightly bizarre analogy: Imagine you are an expert pianist who is blindfolded and seated at a piano (see Fig. 4.15). Jumping up and down on the piano keys are some pesky little gremlins (bear with us, this does have something to do with MRI!). They are very small, so more than one can fit on each piano key. The more gremlins that are on a given key, the louder the sound they make. It is your job to remove the gremlins, but obviously you cannot see them, so how can this be done?

Thankfully, the human ear is quite good at distinguishing different sound pitches or frequencies. Even though the gremlins are all making noise at the same time, you can still hear which frequencies are present. Since the frequency of sound produced by each piano key increases from left to right, the frequency of the sound tells you about the position of each gremlin. Being an expert pianist, you can therefore hear which keys are occupied by gremlins, or in other words, the spatial distribution of the gremlins. Furthermore, the loudness or "amplitude" of the sound at each frequency tells you how many gremlins are on each key. Therefore, just by listening to the noise created by all the gremlins together, you can tell exactly where they are and how many of them there are at each location. You can therefore swiftly dispatch the pesky gremlins and get on with your blindfolded piano playing. The key insight is that you know how exactly frequency maps to position and can therefore build a mental map of how many gremlins are at each location.

So, back to MRI: in this analogy the gremlins are the magnetisation of water molecules that have been excited and the sound they produce is the MR signal. Applying a magnetic field gradient across the slice causes the frequency of the signal produced by the magnetisation to vary with position, just like the piano. Listening to the sound produced by the gremlins is equivalent to recording the total MR signal measured using the RF receive coil. Just like the pianist, the frequencies present in the MR signal tell us the positions of the water molecules (gremlins) along the direction of the applied magnetic field gradient. The amplitude (loudness) of the signal at each frequency tells us the size of the transverse magnetisation at each location. In other words, we have knowledge of the spatial distribution of the transverse magnetisation!

and knowledge of the contribution from each spatial frequency is sufficient to reconstruct an image of the excited slice. This is demonstrated graphically in Fig. 4.16. Points near the centre of k-space represent low spatial frequencies, which give the image its main structure and contrast. Points near the edges of k-space represent high spatial frequencies, which give information about the detailed, high-resolution elements of the image.

From this perspective, frequency encoding corresponds to measuring a single line of k-space and phase encoding corresponds to jumping to a new position in k-space (see Fig. 4.17). Most commonly, a single line is acquired each TR,

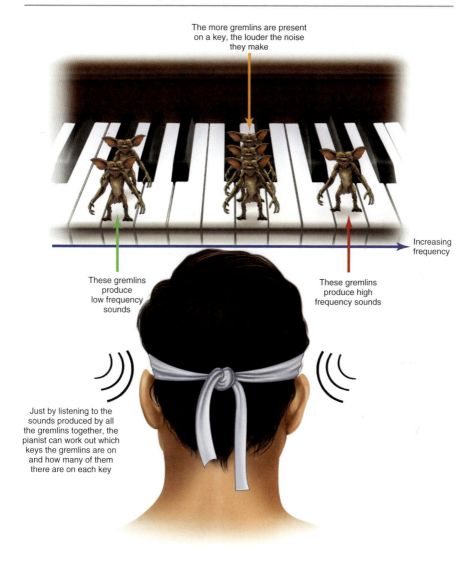

Fig. 4.15 The gremlin analogy for frequency encoding

consisting of a series of measurements made at even intervals along the line. In order to generate an image of the excited slice, all the lines of k-space must be measured before the Fourier transform can be applied to reconstruct the image. The number of pixels in the final image is equal to the number of measurements along the frequency- and phase-encoding axes (i.e. the number of measurements per line and number of lines, respectively). So, for example, an image with 300×200 pixels consists of 200 lines of k-space, each with 300 measurements per line. This property explains why standard MRI acquisitions take such a long time: this image would require 200 RF excitations, each of which is followed by the acquisition of one line of k-space. Many acquisitions (e.g. T2- or PD-weighted) need a relatively long time

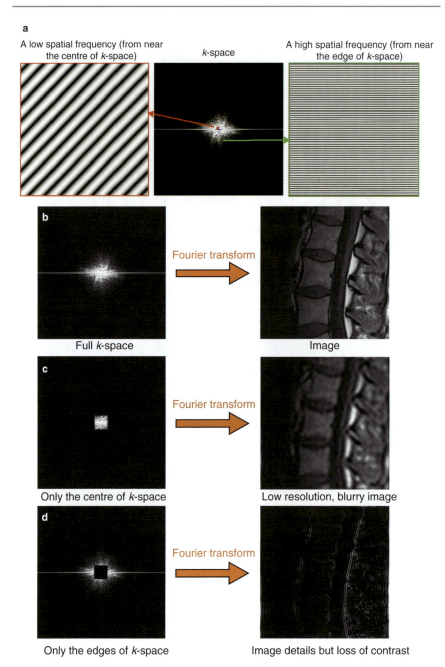

Fig. 4.16 k-space: (**a**) The measured signal at different points in k-space correspond to different spatial frequencies within the image; (**b**) Taking the Fourier transform of the data in k-space yields the MR image; (**c**) Reconstructing an image from just the centre of k-space (the low spatial frequencies) gives a blurry, low-resolution image; (**d**) Reconstructing an image from just the edges of k-space (the high spatial frequencies) retains the high-resolution details (such as edges) in the image, but we lose the overall contrast between different tissue types

4 Magnetic Resonance Imaging (MRI) Methods

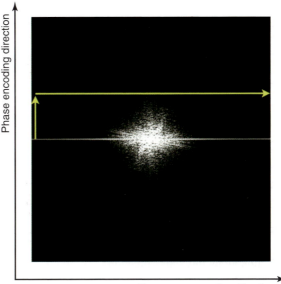

Fig. 4.17 Frequency and phase encoding in k-space: Frequency encoding corresponds to measuring a single line in k-space (*horizontal arrow*). Phase encoding causes us to jump to a new position in k-space (*vertical arrow*), allowing a different line to be measured during frequency encoding

between RF excitation pulses (i.e. a long TR), which means it could take minutes just to produce an image of a single slice. Thankfully there are a number of ways of speeding up the imaging process, as we shall see later, although scan times still tend to be long relative to other modalities such as CT.

There are some important relationships between how signals are measured in k-space and the resulting image. In particular, the field of view (i.e. physical size of the area to be imaged) is determined by how close together points in k-space are measured. Measuring closer together in k-space corresponds to a larger field of view. In addition, spatial resolution is determined by how far out in k-space measurements are acquired. Measuring further out in k-space (at higher spatial frequencies) corresponds to higher resolution images (i.e. the size of each pixel in the image is smaller).

Relationships between how k-space is sampled and the resulting image			
k-space	Image	Relationship
Number of measurements (matrix size)	Number of pixels (matrix size)	The number of measurements in k-space is equal to the number of pixels in the resulting image
Separation of measurements	Field of view (FOV)	Measuring closer together in k-space corresponds to a larger field of view
How far out measurements are acquired (i.e. the maximum spatial frequency sampled)	Image resolution (i.e. the size of each pixel)	Measuring further out in k-space corresponds to smaller pixels (higher resolution images)

One important consequence of the relationships between k-space sampling and the resulting image is wrap-around or aliasing, an artefact that is particularly relevant to spine imaging. As we saw above, the distance between k-space measurements determines the field of view (FOV) of the reconstructed image; however, simply the prescription of a certain k-space measurement scheme does *not* prevent signal contributions from outside the FOV. Given that the slice excitation produces signal from all locations within a given plane, what happens if we prescribe a FOV that is smaller than the extent of the excited slice? Signal is always assigned to some spatial location, but the small FOV introduces ambiguity as to where signal from outside the FOV belongs. As a result, signal from outside the FOV is "wrapped around" into the other side of the image, where it may overlap with other image features, as shown in Fig. 4.18. This problem does not occur in the frequency encoding direction, where we are able to suppress signal from outside the FOV using simple filters. This provides us with our first example of how some knowledge of MRI physics can avoid an image artefact: if there is MR signal outside the desired FOV along one direction, aliasing can be avoided by setting the frequency encoding direction along this same direction.

Imaging more than one slice: 2D multi-slice vs. 3D acquisitions
In this section we have discussed acquiring two-dimensional (2D) images after exciting a single slice. To acquire images of a whole volume, multiple slices can be imaged consecutively to build up a 3D image. However, it is also possible to excite a slab encompassing multiple slices within the subject and encode k-space in three dimensions. In other words, we use frequency encoding along one dimension and phase encoding along the other two dimensions. We can then use a Fourier transform to reconstruct a 3D volume.

In many imaging scenarios, 3D acquisitions offer improved signal-to-noise ratio (SNR). In addition, 3D acquisitions can achieve completely contiguous slices (without the slight gap required in 2D) and thin slices with high fidelity (where thin 2D slices tend to be spatially warped). 3D sequences are useful for cervical spine imaging to reveal foraminal disease accurately and also allow reformatting oblique views en face to the obliquely oriented cervical intervertebral foramina. 3D sequences providing a myelographic effect (see Chaps. 7 and 8) are advantageous in delineating spinal nerve root affection within their intradural and intraforaminal course.

However, 3D acquisitions are somewhat more prone to motion and flow artefacts. In addition, 2D multi-slice acquisitions are often more appropriate for pulse sequences that require a long TR (such as T2 or proton density weighted images). The long time required between successive excitation pulses of the same slice can be utilised to acquire images of other slices, which is not possible if an entire 3D volume is excited each time.

4 Magnetic Resonance Imaging (MRI) Methods   67

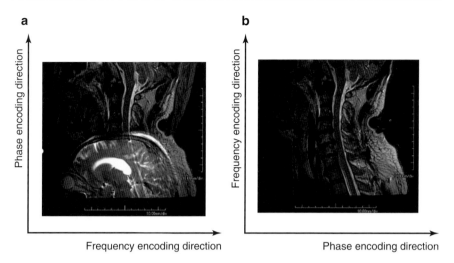

Fig. 4.18 Wrap-around or aliasing: (**a**) Here the phase-encoding direction was selected as inferior-superior, causing signal from the brain to wrap back in to the bottom of the image, obscuring the spine; (**b**) Changing the phase-encoding direction to be anterior-posterior prevents the aliasing from occurring since aliasing does not occur along the frequency encoding direction

4.5.1.4 Readout Methods

In the previous section we discussed how the MR image is generated from a sufficient number of measurements in k-space. We introduced the simplest way to acquire these measurements: by acquiring a single line of k-space after each RF excitation pulse. However, this is only one of many ways of measuring data in k-space. By modifying the way the magnetic field gradients are switched on and off, we can choose any desired trajectory through k-space, acquiring measurements along the way (see Fig. 4.19). Each of these trajectories has various advantages and disadvantages.

Single line readouts are simple and robust, but since only one line of k-space is acquired after each RF pulse, they are only suited to pulse sequences with a short TR, such as T1-weighted acquisitions. In fast spin-echo (FSE, also called turbo spin echo or TSE) readouts, a subset of all of the k-space lines are acquired after the RF excitation pulse, with each line separated by a spin echo. As a result the centre of k-space, which dictates the tissue contrast, is typically acquired with a relatively long effective echo time (TE). Such readouts are therefore often used for T2-weighted images, which require a long TE. They are particularly useful in areas of magnetic field inhomogeneity since the spin-echo pulses prevent signal decay due to T2* effects. Echo planar imaging (EPI) is similar to FSE, but no spin-echo pulses are used and samples are taken in both directions, giving very rapid coverage of k-space. In fact, often all k-space lines are acquired after a single excitation pulse. This makes EPI suitable for high temporal resolution applications like perfusion, functional or diffusion imaging, but it suffers from signal loss and distortion in areas of magnetic field inhomogeneity.

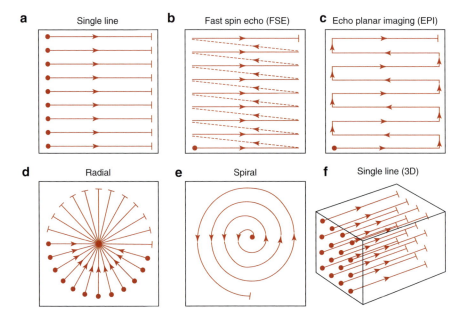

Fig. 4.19 Examples of k-space trajectories: following the RF excitation pulse signals are recorded starting at each circle, following the solid line and ending at the short line at right angles. Only a small number of lines have been shown for clarity. In (**b**) the dashed lines represent movement through k-space without data recording which occur during the spin-echo RF pulses. (**a–e**) Show 2D trajectories for imaging a single slice after excitation, but these can all be used in 3D acquisitions too, as demonstrated using the single line readout in (**f**)

In radial and spiral readouts, k-space samples are not acquired on a regular grid. This introduces some complications for image reconstruction, but these alternative trajectories do offer some advantages. For example, radial readouts are robust to motion artefacts and enable extremely short echo times and some k-space lines can be missed out to reduce the scan time without causing significant artefacts. Spiral readouts cover k-space very efficiently with a short echo time and have reduced sensitivity to flowing magnetisation but suffer from blurring and/or streaking artefacts near magnetic field imperfections.

All of the trajectories described above have corresponding variations that cover k-space in 3D. In Fig. 4.19f, a 3D single line readout is shown where phase encoding occurs along two directions to fill the 3D k-space.

It is worth noting that although certain readout techniques are better suited to certain types of imaging, pulse sequences are essentially modular: any type of readout can be combined with any type of pulse sequence. The pulse sequence type and timing determines the tissue contrast, whereas the readout method is the primary determinant of the total scan time and image artefacts.

4.5.1.5 Acceleration Techniques

As mentioned previously MRI scans often require long scan times (on the order of minutes). This not only reduces patient throughput but can also lead to patient

4 Magnetic Resonance Imaging (MRI) Methods

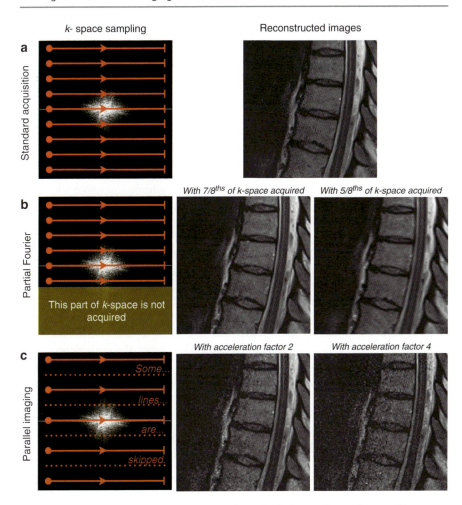

Fig. 4.20 Acceleration techniques illustrated with a single line readout and zoomed images to show changes in image quality: (**a**) In a standard acquisition all lines of *k*-space are acquired (only a small number are shown here for clarity); (**b**) Partial Fourier acceleration involves fully acquiring one half of *k*-space but only partially acquiring the other half. This leads to blurring in the resulting images and/or loss of SNR with severity increasing with the amount of *k*-space not acquired. (**c**) In parallel imaging some lines of *k*-space are skipped (here every other line is skipped corresponding to an acceleration factor of 2). The reconstructed images show non-uniform SNR degradation that worsens at higher acceleration factors. Note the accentuated central canal is blurred in (**b**) resulting in a false myelopathy signal

discomfort, increased motion artefacts and can even preclude certain types of scans requiring fast imaging. In the previous section we discussed some readout methods that acquire many lines of *k*-space after each excitation, dramatically reducing the scan time, but these are not appropriate for all types of acquisition and sometimes further speed up is desirable. A number of techniques have been developed to help accelerate image acquisition. We will discuss two common approaches here, which are illustrated in Fig. 4.20:

- *Partial Fourier*: In most cases there are predictable relationships between signals on opposite sides of outer k-space. Under ideal conditions, only half of k-space needs to be acquired and used to predict the signal from the other half, potentially cutting the acquisition time in two. In practice it is necessary to acquire more than half of k-space to correct for slight errors, giving a more robust image (Fig. 4.20b). The downside of partial Fourier is loss of SNR and/or blurring in the phase-encoding direction.
- *Parallel Imaging*: In recent years RF receive arrays combining multiple, spatially separated coils have gained popularity due to their improved SNR. Each coil element is most sensitive to a region within the subject that it is closest to, so the signals received by each coil element contain some information about where the signal has come from. This additional information means that, with some short calibration steps, some lines of k-space can be skipped (Fig. 4.20c). For example, using a parallel imaging factor of two means that every other line of k-space is not acquired, halving the acquisition time. This is equivalent to increasing the spacing between k-space measurements, which would normally result in reduced field of view and potentially lead to aliasing artefacts. However, the spatial information in the coils can be used to remove this aliasing, leading to a full-FOV image. There are a number of different methods for image reconstruction, the most common of which are SENSE and GRAPPA. In theory the maximum acceleration factor that can be used is equal to the number of coil elements across the phase-encoding direction. However, parallel imaging causes non-uniform degradation of SNR across the image that gets significantly worse with higher acceleration factors.

4.5.2 Image Artefacts

The errors or "artefacts" in MR images can be somewhat unintuitive. For example, motion during an MRI acquisition can cause shifted copies of the true image to appear at a distant location (ghosting) as well as blurring. Getting to grips with the unique way in which MR images are acquired is important for understanding how these artefacts come about. In this section we discuss some of the common artefacts found in spinal images and simple methods for their reduction. In the next section more sophisticated techniques for helping to reduce artefacts and improve image quality are discussed.

4.5.2.1 Susceptibility Artefacts and Metallic Implants
The presence of materials with different magnetic susceptibility to tissue alters the local magnetic field. This occurs at borders between tissue and air or bone, but is most significant near metallic implants. The artefacts are more pronounced for certain types of metal, such as steel, than for others, such as titanium. The alteration of the magnetic field can lead to rapid signal loss (i.e. the $T2^*$ is shortened). In addition, the altered magnetic field interferes with the spatial localisation process, which assumes that the only variation in the magnetic field is caused by the applied

4 Magnetic Resonance Imaging (MRI) Methods

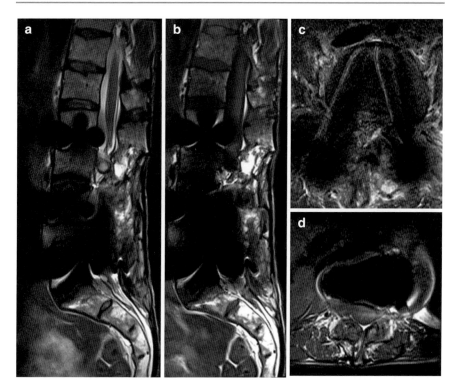

Fig. 4.21 Susceptibility artefacts near a metallic implant. Sagittal (**a**, **b**) and axial (**c**, **d**) images of the lumbar spine after implantation of a dorsal fixateur externe showing severe signal drop out and distortion of the nearby bony and soft tissues. The nerve roots are hardly recognisable (**c**)

magnetic field gradients. As a result, the signal location is miscalculated, leading to distortions in the image. An example of these susceptibility artefacts is given in Fig. 4.21.

The signal loss can be reduced with spin-echo pulse sequences and/or a short echo time (TE). Distortion is most problematic in readout techniques that acquire multiple lines of k-space without interleaved refocusing pulses, such as EPI; alternatives, such as FSE, can significantly reduce distortions, but are not always possible. Increasing the bandwidth of the readout (which equates to increasing the strength of the frequency encoding gradient) increases the speed of the image acquisition process and helps reduce distortion, but at the cost of SNR.

4.5.2.2 Fat Chemical Shift

Although most of the MR signal originates in hydrogen nuclei within water molecules, those bound to fat also contribute. However, due to the differences in chemical binding of hydrogen within water and fat molecules, the hydrogen protons experience slightly different local magnetic fields. This causes the MR signal of fat to have a slightly different frequency to that of water. Since MRI uses frequency to

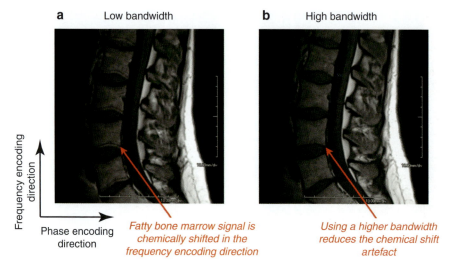

Fig. 4.22 Fat chemical shift artefact: (**a**) The signal from the fatty bone marrow is displaced in the frequency encoding direction due to the chemical shift artefact; (**b**) Using a higher bandwidth reduces the chemical shift

determine spatial location, fat signal is shifted in the image relative to the water signal in the frequency encoding direction, as shown in Fig. 4.22. This shifted signal can cause signal from fatty tissues to overlie other important image features.

This artefact is more significant in pulse sequences that use a low bandwidth. This is because the frequency difference between water and fat is larger relative to the range of frequencies present in the MR signal introduced by the applied gradient. In addition, readout methods like EPI that acquire multiple lines of k-space without interleaved refocusing pulses are particularly sensitive to chemical shift. For these readouts, differences in the MR signals from water and fat accumulate between lines of k-space, giving a large chemical shift, predominantly in the *phase-encoding* direction.

4.5.2.3 Gibb's Ringing (Truncation Artefact)

In order to obtain an image with a certain resolution, we have to collect measurements in k-space out to a certain point, which is further out in k-space for higher resolution images. The truncation of k-space effectively treats the imaged anatomy as if there is no significant signal past this point. This is often not the case, particularly for structures that require high spatial frequencies to represent them properly, such as edges. This over-emphasises the contribution of the spatial frequencies at the edge of the object which were included. The result is "ringing" artefacts at the highest acquired spatial frequencies near sharp transitions in the image, such as boundaries between tissue and air. An example is shown in Fig. 4.23. This artefact is important to be aware of, since ringing appears highly structured and can mimic anatomy (or disease). The artefact can be reduced by acquiring the image again at

4 Magnetic Resonance Imaging (MRI) Methods 73

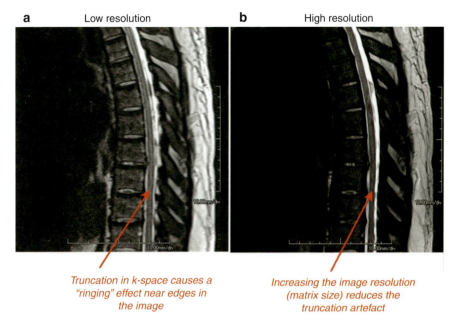

Fig. 4.23 Gibb's ringing or "truncation" artefacts: (**a**) When imaging with a low-resolution, ringing artefacts appear near edges in the image, in this case causing a hyperintense region in the centre of the spinal cord; (**b**) Increasing the image resolution reduces these ringing artefacts

higher resolution or by using processing techniques to attenuate the edges of k-space, smoothing out ringing artefacts at the cost of increased blurring.

4.5.2.4 Patient Motion

Motion is a considerable issue in MRI due to the long time required to form an image. Motion artefacts can be caused by gross motion of the patient or by physiological effects such as swallowing, blinking, breathing or beating of the heart. For many other kinds of imaging, the effect of motion is to blur the moving object, without affecting the rest of the image. This intuitive explanation does not apply in MRI because we acquire data in k-space, where each sample contains information about the entire image. Predicting the effect of patient motion on the resulting images is not simple, because it depends on the type of motion and which parts of k-space are sampled at the time of motion. Generally speaking the result is a combination of blurring and "ghosting", where copies of image features are seen to appear across the image in the phase-encoding direction. Ghosting is more evident if the motion is periodic, such as that caused by cardiac or respiratory effects, or if several k-space lines are acquired per TR. An example of motion artefacts is shown in Fig. 4.24.

Gross patient motion can be reduced by ensuring the patient is comfortable and using appropriate stabilisation to restrict motion where possible. Increasing imaging speed also reduces the chances of significant motion during the course of a single scan. Reduction of artefacts due to physiological motion (e.g. cardiac or respiration) requires more sophisticated methods that are discussed in the next section.

4.5.2.5 Flow Artefacts
Flowing fluid, such as blood or cerebrospinal fluid (CSF), can cause a variety of artefacts in MRI (see Fig. 4.25 for examples):
- *Signal dephasing*: In areas of fast or turbulent flow, the range of velocities within a single voxel can cause the signals from different water molecules to "dephase", leading to signal loss.

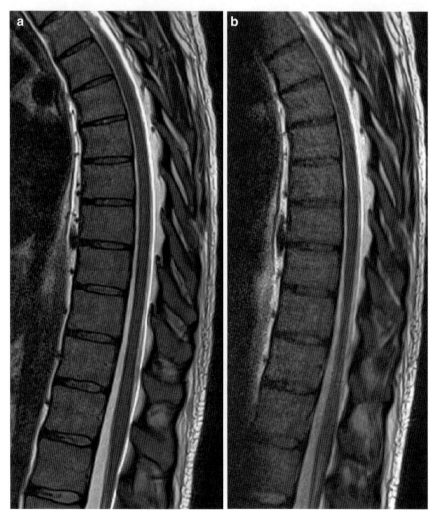

Fig. 4.24 Motion artefacts: in a subject (**a**) without and (**b**) with small movements of their legs. Periodic cardiac motion manifests as ghosting artefacts in the phase-encoding direction, shown by the white arrows (**c**, **d**)

4 Magnetic Resonance Imaging (MRI) Methods

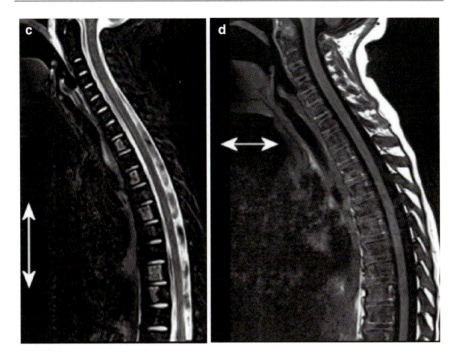

Fig. 4.24 (continued)

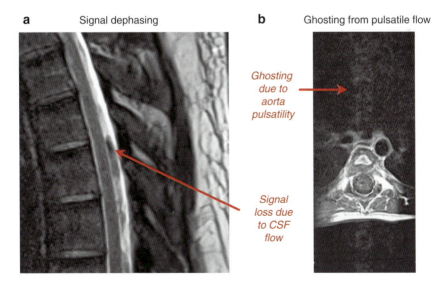

Fig. 4.25 Flow related artefacts: (**a**) Signal dephasing due to turbulent flow within CSF; (**b**) ghosting from pulsatile flow within the aorta, overlaying the spinal canal

- *Outflow signal loss*: In pulse sequences which use a spin echo to refocus the magnetisation, fluid which has experienced the initial excitation pulse may have moved out of the slice of interest by the time the refocusing pulse is applied. Therefore, the magnetisation is not refocused and the resulting MR signal is significantly decreased. Note that this can cause non-uniform artefacts across the flowing region since areas of faster flow will be more greatly affected.
- *Inflow signal enhancement*: The use of a short TR pulse sequence causes the average or "steady-state" signal to be reduced. However, fresh fluid flowing into the imaging region will not have experienced the previous RF excitation pulses and will therefore produce a larger MR signal. This signal enhancement will be more significant in areas of faster flow.
- *Ghosting from pulsatile flow*: The signal in a large pulsatile artery will fluctuate across the cardiac cycle due to the effects described above. In pulse sequences where k-space is not acquired after a single RF excitation pulse, this will lead to a periodic variation in the acquired MR signal across k-space. The Fourier relationship between k-space and image space dictates that periodic variations in k-space cause signal replication, or ghosting, in the image. In other words, copies of the pulsatile structure appear in other locations throughout the image in the phase-encoding direction. These can overlap with other important features, leading to difficulties in image interpretation.

There are a few simple methods for flow artefact reduction. These include using pulse sequences with a short TE to help reduce signal dephasing. Outflow signal loss can be reduced by using gradient echo sequences, positioning the imaging region parallel to the flow direction or using thicker slices. Reduction of inflow enhancement and pulsatility artefacts require more complex methods discussed in the next section.

4.6 Tricks to Improve Image Quality

The basic pulse sequences described so far in this chapter can produce images with a range of different contrasts. Adjustment of the parameters within these sequences can alter the tissue contrast and help reduce certain artefacts, but in some cases this is not sufficient. In this section we discuss some more complex techniques for improving image quality by reducing artefacts and improving contrast.

4.6.1 Reducing Physiological Fluctuations

As discussed in the previous section, physiological fluctuations, such as those caused by cardiac or respiratory motion, can lead to artefacts in the resulting images. There are a number of methods for dealing with these:
- *Gating*: If image acquisition is confined, or gated, to the same periods within the cardiac or respiratory cycles, then the resulting artefacts are significantly reduced. Electrocardiogram or pulse-oximeter readings can be used to trigger image

4 Magnetic Resonance Imaging (MRI) Methods

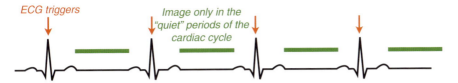

Fig. 4.26 Gating to reduce physiological fluctuations: An example of triggering from the cardiac waveform, to ensure data are always acquired during diastole

acquisition to the cardiac cycle, which helps reduce artefacts from pulsatile behaviour in blood vessels or CSF (Fig. 4.26). Similarly, respiratory bellows allow triggering to the breathing cycle. However, gating typically leads to periods of "dead time" in which no data is acquired whilst the scanner waits for the next trigger, leading to longer acquisition times and reduced efficiency. In addition, differences in the cardiac or respiratory rates between subjects cause differences in the TR and can therefore influence the image contrast, which is often undesirable.

- *Flow compensation*: Signal dephasing due to fast or turbulent flow can be reduced by the addition of "flow compensation" gradients. These additional gradients help refocus the signal from moving magnetisation, bringing back some of the lost signal. These do, however, require some additional time after the RF excitation pulse, meaning that the TE must be extended.
- *Suppression of moving structures*: Removing the signal from fluctuating structures such as the heart, lungs or aorta prevents them from causing artefacts in the resulting images. Such suppression is discussed in the next section.

4.6.2 Suppression of Adjacent Tissues

There are a number of cases where tissues adjacent to the area of interest can cause artefacts that obscure important features. For example, respiratory motion, cardiac motion or pulsatile flow in a large artery can cause ghosting which obscures the spine. Applying a 90° excitation pulse followed by a "spoiler" gradient to the problematic region removes the longitudinal magnetisation and then dephases the resulting signal. This suppresses or "saturates" the problematic region, such that an excitation pulse applied immediately afterward only generates transverse magnetisation and therefore signal from the region of interest.

This technique can be used to saturate regions around the spine before acquiring images, reducing the required field of view. If phase encoding is performed along the direction of reduced FOV, the number of phase-encoding steps can be reduced, speeding up the acquisition. In addition, inflow enhancement artefacts from fluid flowing into the imaging region can be reduced by applying suppression pulses to a region just above or below the slices of interest. This can be useful for reducing the CSF signal in acquisitions where fluid is intended to be dark.

4.6.3 Inversion Recovery

A very powerful technique to manipulate the contrast between different tissues is to apply a 180° "inversion" pulse to the magnetisation before imaging commences. This has the effect of flipping magnetisation initially at its equilibrium position aligned along the z-axis to point in the opposite direction, towards $-z$. The magnetisation then begins to recover back towards equilibrium with time constant T1 (see Fig. 4.27). After waiting a certain time, known as the inversion time (TI), the RF excitation pulse is applied. Due to the different amount of recovery of each tissue, the resulting signal will be inherently T1-weighted. This trick can be used to enhance T1 weighting.

In addition, if the TI is selected in such a way that a tissue with a particular T1 is crossing through the zero point in its recovery, then there is no longitudinal magnetisation for the excitation pulse to act upon, meaning that this tissue produces zero signal. This technique is an example where one knowingly sacrifices SNR (since all tissues have somewhat reduced signal from the inversion) in favour of improved contrast. Common uses of this technique include a short TI to suppress fat (known as Short Tau Inversion Recovery, STIR) and using a long TI to suppress CSF (FLuid Attenuated Inversion Recovery, FLAIR), as shown in Fig. 4.27.

Sagittal T1-weighted FLAIR sequences are often used at 3 T especially for the cervical spine due to the excellent suppression of CSF and better delineation of bony lesions. Sagittal T2-weighted STIR images are also useful for detecting myelon lesions (Fig. 4.28).

4.6.4 Fat Suppression

The MR signal arising from fat can be strong and is particularly problematic if it is chemically shifted on to a region of interest. This makes techniques for suppressing fat highly desirable. In addition, comparison of images with and without the fat signal can help differentiate different types of lesion. Two of the most important methods for suppressing fat are:

- *Spectrally selective saturation*: Fat and water precess at slightly different frequencies (Figs. 4.29 and 4.30). Therefore, if a 90° excitation pulse is applied at the fat frequency in the absence of a magnetic field gradient, then only the magnetisation of fat will be rotated in the transverse plane, with the water magnetisation left unaffected. A strong gradient pulse can then dephase the transverse magnetisation of fat, as described in Sect. 4.6.2. The normal (water) excitation pulse can then be applied. This method works best at higher field strengths where the frequency separation of water and fat is larger. Since it relies on fat processing at a particular frequency, it only works well in areas of good magnetic field homogeneity.
- *Short Tau Inversion Recovery (STIR)*: As described in the section on inversion recovery above, the use of an inversion pulse and a short delay (TI) causes the signal from fat to be suppressed. This method does introduce some T1 weighting which may not always be desirable, and it reduces the longitudinal magnetisation

4 Magnetic Resonance Imaging (MRI) Methods   79

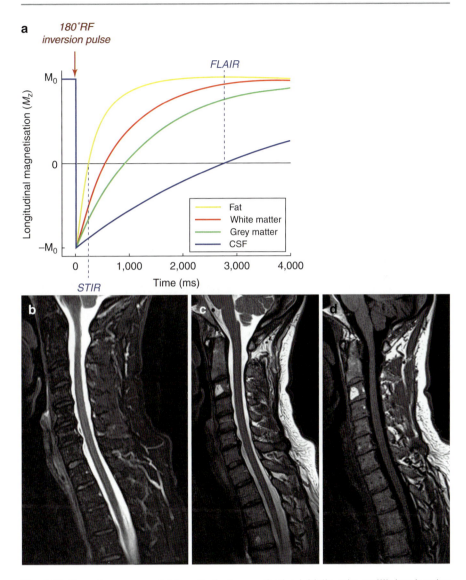

Fig. 4.27 Inversion recovery: (**a**) Longitudinal magnetisation initially at its equilibrium location becomes inverted at time zero and then recovers back towards equilibrium with time constant T1. Fat recovers more quickly than tissue or CSF since it has a shorter T1; (**b**) Applying the excitation pulse at a short inversion time (TI) when fat has zero longitudinal magnetisation (M_z) yields images with no fat signal (STIR); In STIR the fat signal of the haemangioma seen in the T2 weighted image (**c**) is suppressed. (**d**) Similarly, using a long TI can yield images with zero CSF signal (FLAIR, T1-weighted in this case). Note the hyperintense signal of the haemangioma in the body of vertebra C3, which is suppressed in the STIR (**b**)

of the other tissues, which in turn reduces the signal strength and thus the SNR. However, it may be useful in cases where spectrally selective saturation fails, such as in areas of poor magnetic field homogeneity (e.g. over a large field of view) or at low field strengths (Fig. 4.30).

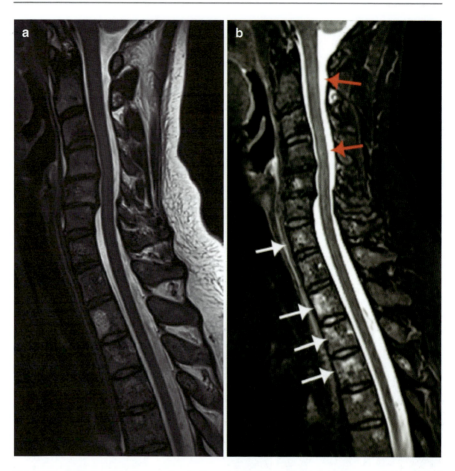

Fig. 4.28 STIR for detecting myelon lesions: (**a**) Sagittal T2-weighted images of the cervical spine show multiple signal inhomogeneities within the bony structures of a patient with multiple bony metastases and secondary progressive multiple sclerosis, but the myelon looks fairly normal; (**b**) Sagittal T2-weighted STIR images depict intramedullary hyperintensities (*red arrows*) and bony metastases are better seen due to their hyperintense signal (*white arrows*)

4.6.5 Contrast Agents

In certain cases the administration of an external agent to enhance contrast in MR images is necessary to distinguish between different types of disease. The most commonly used MRI contrast agents are based on gadolinium (Gd). The primary effect of Gd is to shorten the T1 of the tissue it resides in, although it also shortens the T2 and T2*. The T1 shortening effect leads to an increase, or enhancement, in MR signal in the presence of Gd on T1-weighted images.

Images may be compared pre- and post-intravenous administration of the contrast agent to observe the areas and patterns of signal enhancement. Additionally, images may be acquired rapidly during the injection of the contrast agent in cases

4 Magnetic Resonance Imaging (MRI) Methods

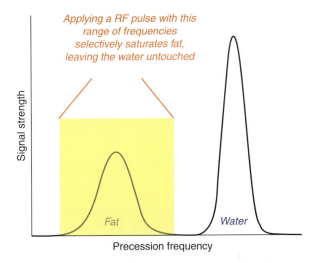

Fig. 4.29 Spectral fat suppression is performed by selectively exciting and then dephasing the magnetisation of fat, which precesses at a different frequency to water

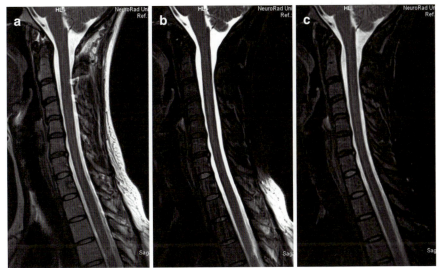

Fig. 4.30 Fat suppression in sagittal T2-weighted images of the cervical spine at 3 T: (**a**) image without fat suppression; (**b**) spectrally selective fat saturation results in insufficient fat suppression at the cervicothoracal junction in this case; (**c**) STIR gives more uniform fat saturation here

where the developing patterns of signal enhancement provide additional information.

Contrast-enhanced scans can be used for a number of different applications, including the identification of tumours, infection and haemorrhage. However, its use is limited in patients with poor kidney function due to concerns about links with nephrogenic systemic fibrosis (NSF) in these patients.

4.7 Suggested Imaging Protocols

MR protocols of the spine should include T1-weighted and T2-weighted sequences in axial and sagittal planes. Axial 2D images angulated parallel to the disc space may better delineate these spaces, but it can also cause areas between the segments to be missed. However, continuous coverage of the segments is preferred to avoid missing pathology in the slice gaps (e.g. herniated disc fragments). Coronal planes are helpful for assessing scoliosis and diseases of the cervicothoracic and lumbosacral plexus, which follows the course of the lateral paravertebral muscles. T2-weighted Short Tau Inversion Recovery (STIR) sequences should be added whenever there is question about oedema.

Considering that the spinal cord has a cross-sectional diameter of only 10–14 mm, high-resolution MRI is required to depict small spinal cord lesions. The voxel dimensions should be less than 50 % of the lesion size in order to avoid significant partial volume effects. However, reducing the voxel volume will also decrease the image SNR, as discussed in Sect. 4.4.6. MR imaging of the spine should go beyond the analysis of pathology by describing in detail the affect on nearby neuronal structures. The differentiation between grey and white matter within the human spinal cord still remains limited, but it is feasible with T2*-weighted images. Distortions of the butterfly-shaped central grey matter may be an indirect sign of spinal cord damage. Furthermore, single nerve roots have to be delineated to assess the affects of pathology. Some suggested spinal imaging protocols are listed in Table 4.3.

> *Some practical tips for MRI of the spine*
> Ensuring patient safety and consistently high image quality are complex topics outside the scope of this chapter, but we provide here some brief pointers to prevent some common problems in spinal MRI:
> - The patient should take off all conducting materials to avoid the risk of burns. Furthermore, the presence of metal, such as that found in trouser and jacket zips, will cause susceptibility artefacts. The patient should wear light clothes to prevent them from overheating.
> - Arms should be positioned alongside the body. Skin-to-skin contact of the arms and between bare legs or feet should be avoided, because induced currents may conduct across the regions of direct skin contact, potentially leading to dangerous heating.
> - Emphasis should be placed on patient comfort and pain relief to minimise movement artefacts.
> - The coil elements should be positioned as close as possible to the anatomical region of interest to optimise the signal-to-noise ratio. A support pad under the knees decreases the lordosis of the lumbar and cervical spine, increasing their proximity to receive coils built into the table.
> - The middle of the region of interest should be adjusted to the centre of the magnet to help maximise magnetic field homogeneity. For the lumbar spine light beam localisers should be adjusted 5 cm above the iliac crest.

4 Magnetic Resonance Imaging (MRI) Methods

Table 4.3 Proposed MR imaging sequences based on clinical symptoms

Clinical question	Sequence type				
	T2-weighted FSE	T1-weighted spin echo	T2*-weighted multi-echo (e.g. MEDIC, MERGE)	T2-weighted STIR	Other sequences
Radiculopathy	Sagittal	Sagittal	Axial (caveat: stenosis of intervertebral foramina is overestimated)	Sagittal; coronal to see nerval plexus	Oblique 2D or 3D T2-weighted images with reformats perpendicular to neural foramina
	Axial	Axial			
Myelopathy	Sagittal	Sagittal	Axial (caveat: bony stenosis of spinal canal is overestimated)	Coronal to see scoliosis	3D T2-weighted myelography (see Chap. 7)
	Axial	Axial			
	Coronal to see scoliosis	Coronal to see scoliosis			
Myelitis	Sagittal	Sagittal with and without contrast agent	Axial	Sagittal	
	Axial	Axial with contrast agent		Coronal to see adjacent tissue changes	
Spinal cord injury	Sagittal	Sagittal	Axial to see haemorrhage	Sagittal	
	Axial	Axial		Coronal to see adjacent tissue changes	
Vascular myelopathy	Sagittal	Sagittal with and without contrast agent			Diffusion weighted imaging and time-resolved contrast-enhanced angiography (see Chap. 5); 3D T1-weighted sequence with fat saturation; 3D T2-weighted imaging
		Axial with contrast agent			
Intradural tumour	Sagittal	Sagittal with and without contrast agent	Axial to see haemorrhage		Diffusion weighted imaging and diffusion tensor imaging (see Chap. 5)
	Axial	Axial with contrast agent			
Extradural tumour	Sagittal	Sagittal with and without contrast agent		Sagittal	
		Axial with contrast agent		Coronal to see adjacent tumour spread	

The use of multichannel coils allows the examination of the whole spine at once. This strategy allows for fast screening of the spine to locate the pathology. However, it has to be borne in mind that the spinal cord is a small structure requiring high-resolution, small field-of-view protocols in most cases. Exact numbering of the vertebral levels is always required, which is challenging for thoracic spine pathologies and also for lumbar radiculopathies. Sagittal imaging the whole spine is the method of choice to count the segments top-down.

Further Reading

Korzan JR, Gorassini M, Emery D, Taher ZA, Beaulieu C (2002) In vivo magnetic resonance imaging of the human cervical spinal cord at 3 Tesla. J Magn Reson Imaging 16(1):21–27

Shapiro M (2012) Imaging of the spine at 3 tesla. Neuroimaging Clin N Am 22(2):315–341. Review

Advanced MRI Methods

5

Thomas W. Okell, Elke Hattingen, Johannes C. Klein, and Karla L. Miller

Contents

5.1 Magnetic Resonance Angiography (MRA) 85
5.2 Diffusion Imaging 88
5.3 CSF Flow Measurements 91
Further Reading 91

In the previous chapter we discussed imaging methods that use relatively standard techniques available on most clinical MRI scanners. In this chapter we focus on cutting edge techniques for spinal MRI.

5.1 Magnetic Resonance Angiography (MRA)

Visualisation of the spinal arteries can be important in patients with vascular malformations or for pre-surgical planning. The inflow enhancement effect described in Sect. 4.5.2.5, which can be the source of image artefacts, is utilised in time-of-flight angiography to provide contrast between tissue and inflowing blood within arteries.

T.W. Okell (✉) • K.L. Miller
FMRIB Centre, Nuffield Department of Clinical Neurosciences,
University of Oxford, Oxford, UK
e-mail: tokell@fmrib.ox.ac.uk

E. Hattingen
Institute for Neuroradiology, Goethe-University,
Schleusenweg 2-16, D-60528 Frankfurt, Germany
e-mail: elke.hattingen@kgu.de

J.C. Klein
Brain Imaging Center (BIC), Department of Neurology, Goethe-University,
Schleusenweg 2-16, D-60528 Frankfurt, Germany
e-mail: klein@med.uni-frankfurt.de

This technique works well for fast flowing arteries such as those supplying the brain. However, the spinal arteries are very small and the blood flow is relatively slow, so time-of-flight angiography does not visualise them clearly. For example, the great anterior radiculomedullary artery (artery of Adamkiewicz), which is the largest intradural blood vessel, measures only 0.5–1.0 mm in diameter, and the anterior spinal artery, running along the anterior surface of the spinal cord, has a diameter of only 0.2–0.8 mm. Spinal MRA therefore requires a technique which is sensitive to slow flowing blood and allows high-resolution images to be obtained.

In addition, spinal veins typically have a larger calibre than the adjacent arteries. Therefore, the intradural spinal vessels that are depicted on standard thin-sliced MRI are generally veins. However, pathologically enlarged intradural arteries may be misinterpreted as veins, especially as the great radiculomedullary vessels, both the inlet arteries and the outlet veins, share the typical hairpin-like configuration. It is therefore desirable for MRA techniques to allow differentiation between arterial and venous vessels.

As mentioned in Sect. 4.6.5, the administration of a gadolinium-based contrast agent reduces the T1 of blood, causing it to become hyperintense on a T1-weighted image. This allows blood vessels to be identified clearly against the background tissue without relying on rapid blood inflow and the high signal strength enables good spatial resolution to be obtained. Contrast-enhanced (CE) MR angiography (MRA) relies on three-dimensional (3D) spoiled gradient-echo pulse sequences with short TE and TR. The shortest possible TE (2–8 ms) minimises the rapid $T2^*$ signal decay of the blood caused by the presence of the gadolinium-based contrast agent, yielding the highest possible signal from blood. A short TR (<10 ms) suppresses non-enhanced background tissue signal intensity from the spine, soft tissue and spinal cord, providing better contrast for the vessels of interest.

Basically two methods of data acquisition can be distinguished: (1) standard 3D CE-MRA, with a long acquisition time (several minutes per 3D volume) and high spatial resolution, and (2) dynamic (time-resolved) 3D CE-MRA, requiring high temporal resolution (several seconds per 3D volume) by special k-space sampling schemes. In standard 3D CE-MRA, optimal vessel contrast requires careful timing between sampling the centre of k-space and arrival of the contrast bolus in the vessels of interest.

The advantage of time-resolved MRA is that the contrast bolus is tracked during arteriovenous passage so that bolus timing is not required. A strong bolus technique utilising a short high-flow injection allows depiction of the first passage of the contrast agent, enabling differentiation between intradural arteries and veins. However, this presents the challenge of acquiring high spatial resolution images every few seconds.

Early time-resolved CE-MRA techniques used modified k-space trajectories, such as "keyhole" strategies, in combination with parallel imaging, to speed up image acquisition. Keyhole techniques frequently sample the inner portions of k-space, which contain most of the contrast information, whereas the outer edges of k-space are only sampled once. Further advances, like time-resolved imaging of contrast kinetics (TRICKS) or time-resolved angiography with interleaved stochastic trajectories (TWIST), sample the outer edges of k-space more frequently to gain improved spatial information.

5 Advanced MRI Methods

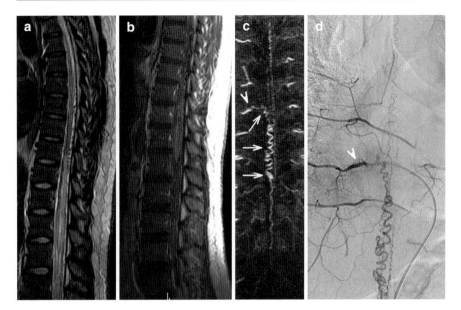

Fig. 5.1 An example of high-resolution CE-MRA in a patient with a spinal dural arteriovenous fistula (SDAVF, more details are given in Chap. 19): a centromedullary edema with faint enhancement and perimedullary dilated vessels are shown on conventional T2-weighted (**a**) and fat-saturated T1-weighted images (**b**). MIP reconstructions of the first-pass CE-MRA images clearly depict the early venous filling (**c**, *arrows*) confirming the shunt of the SDAVF. The level of the radiculomeningeal artery supplying the shunt is also demonstrated (*arrow head*) and was later proven by selective X-ray angiography (**d**) (Courtesy of Timo Krings, Professor of Radiology, Diagnostic and Interventional Neuroradiology, Toronto Western Hospital & University Health Network)

The final image quality obtained in CE-MRA also depends on the post processing, which can be time-consuming and complicated. Tools to aid visualisation include multi-planar and curved reformatting (MPR) combined with subsequent maximum intensity projection (MIP), but these should be performed by neuroradiologists.

The most useful application of spinal MRA is the imaging of arteriovenous (AV) shunts of the spinal cord and its meninges via spinal AV malformations (AVMs) and spinal dural AV fistulas (Figs. 5.1 and 5.2). In these patients, there are three major indications for spinal MRA: (1) screening those with clinical and MR imaging signs suggestive of spinal shunts; (2) localisation of feeding arteries and, in some cases, the great anterior radiculomedullary artery (artery of Adamkiewicz), to plan further invasive angiography and interventions; and (3) monitoring patients after therapy.

Even though X-ray based catheter angiography (digital subtraction angiography, DSA) is the gold standard for diagnosing and classifying spinal vascular lesions, information on spinal cord vascular pathology obtained from a preceding CE-MRA scan can facilitate DSA examination. Specifically, knowledge of the feeding arteries, which may originate from the costocervical or thyrocervical trunks, vertebral or any intercostal lumbar and iliolumbar artery, may not only shorten time of

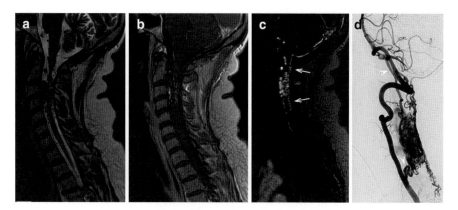

Fig. 5.2 An example of first-pass CE-MRA in a patient with a spinal arteriovenous malformation (SAVM), which appears as a series of multiple flow voids in and around the cervical cord on a T2-weighted image (**a**) with irregular enhancement on a contrast-enhanced T1-weighted image (**b**). First-pass CE-MRA clearly demonstrates the nidus with a plexiform network of arteries and draining veins extending into the subarachnoid space (**c**, *arrows*). The SAVM was confirmed by selective angiography (**d**) which also shows the supplying dilated anterior spinal artery and additional segmental supply from the vertebral artery (*arrow heads*) (Courtesy of Timo Krings, Professor of Radiology, Diagnostic and Interventional Neuroradiology, Toronto Western Hospital & University Health Network)

intervention but also reduce the risk of complications and radiation exposure. However, a single spinal MRA examination can only cover a limited part of the spine, as the craniocaudal extension of the field of view (FOV) should be small enough to allow high-resolution angiograms.

5.2 Diffusion Imaging

Diffusion is the random motion of molecules through a medium. The freedom water molecules have to diffuse depends on their local environment. For example, water within cells is much more restricted than extracellular water. Since diffusion characteristics can change with disease, it is useful to be able to probe this phenomenon. In MRI the signal can be made sensitive to diffusion by the addition of large gradient pulses after the RF excitation pulse, which first encode and then decode the spatial position of the water molecules a short time later. The spatial position of water molecules that diffuse rapidly along the direction of the applied gradient is not properly decoded, leading to dephasing and thus signal loss. Conversely, water molecules that are in restricted environments cannot diffuse very far and therefore the signal strength is not greatly affected by the diffusion gradients. Comparison of images with and without diffusion weighting allows the calculation of an apparent diffusion coefficient (ADC) in each voxel. A high ADC corresponds to larger net displacement of the water molecules (i.e. relatively unrestricted) and therefore low signal strength in the diffusion-weighted image.

5 Advanced MRI Methods

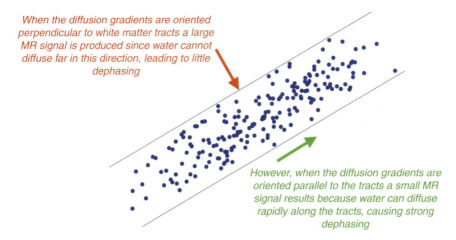

Fig. 5.3 Diffusion tensor imaging (DTI): diagram showing how water diffuses preferentially along the white matter tracts, causing greater signal loss if the diffusion gradient is applied along the tract direction

Diffusion-weighted imaging (DWI) is commonly used to look for ischemia and infarction, where movement of water into cells restricts diffusion and yields a bright signal on a diffusion-weighted image (see Chap. 20). However, it also shows promise in other areas such as identifying active demyelinating lesions and neoplasms.

It has also been discovered that in white matter water diffuses preferentially along the direction of the tracts. Therefore, if the diffusion gradient encodes position along the tract, the water appears to be able to diffuse rapidly, giving a low signal and a high ADC. However, if the diffusion gradient is applied at right angles to the tract axis, then the diffusion appears restricted, giving a high signal on a DWI image and a low ADC (see Fig. 5.3). Collecting images with a variety of diffusion gradient directions allows one to calculate how strongly directional water diffusion is and along what direction. The mathematical description of this directionality is often described by the "diffusion tensor" and the technique is therefore known as diffusion tensor imaging, or DTI.

A number of useful measures can be extracted from the diffusion tensor including the principal diffusion direction, which indicates the direction of white matter tracts (see Figs. 5.4 and 5.5), and the fractional anisotropy (FA), which describes how easily diffusion occurs along the tract direction compared to other directions. Since white matter tracts are inherently directional, FA is thought to relate to white matter integrity and therefore may be a useful marker of disease.

In addition, an advanced computational method known as "tractography" can be applied to DTI data. In essence this technique starts from a "seed" region of interest and follows the principal diffusion direction from one voxel to the next to reconstruct the paths of white matter tracts and determine the connectivity of the seed. This information may be useful in determining whether certain tracts have been disrupted by the presence of a lesion or reduced white matter integrity.

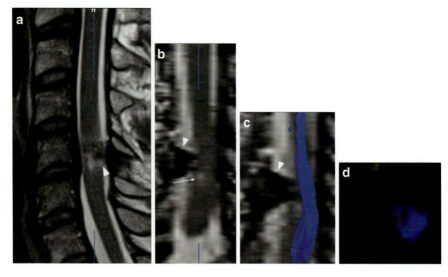

Fig. 5.4 Sagittal (**a**) and reformatted coronal (**b**) T2-weighted images of a patient with cervical spinal stenosis due to a bony spur from the right facet joint (*arrowhead* in **b** and **c**). The spinal cord shows a focal myelopathy signal caudally to the spur (*arrow*). The coronal (**c**) and axial (**d**) colour direction maps (**c, d**) visualise directional information from diffusion imaging, where *blue*, *green* and *red* indicate that diffusion occurs principally along the inferior-superior, anterior-posterior and left-right directions, respectively. Unaffected spinal cord fibres are blue since they run inferiorly/superiorly. The *purple* colour below the level of the spur (**d**) indicates deviation of the fibre directions near the spur

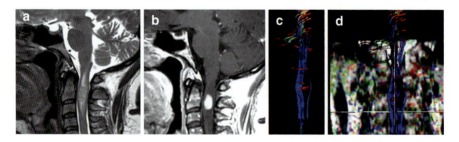

Fig. 5.5 A patient with ependymoma of the cervical spinal cord with adjacent oedema shown by T2-weighted imaging (**a**) and strong enhancement on T1-weighted imaging after contrast agent administration (**b**). The tractography results (**c, d**) show that the fibre tracts are not interrupted, but displaced by the tumour (Reproduced from Setzer M, Murtagh RD, Murtagh FR, Eleraky M, Jain S, Marquardt G, Seifert V, Vrionis FD (2010). Diffusion tensor imaging tractography in patients with intramedullary tumours: comparison with intraoperative findings and value for prediction of tumour resectability. *J Neurosurg Spine* 13(3):371–380, with permission)

5.3 CSF Flow Measurements

The normal flow of cerebrospinal fluid (CSF) can be modified by various diseases, including the presence of obstructing lesions or cavity formation. MRI can be used to study the flow of CSF using a very similar method to diffusion imaging. After the RF excitation pulse, two opposing "velocity encoding" gradient pulses are applied. As in diffusion imaging, these encode and then decode the spatial position of the magnetisation prior to the readout. For diffusion, displacement happens in all directions and every water molecule is displaced by a random amount, so the result is a range of "decoding errors" that lead to dephasing and therefore signal loss. For coherent flowing fluid (e.g. CSF or blood), all molecules are displaced by roughly the same amount, so they all have about the same "decoding error".

We can make our MRI measurements sensitive to this decoding error by recording the "phase" of the MRI signal. The measured phase offset is proportional to the displacement of the water molecules. By knowing how long the velocity encoding gradients were applied for, we can infer the velocity as the displacement divided by the encoding time. This technique is termed "phase contrast" and can be used to quantify flow velocities in CSF or blood. Note that the velocity encoding gradient pulses are relatively small compared to those used in diffusion imaging, so the MR signal is sensitised to macroscopic rather than microscopic scale motion.

In the same manner as diffusion imaging, the MR signal is only sensitised to motion along the direction of the applied gradients. Since most CSF flow is superior-inferior in the spine, applying velocity encoding gradients in this direction alone may be sufficient for most applications, but measurements in all three directions can be made if necessary. One additional consideration is that phase-contrast flow measurements must be cardiac gated to capture these pulsatile flow patterns. Typically a number of images are acquired at different points throughout the cardiac cycle so the full range of flow behaviour can be observed.

Further Reading

Pattany PM, Saraf-Lavi E, Bowen BC (2003) MR angiography of the spine and spinal cord. Top Magn Reson Imaging 14(6):444–460. Review

Vedantam A, Jirjis MB, Schmit BD, Wang MC, Ulmer JL, Kurpad SN (2014) Diffusion tensor imaging of the spinal cord: insights from animal and human studies. Neurosurgery 74(1):1–8

resonance imaging (MRI) – with usual magnetic field strengths between 1.0 and 3 T – by using a spine coil. The phase-difference images of CSF flow studies contain three important points: flow velocity, flow direction with respect to the frequency-encoded axis and phase of CSF pulsation. So CSF flow studies are a suitable method for detecting arachnoid adhesions, which cause blockades of CSF pulsation in patients with idiopathic syringomyelia. Furthermore, CSF flow studies are used to diagnose spinal arachnoid cysts and to display typical phase-shifts within the cyst in relation to the bordering subarachnoid space.

This chapter explains the physiological and technical principles of spinal CSF flow studies and gives a short overview of their field of application.

6.2 Physiological Principles

The motion of cerebrospinal fluid (CSF) along the spinal canal is of a pulsatile character. The arterial pulse wave during systole leads to an increase of the volume of the brain and the spinal cord which results in a passive movement and compression of the ventricles and the subarachnoid CSF spaces because of fluid shifting. Consequently, CSF is pressed through the craniocervical junction into the subarachnoid space (SAS) of the spinal canal during systole and a wave-like CSF pulsation in the craniocaudal direction can be measured. During diastole the spinal CSF pulsation switches to a caudocranial direction because of relaxation of the brain and the spinal cord with consecutive widening of the CSF spaces. Normally the spinal CSF pulsation works in a meander-like way, so main flow is found at anterior SAS of the cervical spine and at dorsal SAS of the dorsal spine. Flow velocity decreases from cranial to caudal with a maximum flow at cervical spine and a very low residual flow at lumbar spine. Under normal conditions the signal of spinal CSF pulsation appears homogenous without evidence of any interruptions.

6.3 Technique

6.3.1 Phase Contrast MRI

CSF flow studies are based on the technique of phase-contrast angiography. The aim of the sequence is to assess a reproducible phase difference between those protons, which are in motion, and the static ones. To avoid disturbing overlays by anatomical structures, the sequence produces a flow-sensitive image and a flow-compensated image, which are later subtracted from each other. To create the phase difference between the protons, a bipolar gradient is needed. Overall the sequence results in three different images (Fig. 6.1): a gradient-echo image (contains anatomical information about static tissue), a phase-contrast amount image (shows only the protons in motion) and a phase-difference image (velocity-encoded image to evaluate CSF pulsation). The degree of phase-difference of the protons in

6 CSF Dynamics

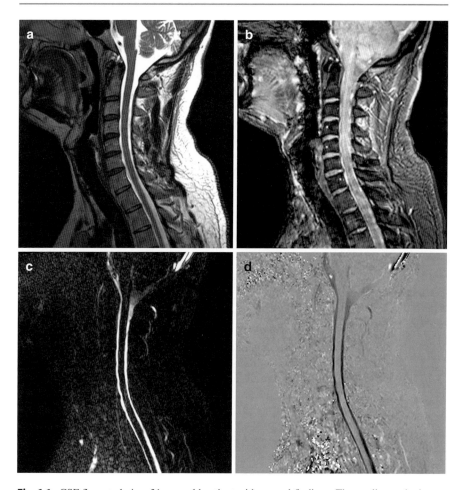

Fig. 6.1 CSF flow study in a 31-year-old patient with normal findings. The gradient-echo image (**b**) contains anatomical information on static tissues (compare with the T2-weighted image **a**). The phase-contrast amount image shows only the protons in motion (**c**). The velocity-encoded phase-difference image is used to evaluate CSF pulsation (**d**). In this case CSF pulsation appears homogenous without any signs of blockades or phase shifts

motion is proportional to flow velocity. So in the phase-difference image the signal intensity (SI) correlates directly with the vector of flow velocity in the direction of frequency-encoded axis. The degree of phase-difference ranges from +180° to −180° and is displayed by a grey tone scale. For static protons, a mid-grey tone with an intensity of 0 is defined. Usually the gradient is performed in the following manner that it causes spin acceleration (up to +180°) and an increase of signal intensity (up to the maximum SI white) for all protons moving in a caudocranial direction. In the opposite direction, the gradient leads to a spin deceleration (up to −180°) and a decrease of SI (up to the minimum SI black). In the case of exceeding of the predefined maximum flow velocity the signal is cut off and reflected to the opposite side, so the wrong flow direction is recorded (black signal instead of white signal and vice versa). This phenomenon is called aliasing and is also known in duplex sonography.

The maximum flow velocity can be adjusted by choosing a suitable echo time (TE). For longer TE the measurement sensitivity increases and thus lower flow rates can also be displayed, but aliasing is reached faster. So for higher flow velocities a shorter TE is needed to decrease measurement sensitivity.

In conclusion, the phase-difference images contain three aspects: flow velocity, flow direction with respect to the frequency-encoded axis and phase of CSF pulsation.

6.3.2 Triggering of CSF Flow Studies

To trigger CSF flow studies, both ECG and peripheral pulse sensor can be used. ECG triggering is more precise, but derivation of an adequate ECG signal can be difficult in some patients at MRI. In such cases peripheral gating by a pulse sensor represents a suitable alternative. Prospective ECG triggering includes the disadvantage of a partial data loss at diastole because the end of the cardiac cycle is not exactly defined and has to be determined prospectively. At retrospective gating, cardiac cycle and CSF pulsation are recorded separately and the required data subsequently divided into the cardiac cycle. So retrospective gating prevents data loss and is more suitable for daily practise.

6.3.3 Practical Tips

In principle, spinal CSF flow studies can be realised at all MRI with the usual magnetic field strengths between 1.0 and 3 T by using a spine coil. To ensure a strictly sagittal position of the CSF flow study in the middle of the spinal canal, additional coronal T2 weighted sequences should be performed for measurement planning. To receive an adequate flow signal and to avoid aliasing, a suitable maximum flow velocity (Vmax) has to be chosen. Common settings are values of Vmax between 3 and 8 cm/s. For examinations of the cervical spine it is advisable to start with a Vmax of 8 cm/s. Examinations of the dorsal spine should be started with a Vmax of 5 cm/s. In cases of aliasing the CSF flow study should be repeated with a higher Vmax of 8 cm/s. If the flow signal is too low, sensitivity of CSF flow study has to be increased by lowering the Vmax. Depending on the software, some MRI scanners enable axial CSF flow studies with the possibility of automated quantitative analysis of flow velocity by using region of interest measurements.

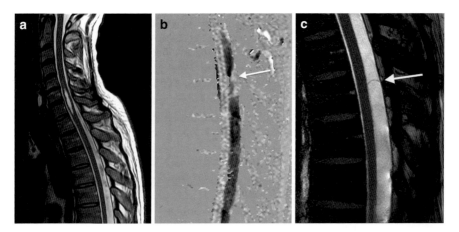

Fig. 6.2 Sagittal T2-weighted sequence shows a 53-year-old patient with cervical syringomyelia at C6-7 level (**a**). Thoracic CSF flow study reveals a blockade of CSF pulsation at the Th5 level with interruption of flow signal (*white arrow*, **b**). At the ECG-gated cine BFFE sequence an arachnoid adhesion at dorsal subarachnoid space is found (*white arrow*, **c**)

6.4 Indications for CSF Flow Studies

Arachnoid adhesions are a common underlying cause for the development of idiopathic syringomyelia, because they can cause blockades of the pulsation of CSF in the spinal subarachnoid space. Because of their movement by CSF pulsation it is nearly impossible to visualize those thin arachnoid membranes directly using standard MRI sequences. So CSF flow studies can be used to diagnose such arachnoid adhesions indirectly by detecting concomitant CSF pulsation blockades (Fig. 6.2). In rare cases, blocking arachnoid adhesions are also found in patients with symptoms similar to syringomyelia but without evidence of syringomyelia. By performing additional retrograde ECG-gated cine BFFE sequences at the height of CSF pulsation blockades, underlying arachnoid adhesions can be visualized directly to facilitate planning of microsurgical adhesiolysis. Nevertheless, correlation of the findings with CSF flow studies remains important, because not all arachnoid membranes detected by cine BFFE sequence cause a relevant blockage of the CSF pulsation.

Spinal arachnoid cysts usually do not induce complete blockades of the CSF pulsation; instead CSF gets tangled within the cyst like in a sail. So CSF flow studies show typical phase-shifts within the cyst in relation to the bordering SAS (Fig. 6.3). In the rare case of an extradural arachnoid cyst, CSF flow studies are very helpful in displaying CSF pulsation within the cyst to verify communication with the SAS.

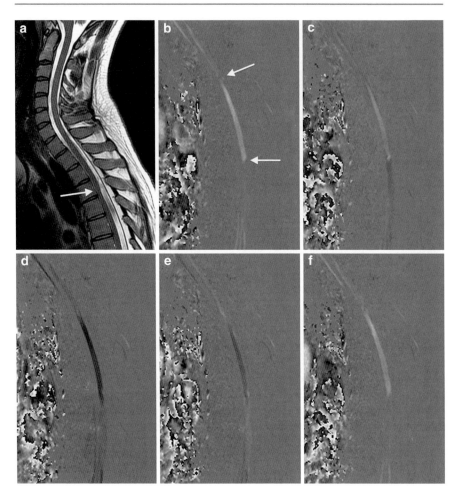

Fig. 6.3 A 27-year-old patient with an arachnoid cyst of the dorsal spine at the Th4-8 level. At T2-weighted sequence a widening of the posterior subarachnoid space as well as compression of the spinal cord is found (*white arrow*, **a**). CSF flow study reveals a phase shift of CSF pulsation within arachnoid cyst during cardiac cycle (**b–f**). Proximal and distal end of the arachnoid cyst is marked by *white arrows* (**b**). An ECG-gated cine BFFE sequence shows arachnoid membranes at proximal and distal ends of the arachnoid cyst (*white arrows*, **g**)

6 CSF Dynamics

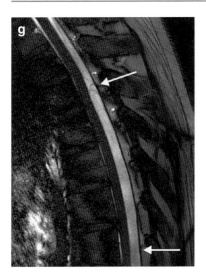

Fig. 6.3 (continued)

Contrast-Enhanced MR Myelography

7

Elke Hattingen and Jürgen Beck

Contents

7.1	Introduction	102
7.2	Contrast-Enhanced MR Myelography	102
7.3	Technique	102
7.4	MR Imaging Protocol	103
7.5	MR Findings in CSF Leakage	103
7.6	Pitfalls of Contrast-Enhanced MR Myelography	103
Further Reading		105

Abbreviations

CSF	Cerebrospinal fluid
FAT SAT	Fat saturation
GD	Gadolinium-based
MRI	Contrast agent with diethylenetriaminepentacetate
SIH	Spontaneous intracranial hypotension
SPAIR	Spectral selection attenuated inversion recovery
SPIR	Spectral presaturation inversion recovery
MRI	Magnetic resonance imaging

E. Hattingen (✉)
Institute for Neuroradiology, Goethe-University,
Schleusenweg 2-16, D-60528 Frankfurt, Germany
e-mail: elke.hattingen@kgu.de

J. Beck, MD
Department of Neurosurgery,
Bern University Hospital, Bern, Switzerland

7.1 Introduction

Basically there are two different methods to perform MR myelography, with and without application of intrathecal gadolinium-based contrast agent. The myelographic effect of 3D T2w sequences was just mentioned in chapter 4. The indication to apply intrathecal contrast agent is the detection of CSF leakage through the spinal dural sac in patients with spontaneous intracranial hypotension (SIH). Detection of dural leaks is important both in approving SIH and in determining the best treatment strategy. In contrast-enhanced (CE) MR myelography, hyperintense signal outside the intrathecal space in T1w sequences with spectral fat saturation (SPIR, fat sat) is usually considered as CSF leakage.

7.2 Contrast-Enhanced MR Myelography

MR myelography with intrathecal gadolinium-containing contrast agent is a useful method to prove and to localize CSF leaks in patients with debilitating symptoms of spontaneous intracranial hypotension. The localization of the leakage allows for the targeted epidural blood patches. The advantage over CT myelography is the avoidance of high radiation dose which results from scanning the whole spine with thin section thickness. The usefulness and high sensitivity of contrast-enhanced MR myelography have been reported in small case series. Although larger case series revealed the relative safety and utility of low-dose intrathecal application of gadolinium-containing contrast agent, any intrathecal injection of gadolinium contrast remains an off-label use. The safety of this intervention is only relative, since intrathecal gadolinium at higher doses is neurotoxic. Thus, contrast-enhanced MR myelography should only be applied for last opportunity in those patients in whom non-enhanced MR myelography failed to show the leakage. Patients should have the classical and debilitating symptoms of SIH (orthostatic headaches, low CSF pressure) and classical MR features of pachymeningeal enhancement, epidural effusions, and/or sagging of the brain. Further, a clear and frank discussion should be performed with the patient including explanation of the off-label use and the potential risk of neurotoxicity.

7.3 Technique

1. Fluoroscopic-guided lumbar puncture by using a 22-gauge spinal needle, with intrathecal location confirmed by using 0.5–1.0 mL of iodine contrast agent (optional)
2. Instillation of 0.3–0.4 ml (max 0.5 ml) of gadopentetate dimeglumine (0.5 mmol/ml Magnevist; Bayer Schering Pharma, Berlin, Germany) into the thecal sac, diluted in 5 mL of sterile 0.9 % saline
3. MR imaging performed within 15–30 min after intrathecal gadolinium administration

7.4 MR Imaging Protocol

The protocol consists in T1-weighted images with spectral fat saturation to visualize the high signal of the Gd-contrasted CSF. Spoiled gradient sequences are faster, but these sequences are susceptible to artifacts from bony structures. In our institution, we prefer spin-echo sequences.
1. Sagittal T1-weighted images are mandatory and should cover the lateral portions of the neuroforamina (increase the slice number!).
2. Axial slices should cover the mostly affected spinal levels at the craniocervical and cervicothoracal junction as well as any level which shows suspicious findings in sagittal planes.
3. Coronal planes are optional. They may be helpful in detecting multiple dilatation of the neuronal sheets.

7.5 MR Findings in CSF Leakage

It is not trivial to diagnose CSF leakage, since there is no study in healthy patients to compare with. In particular, CSF is normally reabsorbed via the sheets of the nerve roots. Therefore, small collections of CSF around the sheets may be physiological. It is even imaginable that even a small backward diffusion of contrast agent into the epidural space is not necessarily pathological. Diluted Gd-containing contrast agent (about 38 mg/ml) has a lower concentration compared to the iodinated contrast medium (about 240 mg/ml), facilitating diffusion of these molecules. Frank accumulation of contrast agent in the epidural space might be more specific for CSF leakage (Fig. 7.1). Further, CSF leakage at the craniocervical junction often yields pronounced enhancement of the soft tissue (Fig. 7.2). However, it only indicates that the leakage should be near the collection, but the dural hole is seldom discernible. Likewise, early MR scans may be more sensitive in cases with large dural tears but may fail in small leakages, whereas in delayed MR scans contrast agent may be moved away from the origin of leakage.

7.6 Pitfalls of Contrast-Enhanced MR Myelography

1. Only examinations with full opacification of the thecal sac including the foramen magnum should be assessed. Cases with incomplete filling should be reevaluated with a delayed MR examination.
2. Artifacts at the cervicothoracic junction consistently occur due to the failure of spectral fat saturation. These artifacts occur in regions with large air-tissue interfaces due to the field inhomogeneity and yield signal increases imitating leakage of contrast agent. The use of more sophisticated fat suppression techniques (spectral selection attenuated inversion recovery, SPAIR) or preceding acquisition of non-enhanced T1-w images may help to minimize misinterpretations.

Fig. 7.1 Young female with symptoms of spontaneous intracranial hypotension. Sagittal T1-weighted image with spectral fat suppression (**a**) after intrathecal application of contrast agent shows accumulation of CSF (*bright*) in the thecal sac and in the ventral epidural space. Notice the small dural membrane between these two spaces. Axial T1-weighted image with spectral fat suppression (**b**) shows the pronounced collection of contrast agent along the left sheet of the nerve root

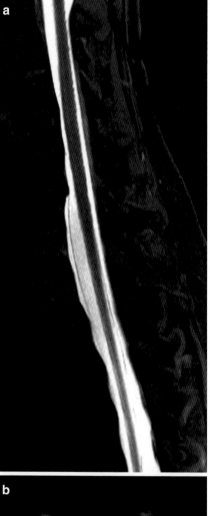
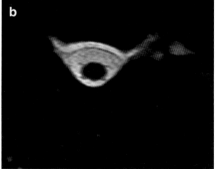

Fig. 7.2 Sagittal T1-weighted image with spectral fat suppression after intrathecal application of contrast agent in a patient with symptoms of spontaneous intracranial hypotension after chiropractic maneuver. Frank CSF collection is seen in the dorsal soft tissue. Note the dorsal dural membrane bordering upon the spinal canal

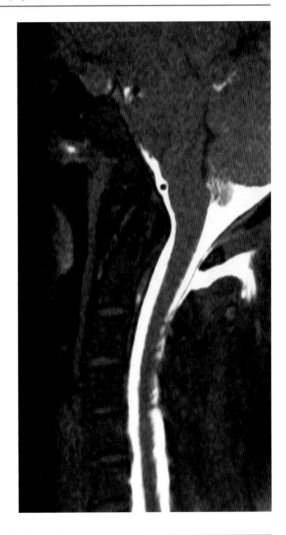

Further Reading

1. Akbar JJ, Luetmer PH, Schwartz KM, Hunt CH, Diehn FE, Eckel LJ (2012) The role of MR myelography with intrathecal gadolinium in localization of spinal CSF leaks in patients with spontaneous intracranial hypotension. AJNR Am J Neuroradiol 33(3):535–540
2. Hattingen E, DuMesnil R, Pilatus U, Raabe A, Kahles T, Beck J (2009) Contrast-enhanced MR myelography in spontaneous intracranial hypotension: description of an artefact imitating CSF leakage. Eur Radiol 19(7):1799–1808
3. Tali ET, Ercan N, Krumina G, Rudwan M, Mironov A, Zeng QY, Jinkins JR (2002) Intrathecal gadolinium (gadopentetate dimeglumine) enhanced magnetic resonance myelography and cisternography: results of a multicenter study. Invest Radiol 37(3):152–159

Myelography and Post-myelographic CT

8

Elke Hattingen and Stefan Weidauer

Contents

8.1 Introduction 107
8.2 Procedure and Imaging Features 108
8.3 Contraindications 111
References 113

Abbreviations

CSF   Cerebrospinal fluid
CT   Computed tomography
GD-DTPA Gadolinium-based MRI contrast agent with diethylenetriaminepentacetate
MRI   Magnetic resonance imaging
PT   Prothrombin time
PTT   Partial thromboplastin time

8.1 Introduction

Myelography refers to the examination of the contents of the thecal sac after administration of intrathecal water-soluble nonionic contrast agent.

This examination is usually performed to assess for herniated nucleus pulposus or spinal canal stenosis and to determine the level of spinal cord compression from

E. Hattingen (✉)
Institute for Neuroradiology, Goethe-University,
Schleusenweg 2-16, D-60528 Frankfurt, Germany
e-mail: elke.hattingen@kgu.de

S. Weidauer
Department of Neurology, Sankt Katharinen Hospital,
Seckbacher Landstr. 65, D-60389 Frankfurt, Germany
e-mail: stefan.weidauer@sankt-katharinen-ffm.de

bony disease or trauma. Also traumatic nerve root injuries with possible extravasation of contrast medium, arachnoiditis, and different types of arachnopathy can be diagnosed with myelography. In addition, extradural neoplasms and intradural tumors, the latter divided into intramedullary and extramedullary location, may be diagnosed by myelography, when the compartment of the CSF is constricted [1, 2].

Today, myelographic examinations are mainly replaced by CT and MR imaging. However, myelography combined with post-myelo-CT is still indicated in patients with contradictions for MRI. Furthermore, myelography yields additional information about the bony structures, functional stenosis, and instabilities with pathological mobility of neighboring vertebra of the spinal canal. The intrathecal application of contrast agent allows accessorily the assessment of dynamic CSF processes in case of intradural cysts, myelon herniation, and CSF leakages. Apart from x-ray myelography, contrast-enhanced MR myelography with intrathecal application of 0.5–1.0 ml contrast agent (0.1 mmol/kg Gd-DTPA) was introduced to diagnose and localize CSF leakage (Chap. 7).

In addition, the lumbar puncture enables for CSF analysis (e.g., cells, protein content, lactate, glucose) and to measure the CSF opening pressure. Normal adult opening pressure is between 7 and 15 cm fluid, although in young adult it can be slightly higher with a normal opening pressure below 18–20 cm fluid. Herein a short introduction of the method, most important contraindications and complications, and in addition some concise imaging findings of myelographic examinations in selected pathologies will be presented. The detailed description of the whole procedure and pathological diagnostic findings goes beyond the scope of this chapter.

8.2 Procedure and Imaging Features

Very often, myelography is performed in the lumbar spine using a mid-sagittal or parasagittal approach. The puncture should be performed at levels L3/4 and L4/5, being aware that the conus medullaris is normally positioned at level L1/2. Only nonionic contrast medium can be injected. The spinal CSF volume is about 75 ml so that the volume of 15–17 ml should not be exceeded. The adult dose limit for myelography is 3 g total of iodine (i.e., 17 ml of 180 mg I/ml or 10 ml of 300 mg I/ml contrast agent). The 300 mg I/ml concentration is used for lumbar puncture to perform cervical, thoracic, or combined myelograms.

The myelograms exhibit the spinal cord, the conus medullaris, the cauda equine, and the radices in a negative contrast to the enhanced CSF. Therefore, the assessment of imaging findings is notably based on filling defects and/or compression of the CSF space, and in addition displacement of above-mentioned structures should be analyzed. The myelograms should show the entire extent of the lumbar spine including the very distal caudal thecal sac in the sacral region. The exact location and documentation of pathological findings should be documented, and therefore unequivocal landmarks of levels, e.g., the os sacrum along with the lowest rib, are necessary even for thoracic pathologies. Standard lumbar examination includes posterior–anterior (p.a.) and oblique (about 15–25°) projections in a prone position. Examination of the thoracic and cervical part of the spine needs ascension of contrast agent, and a dorsal position of the patient is favorable. The assessment of pathological mobility of vertebral structures or position dependency of spinal canal narrowing requires additional imaging in flexion/extension and in upright/horizontal position [3, 4].

8 Myelography and Post-myelographic CT

Analysis of myelograms could differentiate three types of contrast reliefs [1, 2]:
1. Extradural processes may cause a sand glass-like constriction or even a stop of contrast medium dispersion in the thecal sac. In lumbar stenosis, imaging in upright position may accentuate extradural compression (see Figs. 8.1 and 8.2).

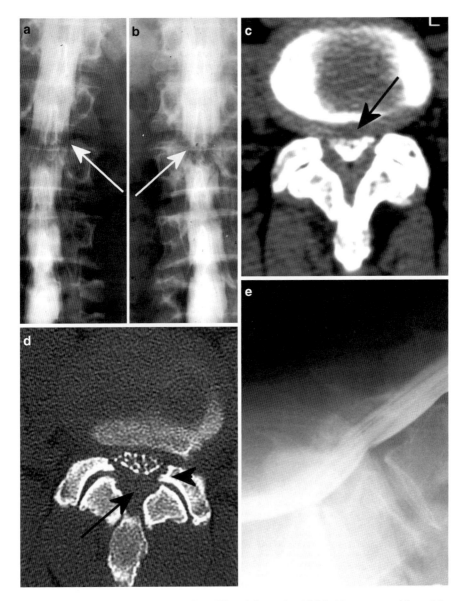

Fig. 8.1 (a–f) Waist-like contrast medium filling defect at level L2/3 (a), accentuated in upright position (b) due to degenerative lumbar spinal canal stenosis (*arrow*) in a patient suffering from claudicatio spinalis. (c, d) Axial post-myelo-CT at level L4/5 showing severe stenosis and consecutive slight enhancement of the thecal sac; constriction of the dural sac from anterior (medial disk protrusion; c, *arrow*) and dorsolateral due to thickened ligamenta flava (d, *arrow*) and degenerative alterations of the intervertebral articulations (d, *arrowhead*). (e, f) Myelography in upright position (lateral projection) exhibits severe increase of dural sac compression in retroflexion (e, f: anteflexion)

Fig. 8.1 (continued)

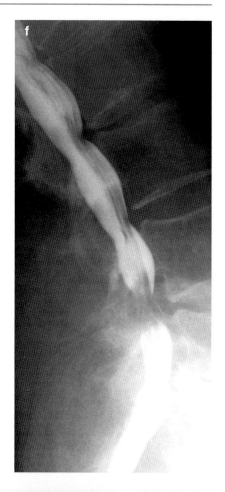

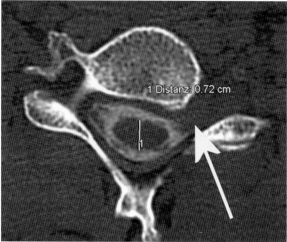

Fig. 8.2 Post-myelo-CT axial at level C6/7 illustrating a filling defect of the radicular pouch C7 left sided (*arrow*) due to a lateral intraforaminal disk herniation at the segment C6/7

Fig. 8.3 (a, b) Dorsal shift of the lower thoracic spinal cord due to intradural extramedullary tumor, i.e., meningioma, at level Th10/11 with ventral adhesion; note ovoid-shaped contrast filling defects. However, method of choice nowadays is spinal MRI; (b): sag. T2WI showing a meningioma at level Th11

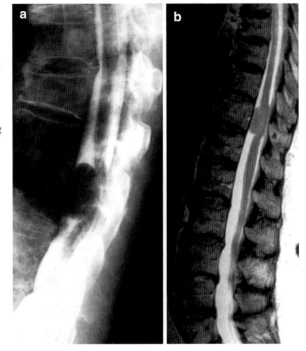

2. Intradural extramedullary space-occupying lesions result in ovoid-shaped defects in lateral and p.a. projection and possible shift of the spinal cord. Due to the extent of such lesions, myelograms may also show a stop of contrast medium distribution going ahead with tapered margins (see Fig. 8.3).
3. Intradural intramedullary space-occupying lesions cause enlargement of the spinal cord resulting in narrowing of the lateral thecal edges (Fig. 8.4). However, small intramedullary lesions with slight volume effects are not visible on myelograms.

8.3 Contraindications

Important contraindications are coagulopathy, increased intracranial pressure especially due to space-occupying lesions, and infection at the puncture site. Laboratory tests (platelets, prothrombin time [PT], partial thromboplastin time [PTT]) should be tested before lumbar puncture at least in patients with history of bleeding abnormalities and in patients with antiplatelet agents or anticoagulant treatment. However, some practitioners do not believe that routine laboratory testing is necessary before myelography in healthy outpatient and binding guidelines for management of myelography patients are unavailable.

Heparin should be held for 4 h prior to the procedure and can be restarted 2 h after lumbar puncture. Coumadin should be held until PT is normal (for 3–4 days),

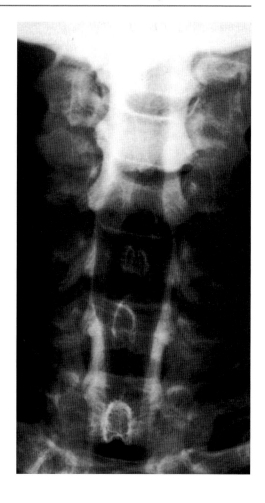

Fig. 8.4 Cervical astrocytoma (WHO grade II) in a 49-year-old man suffering from progressive sensible sensation deficits in the legs over 12 months. Myelography shows enlargement of the cervical spinal cord (p.a. projection) with narrowed thecal edges at levels C4/5–C5/6

platelets should be above 50,000, and acetylsalicylic acid should be discontinued before myelography. It is still debatable if other drugs like metformin, nonsteroidal anti-inflammatory drugs (NSAIDs), and potentially epileptogenic drugs should be discontinued. Creatinine is usually not checked prior to the myelography. If the patient has a very poor renal function and there is no other option to examine the spinal canal and spinal cord, one could time the myelography to precede dialysis. However, the risk of contrast-induced nephrotoxicity is very low in myelography due to administration of small volumes of contrast agent.

In myelography patients, complications are relatively uncommon, especially with the current nonionic water-soluble intrathecal contrast agents. While seizures had been reported to occur in up to 0.6 % of myelography examinations performed with metrizamide, they rarely occur with the use of newer contrast agents. Contrast reactions, hemorrhages, infections, and spinal cord or conus medullaris injuries caused by false injection are rare but potentially serious complications.

The most common harmless complication is the post-myelography headache due to CSF loss at the site of lumbar puncture with consecutive lowering of the intrathecal pressure. Meningeal reactions, e.g., orthostatic headache, vomiting, vertigo, and neck pain, are observed. This complication is minimized by using a small needle. Further, needle position parallel to the longitudinal fibers of the thecal sac may reduce dural injury, i.e., to orient the bevel during the lumbar puncture in order to separate the fibers rather than cut them. One limiting factor for needle caliber is the viscosity of the injected contrast material. However, in some patients, CSF leak persists, and a rare complication is bilateral cerebral subdural hematomas and engorgement of epidural veins due to permanent CSF low-pressure syndrome. Adequate therapy will be blood patching most suitable at the level of CSF leakage.

References

1. Bradač GB, Kaernbach A (1981) Neue Aspekte in der Myelographie. Schering AG, Berlin
2. Thurn P, Friedmann G, Lackner K, Prömper C, Schroeder S (eds) (1986) Computertomographie der Wirbelsäule und des Spinalkanals. Enke, Stuttgart
3. Benini A (1992) Clinical aspects, pathophysiology and surgical treatment of lumbar spinal stenosis. Schweiz Rundsch Med Prax 81:395–404
4. Wildermuth S, Zanetti M, Duewell S, Schmid MR, Romanowski B, Benini A, Böni T, Hodler J (1998) Lumbar spine: quantitative and qualitative assessment of positional (upright flexion and extension) MR imaging and myelography. Radiology 207:391–8

Part III
Malformations of the Spine

Malformations of the Spine

9

Luciana Porto

Contents

9.1	Introduction	117
9.2	Craniocervical Junction Anomalies	118
9.2.1	Malformations of the Occipital Bone	122
9.2.2	Malformations of the Atlas	125
9.2.3	Malformations of the Axis and Odontoid Process	126
9.2.4	Instability Associated with Representative Inherited Syndromes	129
9.3	Spina Bifida	134
9.3.1	Closed Spinal Dysraphism	139
9.3.2	Meningocele	140
9.3.3	Open Spinal Dysraphism	148
9.4	Miscellaneous Malformations of the Spine	152
9.4.1	Tethered Cord and Fibrolipomas of the Filum Terminale	152
9.4.2	Caudal Regression Syndrome	154
Further Reading		156

9.1 Introduction

Spinal dysraphisms are a heterogeneous group of malformations, which may involve the vertebral column and the neuroaxis. The involvement of mesodermal structures is common and variable. The focus investigating these children should lie on the neural tissues. When a malformation is found, full and detailed mapping of the entire malformation should be performed to facilitate surgical planning.

L. Porto
Institute for Neuroradiology, Goethe-University,
Schleusenweg 2-16, D-60528 Frankfurt, Germany
e-mail: luciana.porto@kgu.de

- The conus at term birth: L2/L3. By 8 weeks, the cord has ascended to the adult level at the L1/L2 intervertebral space.
- The pediatric cervical spine is more prone to instability.

Two embryological processes are involved in the formation of the spinal cord. The upper part of the cord up to mid-lumbar enlargement occurs by neurulation. The smaller distal lumbar portion of the cord, the conus medullaris, and the filum terminale are formed by canalization and regressive differentiation. Although nervous tissue abnormalities are not always associated with musculoskeletal anomalies, congenital spine abnormalities may involve mesodermal as well as neuroectodermal structures. In the early embryonic phase, the cutaneous ectoderm is attached to the neuroectoderm. The disjunction between neural and cutaneous ectoderm is critical. If it fails, mesenchymal tissue becomes enclosed within the neural tube.

Because of the relatively rapid fetal growth in the caudal direction, the conus lies at birth at the vertebral segment L2/L3. By 8 weeks after birth, the cord has ascended to the adult level at the L1/L2 interspace.

The pediatric cervical spine is more prone to instability due to weak cervical musculature, disproportionately large head size, and incomplete ossification of the dens. In addition, the immature spine is hypermobile due to laxity of the ligaments, and it has small and thin facet joints making the atlas–axis region prone to injury. Therefore, children younger than 11 years of age are more likely to have ligamentous injuries rather than fractures of the upper cervical spine. In contrast, teenagers more often sustain injuries to the lower cervical spine. MRI is irreplaceable when evaluating "spinal cord injury without radiographic abnormality" (SCIWORA); it helps evaluating the spinal cord, discs, and ligaments.

Unfortunately, the evaluation of the pediatric cervical spine, particularly the craniocervical junction (CCJ), can be very difficult because of the presence of synchondroses, variants, and injuries that are found in this age group only. Therefore, knowledge of the anatomy is prerequisite to evaluate imaging correctly.

9.2 Craniocervical Junction Anomalies

The CCJ consists of the occipital bone, foramen magnum, clivus, atlas, axis, and the ligaments of the atlantooccipital and atlantoaxial articulations. The CCJ is, as other transitional zones, host to many variants, anomalies, and malformations; therefore, it is considered an unstable zone. The upper part (C1 and C2) is responsible for most of the rotational mobility of the cervical spine, but the cervical bones and joints are intrinsically unstable; therefore, the ligaments are structurally responsible for upper cervical stability. C1–C2 instability is present in up to 50 % of congenital atlantooccipital anomalies.

Basilar invagination is typically caused by occipital bone anomalies and atlantooccipital non-segmentation.

9 Malformations of the Spine

In case of a CCJ anomaly, important areas, such as the brainstem, spinal cord, and their arteries, can be affected and become compressed from posterior displacement of the odontoid process. The symptoms of patients with CCJ abnormalities are inconsistent. Neurological symptoms may occur late; they usually develop insidiously and progress slowly, becoming symptomatic as late as in the second or third decade of life. Since the associated C1–C2 instability progresses with age, patients show slow progression. Patients can be completely asymptomatic in the newborn period and early infancy, especially in connective tissue disorders associated with ligamentous laxity and in congenital anomalies, posing a diagnostic challenge.

Imaging

- MRI is the ideal method to evaluate the neural structures, ligaments, and soft tissues, while computed tomography (CT) can be used to evaluate the osseous structure of the CCJ. However, dose considerations limit the use of CT.
- Radiological imaging can be confounded by incomplete ossification of the bone (due at 9 years of age). Still, conventional radiographs remain the main diagnostic tool to evaluate pediatric cervical instability. Certain standards should be followed to obtain good RX in pediatric patients.
- When possible, RX should be taken sitting or standing. If supine RX is performed, the shoulders should be lifted from the table by a support (avoiding cervical hyperlordosis).
- RX should be perpendicular and taken from the farthest possible distance from the patient (min. 2.75 m).
- Lateral and open mouth odontoid views should be performed only after 5 years of age.

The atlantodens interval (ADI) is the space between anterior surface on the dens and posterior surface of anterior ring of C1 (Fig. 9.1a). ADI greater than 5 mm on lateral radiographs indicates instability; this value is higher than in adults (3 mm) because of the thicker cartilage of both the dens and the ring of C1. Still, an ADI of 5 mm or more can occur in children without disruption of the transverse ligaments. The risk of associated neurological problems is evaluated with the measurement of the space available for the cord (SAC), as measured between the posterior surface of dens and the anterior surface of the posterior arch of C1. A SAC of less than 14 mm is considered abnormal, and a value of less than 13 mm is probably an indication of cord injury. As a rule of thumb, the so-called Steel's rule of thirds can be easily applied, stating that at least one-third of the spinal canal should be left for the cord. The rule does not change during growth of the cervical spine.

Normal physiological displacement can be found in children at the level of C2–C3 and to a smaller degree at the level of C3–C4 up to 7 years of age. In addition, dentocentral synchondrosis (visible up to 11 years of age) and ossiculum terminale (appears after 5, mostly after 8 years of age) may be confused with odontoid tip fracture. Be aware that normal wedging of the C3 is seen in 7 % of younger children.

Fig. 9.1 Atlantoaxial instability and basilar invagination. (**a**) Atlantoaxial instability is determined by the atlantodens interval (*ADI*) and the space available for cord (*SAC*) (**b**): basioccipital hypoplasia associated with Chiari I malformation. There is a protrusion of the dens's tip above McGregor's line (this *line* is drawn from the hard palate to the base of the occipital bone), so-called basilar invagination with impression on the brainstem. Wackenheim's clivus baseline (which should fall tangent to the dorsal surface of the odontoid process) falls too posterior, compatible with a posterior craniocervical dislocation

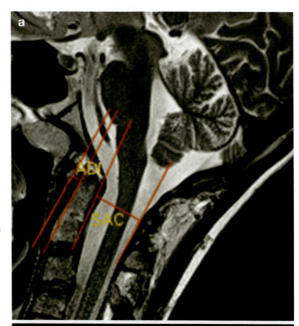

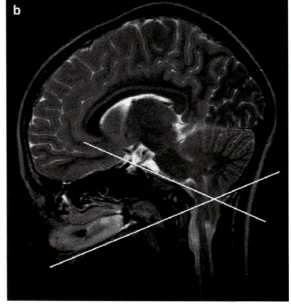

9 Malformations of the Spine

- Cervical instability is frequently discovered incidentally in an asymptomatic patient
- CCJ anomalies, in particular congenital atlantoaxial dislocation, can be missed in children if not looked for.
- If trauma is not present, rule out congenital anomaly, skeletal and metabolic dystrophy, as well as rheumatoid arthritis. Typical syndromes associated with CCJ anomalies are Klippel–Feil and Down syndromes, achondroplasia, mucopolysaccharidoses, and osteogenesis imperfecta.
- Patients with connective disorders should have an MRI around 6 years of age (spine is more fully ossified and modeling has happened).
- Relative motion of more than 5 mm between anterior surface on the dens and the posterior aspect of the anterior ring of C1 indicates surgical intervention in children. This value is higher than the adults (3 mm).
- In children, a distance of less than 13 mm between posterior surface of dens and anterior surface of the posterior arch of C1 is considered abnormal.
- Basilar invagination is the protusion of dens tip more than 0.5 cm above McGregor's line. It is typically caused by occipital bone anomalies and atlantooccipital non-segmentation.
- Platibasia is the displacement of the upper cervical vertebrae with an increase of the basal angle, >150°.
- Pseudo-"physiological subluxation" at the level of C2–C3 and to a smaller degree at the level of C3–C4 is normal findings up to 7 years of age.

In general, the best diagnostic clue in imaging (MRI and/or CT) for CCJ anomalies is the flattening or malformation of the clivus, anterior ring of C1, or odontoid process. Flexion–extension MRI is often necessary to fully evaluate the pathology.

Chen and Liu (2009) described a simplified classification for malformations of the CCJ, as follows:
- Malformations of the occipital bone
- Platybasia
- Basilar invagination (basioccipital hypoplasia)
- Condylar hypoplasia
- Condylar dysplasia
- Malformations of the atlas
- Occipital atlas assimilation
- Aplasia and hypoplasia of the atlas
- Atlas arch anomaly
- Malformations of the axis and odontoid process

- Aplasia or hypoplasia of the dens
- Persistent ossiculum terminale
- Os odontoideum
- Klippel–Feil anomaly
- Instability associated with childhood diseases
    (a) Down syndrome
    (b) Neurofibromatosis
    (c) Juvenile rheumatoid arthritis
    (d) Mucopolysaccharidoses
    (e) Achondroplasia
    (f) Osteogenesis imperfecta
    (g) Spondyloepiphyseal dysplasia
    (h) Larsen syndrome
    (i) Others

9.2.1 Malformations of the Occipital Bone

- Platybasia
- Displacement of the upper cervical vertebrae with an increase of the basal angle (normal <150°)
- Basilar invagination
- Refers to the cranial displacement of the foramen magnum with radiological protusion of the dens tip more than 0.5 cm above McGregor's line

The lower part of the clivus is formed by the basiocciput, and malformations of the occipital bone, such as basioccipital hypoplasia (Fig. 9.1b), can cause platybasia, basilar invagination (upward migration of the cervical spine into the foramen magnum), condylar hypoplasia, and condylar dysplasia. *Platybasia* can cause bony impingement on the brainstem (Fig. 9.1b) and obstructive hydrocephalus if it is associated with basilar invagination. Basilar *invagination* is associated with not only platybasia but also occipitalization of C1, fused upper vertebrae, Klippel–Feil syndrome, Chiari malformation (Fig. 9.1b), and skeletal dysplasias, mainly achondroplasia. In children, due to the greater laxity of the cervical spinal ligaments, basilar invagination can be attributable to trauma or bone softening (Fig. 9.2), as, for example, in rheumatoid arthritis. Other diseases with potential risk for basilar invagination are osteoporosis, hyperparathyroidism, osteomalacia, rickets, renal osteodystrophy, and Hurler syndrome.

Wackenheim's clivus baseline is useful for assessment of cervical instability in children with Down's syndrome and also in the assessment of traumatic injuries.

9 Malformations of the Spine

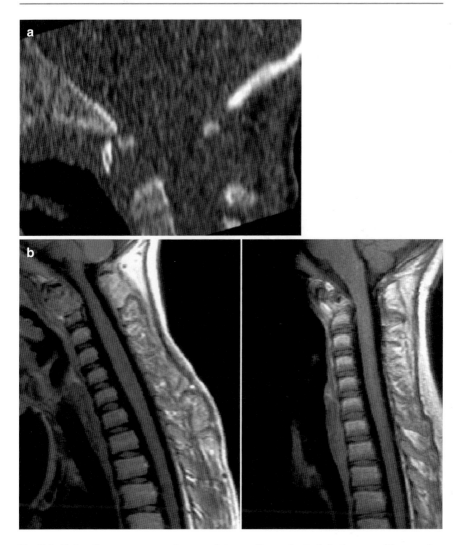

Fig. 9.2 Farber disease, a very rare lysosomal storage disease due to defective ceramidase causing accumulation of lipids leading to abnormalities in the joints, liver, throat, tissues, and central nervous system. (**a**) Sagittal CT shows a soft tissue mass eroding much of the dens axis (C2) pretransplant. (**b**) T1-w after contrast before (*left image*) and after (*right image*) bone marrow transplantation. There is a large soft tissue mass (C2 level) which extends into the spinal canal. Note the skin nodules over spinous processes pre-transplant. *Right image*: clear improvement after therapy

It runs from the posterior surface of the clivus and normally is tangential to the posterior margin of the dens. If the line falls far of the posterior limits of the odontoid, a posterior dislocation is present. If the line intersects the anterior or middle body or the base of the odontoid, an anterior dislocation is diagnosed (Fig. 9.3).

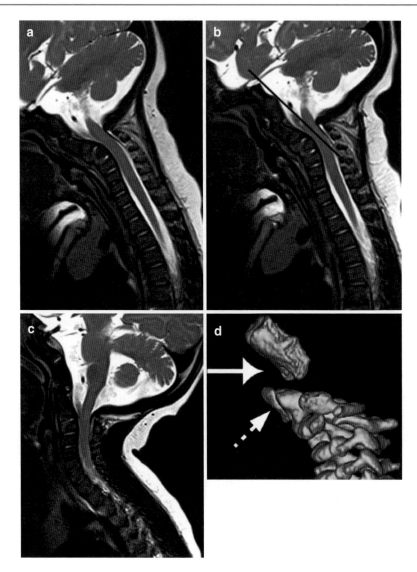

Fig. 9.3 Newborn child with incidental finding: atlantodental occipital subluxation. (**a**) Midsagittal T2-w MRI in flexion. The MR image best reveals the narrow spinal canal with compression of the spinal cord at the C1–C2 level, especially in anteflexion. (**b**) Midsagittal T2-w image in neutral position. The Wackenheim's clivus baseline intersects the body of the odontoid, well matched with an anterior craniocervical dislocation. (**c**) Midsagittal T2-w image in extension. Note that the narrowing of the spinal canal at the C1 level in flexion and neutral positions reduces in extension. (**d**) The CT scan with 3D sagittal reconstruction at the time of presentation showed an anterior displacement of unfused dens (*dotted arrow*) relative to the occipital condyles (*straight arrow*). Note the two separate ossification centers of the odontoid, so-called bifidus; normally the ossification centers fuse by the 7th fetal month. (**e**) CT scan with 3D coronal reconstruction. The neural arch is present (*star*) but unfused posteriorly. (**f**) CT scan with sagittal reconstruction. Notably, the anterior arch is not ossified in this child, which is the case in 80 % of the newborns. Besides, no unification of the posterior synchondrosis of the spinous processes is seen, which is also normal for a newborn. Therefore, during the newborn period, it is difficult to evaluate malformations, such as atlas hypoplasia, or more specifically hypoplasia of a non-united posterior arch, due to the lack of ossification, presence of synchondroses, and variants. As a differential diagnosis, one should include traumatic delivery. A control evaluation at 3 years of age is necessary

9 Malformations of the Spine

Fig. 9.3 (continued)

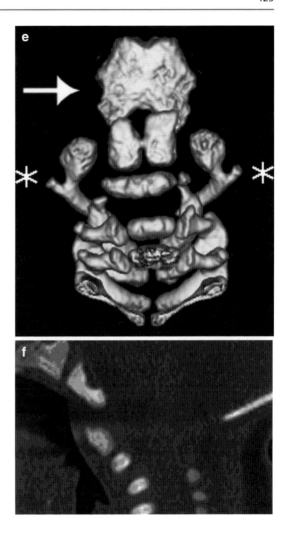

9.2.2 Malformations of the Atlas

- Due to failures of chondrogenesis, the majority of atlas anomalies are posterior arch anomalies.
- Rachischisis: Cleft of the posterior arch located in the midline, found in ca. 4 % of autopsies and in 70 % of children with myelomeningoceles

In children, the knowledge of atlas ossification centers is essential to the diagnosis of clefts, aplasias, and hypoplasias. The atlas has three ossifications sites: its anterior arch and the two neural arches. The anterior arch is ossified at birth in 20 % of children only. Usually, it becomes visible as an ossification center by 1 year of age (varying between 6 months and 2 years). During the 7th fetal week, the neural arches appear. The posterior synchondrosis of the spinous processes unites by 4–6 years of age. The complete fusion of the anterior and neural arches (neurocentral synchondrosis) does not happen before 7 years of age.

Clefts of the atlas arches are more frequent, compared to arch aplasia and hypoplasia. The greatest part of posterior arch clefts is located in the midline (rachischisis). In contrast, anterior arch rachischisis is exceptional, only found in 0.1 % of autopsies. Importantly, clefts of the anterior arch may be a sign of dysraphic anomaly of the meninges and spinal cord. Even though most of the atlas's clefts are incidental findings, its presence may be associated with other malformations of the spine, and more importantly, large clefts with fibrous tissue may present with atlas instability.

Occipital assimilation of the atlas results from a segmentation failure between the skull and the first cervical vertebra, also known as occipitalization of the atlas. The assimilation may involve the anterior arch only, the posterior arch, or both combined. This anomaly is reported as the most common anomaly involving the CCJ, encountered in 0.14–0.25 % of the population. It is always linked to basilar invagination, and there is an increased association to Klippel–Feil anomaly in C1 and C2. In this constellation, atlantoaxial subluxation and dislocation may occur. In an excellent overview, Smoker et al. describe that with the exception of the previously described atlantooccipital assimilation, most of atlas anomalies, when isolated, are not associated with abnormalities of the CCJ.

Half-sided pathology of C1 varies from *hypoplasia* of the lateral mass, up to complete agenesis of the hemiatlas with rotatory instability and basilar impression. In two-thirds of the patients, symptoms are present at birth; others show torticollis later. Partial hemiaplasias may simulate fractures on RXs.

9.2.3 Malformations of the Axis and Odontoid Process

The axis is formed by four ossification centers: one for the odontoid process, one for the body, and two for the neural arches. The odontoid process is formed in utero from two separate ossification centers which fuse by the seventh fetal month (Fig. 9.3d). The body of the axis fuses with the odontoid process around 3–6 years of age. Between 3 and 6 years of age, a secondary ossification center appears at the apex of the odontoid process (os terminale), and fusion of the os terminale with the odontoid process is completed by the age of 12 years.

By 2–3 years of age, the neural arches fuse posteriorly; their fusion to the body of the odontoid process happens between 3 and 6 years of age.

The most frequent congenital anomaly of the axis is malformation of its odontoid process, and this is not associated with basilar invagination. The malformations of the odontoid process range from mild *hypoplasia to complete aplasia*. In odontoid

9 Malformations of the Spine

hypoplasia, a short odontoid process can be recognized. Complete aplasia is particularly uncommon. The presence of a hypoplastic odontoid can be associated with spondyloepiphyseal dysplasia, mucopolysaccharidoses, and metatropic dwarfism. In the rare case of hypoplasia or aplasia, there is a predisposition to atlantoaxial dislocation with cord compression due to the absence of the apical and alar ligaments. Secondary to the hypermobility, patients may present with pannus similar to that seen in rheumatoid arthritis. In addition, there is an association with metatropic dwarfism, spondyloepiphyseal dysplasia, and Morquio syndrome.

The *ossiculum terminale* at the tip of the dens appears between 5 and 8 years and fuses to the dens between 10 and 13 years. The failure of fusion of the terminal ossicle with the rest of the odontoid process is called persistent ossiculum terminale.

- Os odontoideum
- Independent osseous structure located cranially to the axis body with a gap between these two structures. Usually a small hypoplastic dens is present.
- Persistent ossiculum terminale.
- Failure of fusion of the terminal ossicle with the rest of the odontoid process.

When isolated, the persistent *ossiculum terminale* is a stable anomaly and of little clinical significance. In contrast, *os odontoideum* (Fig. 9.4) is associated with a number of congenital conditions, such as Down and Morquio syndromes, spondyloepiphyseal dysplasia, Klippel–Feil anomaly, and Laron syndrome. If the os odontoideum is associated with ligament weakness, patients present with atlantoaxial instability (Fig. 9.4) with compression of the spinal cord. The hypermobility at C1–C2 level may cause transient occlusion of the vertebral artery. Patients with a gap between the os odontoideum and the axis body should be carefully assessed with flexion and extension examinations (Fig. 9.4).

Atlantoaxial rotatory subluxation (Fig. 9.5) in children occurs often after a minor trauma; other causes include surgery of the head and neck, following an infection or inflammation of the adjacent neck tissues. Consider anatomical variations in the differential diagnosis, i.e., children with normal atlantoaxial articulation fixed in a vicious rotatory position due to extreme torticollis (Fig. 9.6c). Clinically, children with rotatory subluxation present with new torticollis because of pain. Fortunately, most of the atlantoaxial subluxation resolves spontaneously. But, if an unresolved subluxation remains untreated, plagiocephaly may follow.

Klippel–Feil syndrome (Fig. 9.6) is a rare condition characterized by the congenital fusion of any 2 of the 7 cervical vertebrae. It is the result of a failure of the vertebrae's segmentation.

Be aware that fusion can be missed in infancy due to the incomplete ossification.

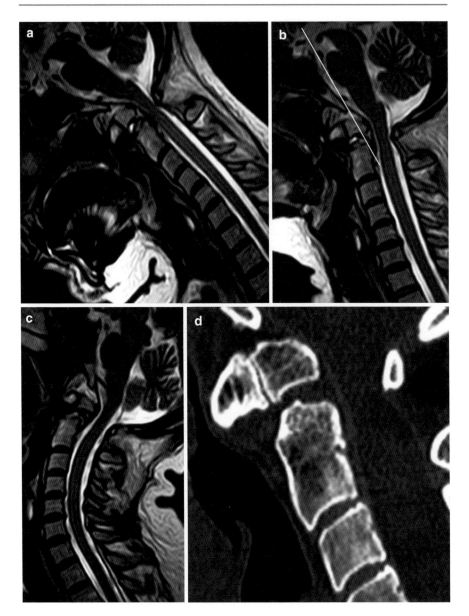

Fig. 9.4 Older patient with os odontoideum and atlantoaxial instability. (**a**) Midsagittal T2-w image in flexion. The MR image best shows the narrowing of the spinal canal with compression of the spinal cord at the C1–C2 level. (**b**) Midsagittal T2-w image in neutral position. The Wackenheim's clivus baseline intersects the body of os odontoideum, compatible with an anterior craniocervical dislocation. (**c**) Midsagittal T2-w image in extension. The narrowing of the spinal canal at the C1 level in flexion positions reduces in extension. (**d**) The CT scan shows the os odontoideum as an independent osseous structure located cranially to the axis body with a gap between these two structures. Note the presence of small hypoplastic dens

Fig. 9.5 Traumatic atlantoaxial rotatory luxation after a car accident. In children, the greater laxity of the cervical spinal ligaments results in more frequent high cervical cord injury

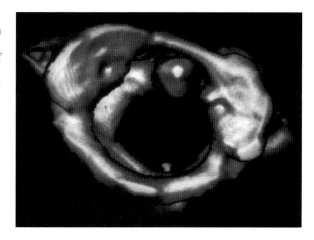

The patient usually presents with a short neck, low posterior hairline, and limited cervical motion.

Classification
- Type 1 (9 %): Extensive cervical and thoracic segmentation anomalies
- Type 2 (84 %): Fusion of 2 or more cervical vertebrae
- Type 3 (7 %): Type 1 or 2 associated with lower thoracic/lumbar anomalies

Approximately 20 % of the patients have a complete or partial diastematomyelia (Fig. 9.6b). Other associated abnormalities may include basilar invagination, odontoid hypoplasia, atlantooccipital assimilation, platybasia, Chiari I, scoliosis, kyphosis, Sprengel's deformity of the scapula with a bridging omovertebral bone, spina bifida, Dandy–Walker, malformations of the kidneys and the ribs, cleft palate, respiratory problems, and heart malformations. There is an increased likelihood for early instability of the CCJ in patients with atlantoaxial fusion or odontoid hypermobility associated with occipitalization of the atlas or with multiple fusion of the cervical vertebrae associated with anomalies of the atlas and odontoid process. It is important to look for instability, progressive degenerative changes, and brainstem compression.

9.2.4 Instability Associated with Representative Inherited Syndromes

9.2.4.1 Down Syndrome

In Down syndrome, a combination of osseous anomalies and lax ligaments contributes to C1–C2 instability. Patients usually present with hypoplasia of the dens without soft tissue dens mass. The prevalence of cervical instability has been estimated at 9–30 % in children with Down syndrome, although only 2.5 % of the patients present with symptomatic instability. This small group, however, has a higher

Fig. 9.6 Klippel–Feil syndrome associated with diastematomyelia. (**a**) Sagittal T2-w image shows multiple segmentation anomalies with congenital fusion. In this patient, there are associated anomalies of the atlas and odontoid process with instability of the CCJ. The Wackenheim's clivus baseline falls far too posterior to the odontoid, compatible with a craniocervical dislocation. (**b**) Almost complete split of the cord into two hemicords within a single dural sac (type II diastematomyelia). No osseous or fibrous septum was seen. (**c**) In the CT images, note the vicious rotatory position of atlanto-axial articulation due to extreme torticollis in this patient with Klippel–Feil syndrome

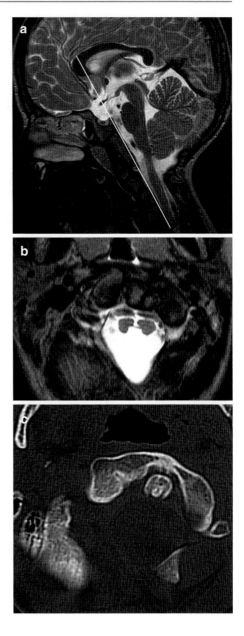

prevalence of associated bone abnormalities, such as os odontoideum, persistent synchondrosis, or posterior rachischisis. As a general rule, children with Down syndrome show no major compression symptoms of the spinal cord. Patients usually present with slowly progressive neurological symptoms, which can eventually lead to a main injury.

9 Malformations of the Spine

Instability can be easily evaluated using Wackenheim's clivus baseline. According to the literature, children with Down syndrome who have no C1–C2 instability will not develop a dangerous instability. Therefore, this group of patients will not need further screening after the age of 10 years. Be aware that this cutoff age can be controversial.

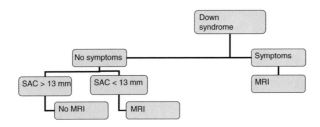

9.2.4.2 Neurofibromatosis

Neurofibromatosis can present with dystrophic changes in the vertebral bodies and dysplasia of vertebral bodies; abnormalities can also be secondary to pathological alignment. Furthermore, patients may present with focal or acute kyphoscoliosis. RX is important to quantify and to follow-up the scoliosis, while MRI is the ideal method to evaluate cord compression and nerve pathology in patients with severe cervical kyphosis. Although instability is rare, the strategy is similar as in the diagram above for Down's syndrome.

9.2.4.3 Juvenile Rheumatoid Arthritis

> Juvenile rheumatoid arthritis is an important differential diagnosis to CCJ variants and anomalies.

Rheumatoid arthritis (Fig. 9.7) is a systemic disease characterized by persistent synovitis, which can affect the joints of the cervical spine.

The incidence of cervical involvement ranges from around 40 to 80 % of cases, depending on the duration of the disease. Typically, the cervical spine is involved in the beginning of the disease and shows erosive synovitis, ligamentous subluxation, osteopenia, and vertebral fractures. Patients usually develop C1–C2 subluxation within 2 years of disease onset, and spontaneous clinical remission is uncommon.

Imaging

Patients usually present with enhancing "pannus" best seen on T1-w MRI (Fig. 9.7). C1–C2 subluxation is best seen with CT reconstructions. To evaluate instability, dynamic flexion–extension plain films or T2-w MRI are invaluable.

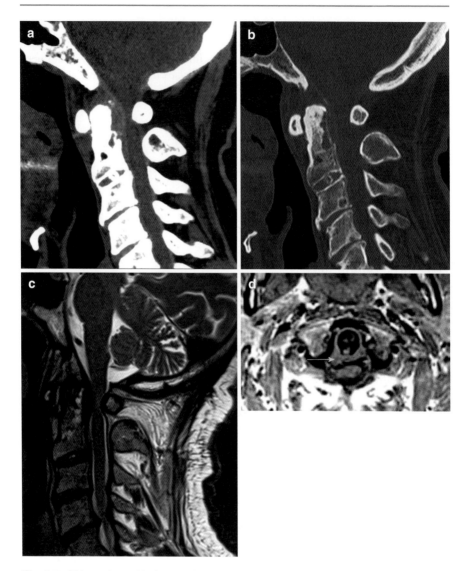

Fig. 9.7 Older patient with rheumatoid arthritis with cervical involvement. (**a**, **b**) Atlantoaxial joint CT in sagittal reformatted images: gross bone erosions of odontoid process and synovial joints, associated with joint instability (**c**, **d**) Sagittal T2-w and axial T1-w images, respectively, show the synovial pannus (*yellow arrow*) and cord compression by the odontoid process. MRI can assess the relationship of the occiput, atlas, and axis, and it is useful in depicting the extent of subluxation and the compression of the spinal cord

9.2.4.4 Mucopolysaccharidoses

Deformities of the spine are caused by deposits of glycosaminoglycans in the tissues surrounding the spinal cord, which can result in spinal cord compression. In the case of mucopolysaccharidosis IV, also called Morquio syndrome, the "os odontoideum" is invariably present; this is due to a partially cartilaginous dens. On top, the anterior ring of C1 can be unstable because of failure in the ossification process. All these components associated with pannus lead to C1–C2 instability classically described in Morquio syndrome. However, odontoid hypoplasia and associated soft tissue thickening have been shown to reverse after bone marrow transplantation.

In Hurler syndrome (MPS 1H), another type of mucopolysaccharidosis, narrowing of the craniocervical junction, thickening of the dura mater, and odontoid dysplasia are seen (Fig. 9.8). It seems that stem cell transplantation has an early and positive impact in children with Hurler syndrome and narrowing of the craniocervical junction, influencing the development of the odontoid.

9.2.4.5 Achondroplasia
Achondroplasia is a condition characterized by short-limbed dwarfism with affection of the spine. Areas with endochondral ossification are affected, and, therefore, the skull base and foramen magnum are underdeveloped. The small foramen magnum shows a typical "teardrop" configuration, and the odontoid is usually dysplastic. Patients can also present with basiocciput hypoplasia, decrease of the basal angle, and thickening of the posterior rim of the foramen magnum.

9.2.4.6 Osteogenesis Imperfecta
Osteogenesis imperfecta is a disorder of collagen with secondary bone fragility. Patients can present with CCJ deformity, which is usually asymptomatic. As a result of recurrent microfractures, infolding of the occipital condyles can occur, leading to cranial settling with platybasia and basilar invagination. In this scenario, brainstem or lower cranial nerves compression is to be expected.

9.2.4.7 Spondyloepiphyseal Dysplasia
Atlantoaxial instability may occur due to odontoid hypoplasia or os odontoideum, resulting in cervical myelopathy.

9.2.4.8 Larsen Syndrome
Larsen syndrome is a rare defect of connective tissue formation characterized by multiple joint dislocations. Spinal anomalies may lead to major spinal instability and spinal cord injury. Atlantoaxial instability is a rare finding in this syndrome and has been reported with other abnormalities of the upper cervical spine including basilar impression and occipitalization of the atlas.

9.2.4.9 Others
Additional causes of cervical instability in children include connective tissue disorders as, for example, Ehlers–Danlos syndrome and inflammatory diseases, such as oropharyngeal infections.

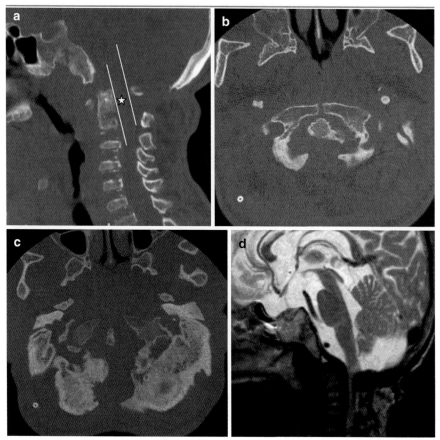

Fig. 9.8 Child with Hurler syndrome (courtesy from Prof. Lanfermann). (**a–c**) Notice the odontoid process is poorly developed with a short C1 posterior arch. SAC (*star*): Note the reduced available space for the cord. (**d**) Associated atlantoaxial instability. Note the typical mucopolysaccharidosis related changes: dilated Virchow–Robin spaces with involvement of the corpus callosum, frontal bossing, and a large J-shaped sella turcica. The Wackenheim's clivus baseline intersects the odontoid anteriorly, well matched with a craniocervical dislocation. In addition, meningeal hypertrophy at C2 level with clear compression of the CCJ and a smaller SAC than expected on the CT scan. The Steel's rule of thirds is violated; less than one-third of the spinal canal is left for the cord

9.3 Spina Bifida

Spinal, usually posterior defect
There are two types: closed and open
- Closed spinal dysraphism (CSD): spina bifida occulta, neural tissue covered by skin, often occurs at levels L5 and S1.
- Open spinal dysraphism (OSD): neural tissue exposed to the environment (myelomeningocele and myelocele).

9 Malformations of the Spine

- Meningocele: large opening of the spinolaminar arch with extrusion of a portion of the meningeal sac, not including the spinal cord.
- Myelomeningocele: large opening of the spinolaminar arch with extrusion of a portion of the meningeal sac with exposure of the neural placode.

Spinal dysraphisms result from an incomplete midline closure. The term spina bifida (Latin: "split spine") relates to a developmental congenital disorder caused by the incomplete closing of the osseous elements of the vertebral canal. Some vertebrae overlying the spinal cord are not fully formed and remain unfused and open. The causes of the neural tube defects are multifactorial. Environment and demographics may play a significant role in predisposing the fetus to a neural tube defect, with several studies showing the link between folic acid deficiency and neural tube defects. Methylenetetrahydrofolate reductase mutations are, for example, associated with abnormal folate metabolism predisposing to open spinal dysraphism (OSD). Additional associations are trisomy 13 and 18.

Imaging
When examining the pediatric patient, it is important to consider the radiation dose. Computed tomography of the spine has a high dose of radiation to the gonads, particularly in females. Therefore, its use should be restricted and carefully evaluated for every individual case. Neurosonography is a good initial imaging modality to evaluate the spinal canal; unfortunately, this method is limited to the neonatal period (up to 3 months) and is very operator dependent, leading to low sensitivity. Still, neurosonography has a clear role in the preliminary evaluation of a suspected spinal malformation; it gives a general idea of the position of the conus and possibly the extent of intraspinal structures, such as lipomas or cysts (Fig. 9.9).
Bony Spine
To evaluate skeleton anomalies, one should start with plain films. CT can be invaluable to understand the complex bone anatomy of segmentation anomalies, particularly in the presence of severe malformations with scoliosis (Fig. 9.10).

It is extremely important to rule out tethering of the cord prior to correction in case of segmentation anomalies with hemivertebrae and block vertebrae. In the same way, scoliosis may be caused by diastematomyelia or other forms of closed spinal dysraphism, requiring preoperative investigation of the spinal cord.

Neuroradiological investigation of the spinal canal and its contents:
MRI is the method of choice: (1) for diagnosis and determining the extent of the malformation, (2) for evaluation of the nerve roots and possible adhesions, and (3) to identify associated variants, i.e., to rule out possible surgical difficulties.
Routine: T1-w spin echo sequences and T2-w MRI, in sagittal and axial planes without contrast.

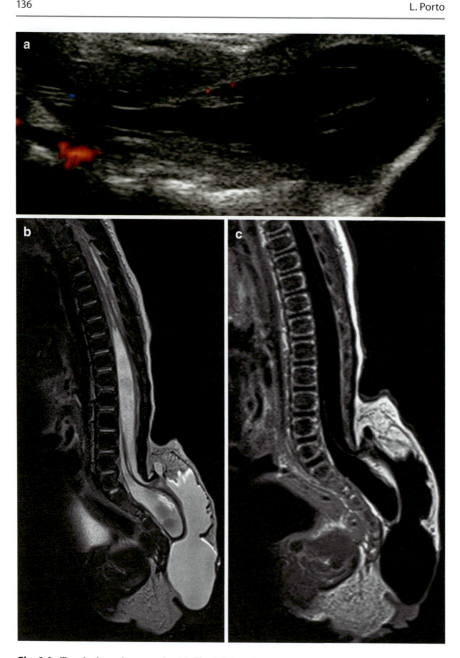

Fig. 9.9 Terminal myelocystocele. (**a**) The US imaging, corresponding to the MRI (9B), shows closed marked cystic dilatation of the distal cord central canal or the ventriculus terminalis. (**b**) Axial T2-w image shows a dilatation of the distal central canal with herniation through a posterior lumbosacral defect. (**c, d**) Sagittal T2-w and T1-w images, respectively, show a disruption of the mesenchyme, but not of the ectoderm, with tethered cord

9 Malformations of the Spine

Fig. 9.9 (continued)

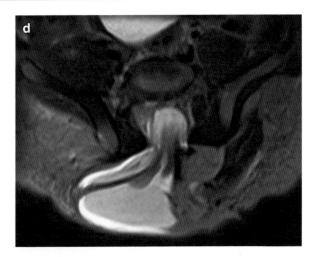

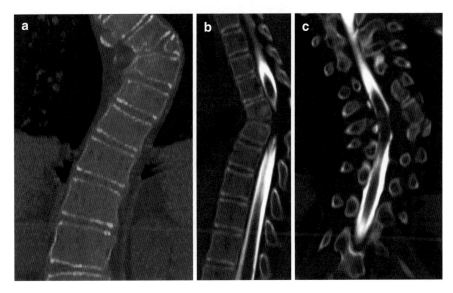

Fig. 9.10 Myelography followed by CT scanning in a patient with severe scoliosis caused by hemivertebrae with displacement of the cord. (**a**) Bone window CT scan with coronal reconstruction. (**b, c**) Myelography

Additional imaging: fat-suppression sequences may be useful in lipomas. Heavily T2-w multislice or single-slice MR myelography may be helpful in demonstrating the sac content with myelographic effect of the hyperintense CSF. If a spinal tumor is identified or infection is suspected, contrast should follow.

Fig. 9.11 Chiari II malformation. Sagittal T1-w image shows the typical posterior fossa deformities with small posterior fossa, low-lying tent, caudalization of the medulla. The cervicomedullary kink can be seen. The corpus callosum is dysplastic; there is a large mass intermedia, a beaked tectum of the midbrain. Note the multiple small malformed gyri (stenogyria)

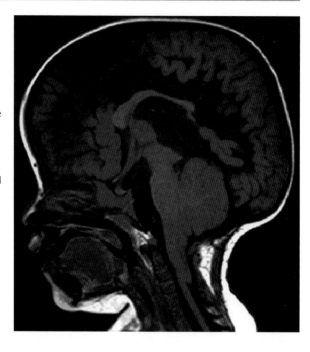

In cases of severe curvature of the spine, the MRI interpretation can be difficult, and a combined evaluation with CT and CT reconstruction is advisable. In exceptional, complex cases with severe deformity, the use of myelography followed by CT scanning can be helpful (Fig. 9.10). The role of the neuroradiologist is to show all components of the malformation in detail, preparing the neurosurgeon for reconstructive surgery.

There are fundamental differences between CSD and OSD. Open spinal dysraphism is strongly associated with Arnold–Chiari II malformation (85–100 %), which is a cerebral dysgenesis characterized by a small posterior fossa. This is simply explained by the association between Chiari II malformation and the leakage of CSF through the spinal defect. The outflow (leak) collapses the primitive ventricular system, preventing the increase of the rhombencephalic vesicle and resulting in a small posterior fossa with cerebellar tonsil herniation (Fig. 9.11). The associated Arnold–Chiari II (Fig. 9.11) may be of varying degree. In the majority of cases (90 %), it is associated with hydrocephalus. Hydrocephalus may develop secondarily to mechanical obstruction due to Chiari II malformation and/or impaired CSF reabsorption. Hydrocephalus may develop in the second trimester of pregnancy, after birth, and sometimes it is seen only after the repair of meningomyelocele. Myelomeningoceles account for more than 98 % of open spinal dysraphisms, whereas myeloceles are rare. In contrast, the occurrence of closed spinal dysraphism with Arnold–Chiari II is rare. Associated cranial abnormalities with OSD include tectal beaking, callosal dysgenesis, and subependymal heterotopias.

9.3.1 Closed Spinal Dysraphism

It is also called spina bifida occulta; occulta is the Latin word for "hidden." This old terminology is not appropriate because isolated defects in the posterior elements of the lumbosacral region are found in 10–24 % of the normal population. The term CSD implies unbroken skin. Therefore, this type of dysraphism is not evident at birth and is normally missed prenatally. CSD are usually not associated with Chiari II malformations; therefore, no prenatal surgery is necessary. Embryologically, it results from a failure of fusion or failure of development of part of the vertebral arch, usually its lamina.

- Closed spinal dysraphism (CSD) is usually asymptomatic, with only a small number of children showing concomitant changes of the spinal neuronal tissue.
- CSD are usually not associated with Chiari II malformations; therefore, no prenatal surgery is necessary.
- Disjunction between neural and cutaneous ectoderm during early fetal life, including various mesodermal components such as fibrotic bands with lipomatous tissue, may tether the cord.
- Cutaneous manifestations of an underlying malformation are common.

Lumbosacral skin indentation, hyperpigmentation, nevus, subcutaneous lipoma (Fig. 9.12), patch of hair growth, or dermal sinus are all findings that should prompt further evaluation. Preliminary screening can be performed in newborns with neurosonography, but be aware of the age dependent conus level. The tip of the conus lies between L2 and L4 in babies aged between the 30th and 39th postmenstrual week. On sonography, it is essential to rule out a spinal mass lesion and/or tethered cord. Typically, reduced mobility of the spinal cord and filum terminale associated with an increased thickness of the filum terminale (over 2 mm) suggests cord tethering. In the presence of cutaneous manifestations, MRI and plain films should follow, with or without positive findings in sonography, because this method is very operator dependent.

Although, in the postnatal phase, CSD are mostly asymptomatic; they may cause neurological, urological, and orthopedic problems in children and young adults. These patients typically develop first neurological symptoms at age 3 or during the rapid somatic growth phase (adolescent growth spurt or at school age 4–8 years).

In CSD, focal damage to the spine and its contents can occur during early fetal life. Presumably, the subsequent repair process disturbs the disjunction between neural and cutaneous ectoderm and includes various mesodermal components such as fibrotic bands with lipomatous tissue tethering the cord. The growth of this abnormal mesodermal tissue will lead to a low position of the conus. The mesenchymal

Fig. 9.12 "Taillike" lipoma

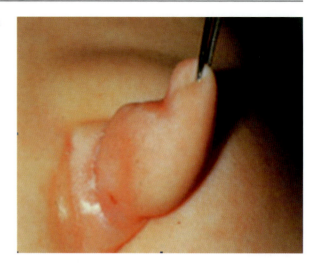

origin almost certainly explains the variations of malformations associated with CSD. Therefore, multiple mesenchymal anomalies can be found in the same patient, and these are not limited to the area of the cutaneous manifestations. Adhesions between the cord and dural sac can be caused by a lipoma attached to the filum terminale, by lipomyeloschisis, or by a thickened filum terminale with fibrotic or fat components. Other malformations associated with CSD are split notochord syndrome, terminal myelocystocele, intraspinal enteric cysts, dorsal dermal sinus, and diastematomyelia.

Dermal sinuses are typically oriented from dermal caudal to cranial intraspinal. It has a tract lined by epithelium and can communicate to the central nervous system (CNS) resulting in (Figs. 9.13 and 9.14a) an increased risk for meningitis. Caudal pits at the sacral level and below usually do not communicate with the subarachnoidal space, which ends at the level of S2. The typical dermal sinuses are found more cranially and end intradurally, and these can be associated with dermoid cysts or teratomas. An early surgical intervention is indicated. Otherwise, progressive neurological deterioration results from cord tethering (Fig. 9.13b), epi- or dermoid enlargement (Fig. 9.14b), and compression of the cord or cauda equina. Further possible complications are meningitis and abscess leading to sequelae.

9.3.2 Meningocele

- Closed sac extending through posterior or anterior bone defect.
- MRI is the best method with patient prone not to compress the sac.
- Look for associations: low cord, thick filum terminale, split cord, epidermoid, lipoma, hydromyelia, and Chiari I (Fig. 9.15) are possible due to hydrodynamic imbalance. Also vertebral anomalies: segmentation disorders, hemivertebrae, or Klippel–Feil anomaly.

9 Malformations of the Spine   141

Fig. 9.13 Dermal sinus. (a) At 2 days. Sagittal T2-w image MR shows a hypointense linear sinus tract (*arrow*) extending from the skin surface. (**b**) At 7 weeks. After surgery sagittal T2-w image MR shows a much smaller tract (*arrow*) extending from the surface, through posterior elements into the thecal sac. Although the low position of the conus is normal at birth (first MRI image at 2 days), it should have ascended to the normal adult level (L1/L2 interspace) at 7/8 weeks. The persistent low conus at the second image implies tethering; note the adhesion of the conus dorsally

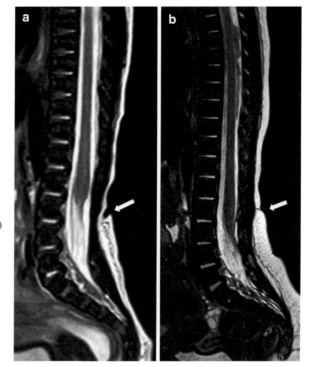

- Look for possible surgical difficulties: entrapped roots attached to the sac, tethered cord, or intraspinal mass outside the sac. Exclude also subcutaneous tracts or fistulas.
- Complications may occur in "simple" meningoceles. Look for malformations!

Note that the simple meningocele (without myelocele) is not associated with Chiari II malformation. It is usually covered by a layer of epidermis covering the meninges. Therefore, no increase in the AFP is seen.

The meningocele is more common at the lumbar and sacral locations but can also occur at the cervical level (Fig. 9.15). In fact, it can be found anywhere along the spine. The frequency of meningocele is 1 in 10,000 births.

Because this kind of lesion does not involve the spinal cord, no neurological symptoms are present. Treatment usually follows due to cosmetic reasons. Meningocele is lined by arachnoid; in this way, arachnoid adhesions may obstruct the neck of the sac. The CSF-filled sac herniates through a posterior spinal defect, but the spinal cord does not enter the sac. Occasionally, the filum terminale or nerve roots herniate (Fig. 9.16).

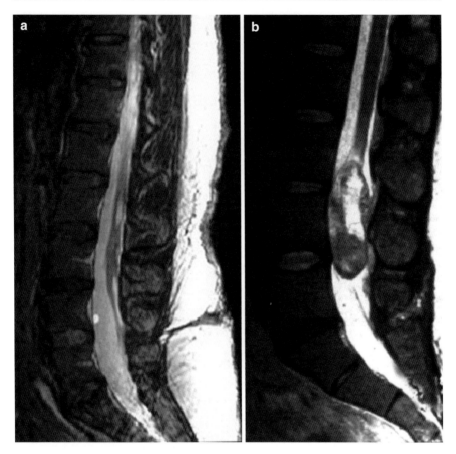

Fig. 9.14 Dermal sinus and dermoid. (**a**) Patient **a**: Sagittal T2-w image MR demonstrates lumbar skin dimple (*white arrow*) with a persistent connection, dermal sinus tract containing a small dermoid (*black arrow*). The low-lying spinal cord is fixed to dorsal lipoma (*block white arrow*). (**b**) Patient **b**: Sagittal T2-w image MR shows a heterogenous, mixed intensity mass in the region of conus medullaris und cauda equina. Note the expanding of the cord. The hyperintensity (*block white arrow*) was due to fat in the dermoid

9.3.2.1 Lipomyelomeningocele

- Mesenchyme is incorporated into neural folds.
- Twenty to fifty-six percent of CSD. Not associated with Chiari II. The brain is typically normal.
- The deep portion of the lipoma is adherent to the placode, but the roots do not travel through the lipoma.
- MRI evaluation should assess the relationship between lipoma and neural placode. Rule out any central canal extension of the lipoma. Position of lipoma, placode, and nerve roots in relation to the midline.
- Rule out cord tethering, myeloschisis, terminal hydromyelia.
- Look for possible surgical difficulties: specially rotation of the lipoma with secondary distortion of the nerve roots.

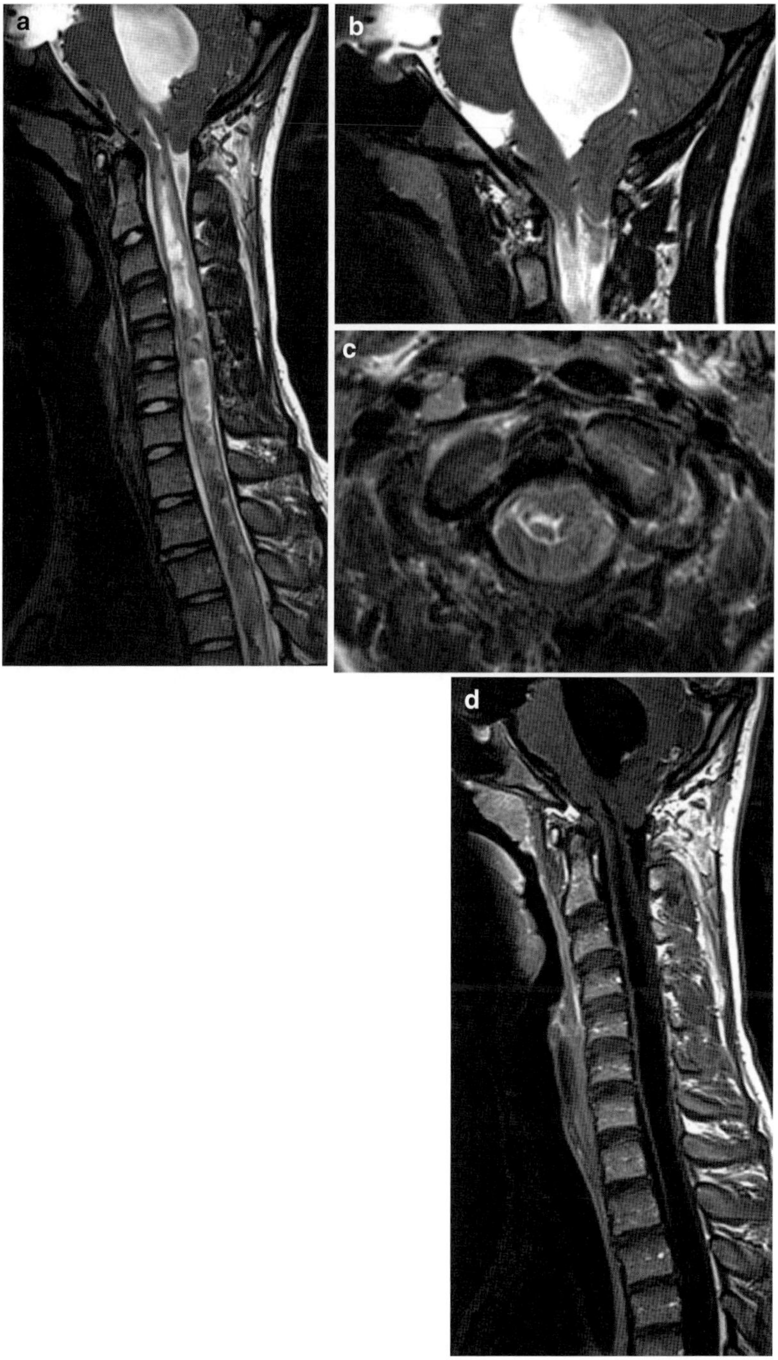

Fig. 9.15 Chiari I malformation. (**a**) Sagittal T2-w image shows herniation of the cerebellar tonsils through the foramen magnum into the cervical spinal canal. There is a large distention of the central canal of spinal cord filled with CSF (i.e., hydromyelia), and also hydrocephalus with the enlarged fourth ventricle is seen. (**b**) The cerebellar tonsils are elongated, and a mild kinking of the medulla is present. (**c**) The tonsillar herniation fills the cisterns. (**d**) Contrast-enhanced T1-w images should be performed to exclude a tumor

Fig. 9.16 Cervical meningocele. Sagittal T1-w image shows nerve roots herniating into sac (*white arrow*). This dysraphism is close and therefore not associated with Chiari II malformation

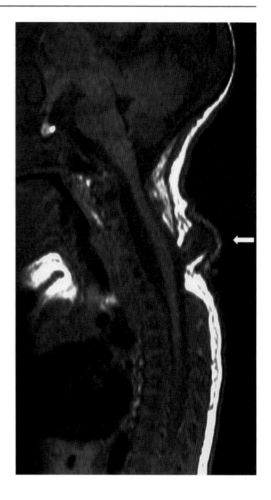

> Re-tethering
> The diagnosis of re-tethering after surgery is clinical; MRI is indicated to rule out complications.

The neural tube forms by infolding and closure of neural ectoderm as it separates from cutaneous ectoderm during the third and fourth weeks. Lipomyelomeningocele is probably a result of premature disjunction. The mesenchyme is exposed with contact to the neural tube. As a consequence, the ependymal lining of the primitive neural tube induces the mesenchyme to form fat. The neural folds remain open, forming a neural placode at the site of premature disjunction. It accounts for 20 % of the skin-covered lumbosacral mass. Unfortunately, lipomyelomeningocele's incidence is not reduced with the supplementation of folate.

Fig. 9.17 Lipomyelomeningocele: sagittal T2-w image reveals an elongated, tethered low-lying spinal cord inserting into a large terminal lipomatous mass contiguous with subcutaneous fat through dysraphic defect

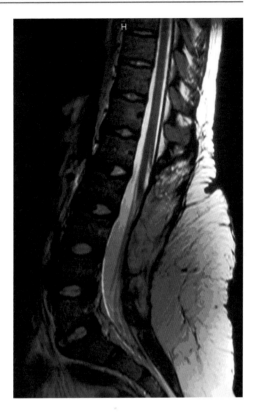

The deep portion of the lipoma is adherent to the placode (Fig. 9.17). The lipoma may spread superiorly along the myeloschisis and may involve the spinal cord. Almost always, there is a low position of the involved spinal cord (Fig. 9.17) which ends at the placode. The roots do not travel through the lipoma. Instead, the motor and sensory roots exit from the ventral surface. With larger meningoceles, the lipoma, which is tethered to the cord, may rotate and then cause distortion of the nerve roots. The repair in the case of asymmetrical lipomas can be difficult with short nerve roots on the lipoma side and elongated roots on the other side, necessitating careful relocation at surgery.

If left untreated, these children usually show irreversible progressive neurological impairment (16–88 %) due to cord tethering and enlarging lipoma (the lipoma grows with the infant). If tethering of the cord is not released early, bladder dysfunction usually persists. The main goal of reconstructive surgery is to untether the spinal cord, to reduce the volume of the lipoma, and to reconstruct the spinal canal, at the same time minimizing scarring and, consequently, the risk of re-tethering. Postoperatively, patients should not deteriorate with longitudinal growth. It is important to know that symptomatic re-tethering is common, weeks or years after surgery.

Imaging
The high signal of lipomas, contrasting to the intermediate signal of the cord, gives an excellent contrast in sagittal and axial T2-w images (Fig. 9.17). T1-w with and without spectral fat suppression confirms the fatty composition of the mass. The most common differential diagnosis is intradural and terminal lipomas. The former, also called juxtamedullary lipoma, is covered by an intact dura, and cutaneous manifestations are unusual.

9.3.2.2 Split Cord Malformation

- Diastematomyelia: spinal cord or canal splitting
- Diplomyelia: RARE, spinal cord or canal duplication; each cord with two anterior and two posterior horns and roots
- Rule out in patients with cutaneous stigmata ("faun's tail" hair patch), intersegmental fusion of posterior elements, and clinical tethered cord
- Look for spur: almost pathognomonic for split cord malformation (SCM): intersegmental laminar fusion + segmentation anomalies
- While osseous spur are visible, fibrous spurs may be occult.

Split cord malformations (SCM) include both diastematomyelia (diastema from ancient Greek means spacing) and diplomyelia. Diastematomyelia (Fig. 9.6) is distinguished from the rare diplomyelia, a more or less complete duplication of the spinal cord. In diplomyelia, there are two separate whole cords, each with two ventral and two dorsal nerve roots.

In the case of diastematomyelia, there is a sagittal division of the cord. Usually, only a short segment is involved with asymmetry in size of the hemicords, each segment is lined by its own pia mater, and each hemicord has a central canal. The cleft can be complete or it may involve only the ventral or dorsal half of the cord. The septum between the two pia-lined hemicords can be an ossified spur (type I, Fig. 9.18c), or a non-ossified fibrous septum can be present within a single dural tube (type II, Fig. 9.6b). This last type is rarely symptomatic, unless hydromyelia and tethering are present.

The length of the split cord is variable and, by necessity, longer than the spur. The cleft is between T9 and S1 in 85 % of the cases. The classical bone spur is not always found in all patients with SCM; patients may present with a partial or complete fibrous bridge between the posterior surface of the vertebral body and the vertebral arch. Hemicords usually reunite below the cleft (ca. 90 %). It should be noted that the spur arises from the laminae and afterward fuses with the vertebral body. Therefore, asymmetry of the two canals may result from the oblique position of the spur or from scoliosis, which rotates the spur.

SCM are usually associated with vertebral body anomalies, such as segmental and fusion anomalies, intersegmental laminar fusion associated with spina bifida (60 %), myelocele/myelomeningocele (15–25 %), hemimyelocele (15–20 %), tethered cord (75 %), thickened filum terminale (40–90 %), hydromyelia (50 %) in one or both hemicords (often above the diastematomyelia), scoliosis (79 %), and Chiari II malformations (15–20 %).

9 Malformations of the Spine

Fig. 9.18 Diastematomyelia with lipoma. (**a**) CT shows bony diastematomyelia (*yellow arrow*) at the upper spine with bony remodeling at the level of the lipoma (*white arrow*). (**b**) Sagittal T1-w image shows a hyperintense mass in the region of the conus medullaris, partially intramedullar. The T1 hyperintensity suggests dermoid or an intradural (juxtamedullary) lipoma. (**c**) The axial CT image shows a large osseous spur dividing the canal

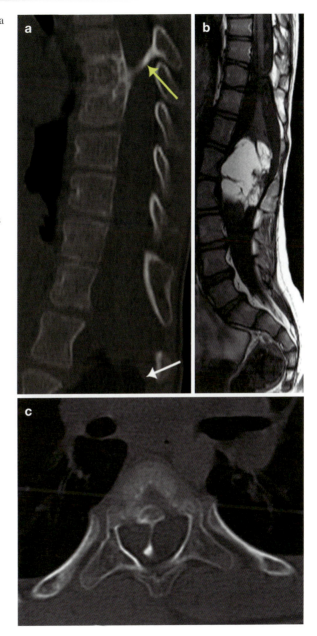

Imaging

MRI is necessary to detect the extension of the cord split, to assess the existence of a fibrous septum and hydromyelia, to determine the level of the conus and to rule out other causes of tethering. It is important to evaluate the nerve roots, which can become adherent to dura and tether the cord. Computed tomography (17C) may show ossified septation and can be very useful for surgical planning.

9.3.2.3 Terminal Myelocystocele

> Important points
> - Closed sac with marked cystic dilatation of the distal cord central canal or the *ventriculus terminalis*
> - MRI is the best method for patients not prone to compress the sac.
> - Look for associations: hydromyelia with low-lying tethered cord. Not associated with Chiari II malformation
> - MRI is performed to determine the extension of hydromyelia and rachischisis and the size of the cysts and to rule out associated anomalies.

Terminal myelocystocele (Fig. 9.9) is a skin-covered uncommon malformation. The distal central canal becomes noticeably dilated and herniates through a posterior lumbosacral defect. It may represent a large persistent terminal ventricle. This anomaly can be difficult to be differentiated from meningomyelocele (MMC) prenatally. Distinguishing myelocystocele from the former, the presence of a thick-walled sac (skin cover), the absence of a true neural placode dorsally, the absence of Chiari II malformation, and the lack of elevated AFP in the maternal blood suggest this diagnosis.

MRI rules out genitourinary malformations. Notably, myelocystocele can be associated with caudal regression syndrome and OEIS syndrome (omphalocele, exstrophy of the bladder, imperforate anus, and spinal anomalies).

The ballooning of the terminal ventricle disrupts the mesenchyme, but not the ectoderm (Fig. 9.9c, d). At the same time, the cyst volume prevents the ascent of the cord with tethered cord.

9.3.3 Open Spinal Dysraphism

This entity is commonly located in the lumbosacral region (80–90 %), a location associated with the final component of neural tube closure. The incidence of OSD is of 0.5–1 in 1,000 live births. Typically, it presents with an increased interpeduncular distance, wide spinal canal, and absence or incomplete closure of the vertebral arches. Other neurological defects may be associated in the patient, such as hydrocephalus, diastematomyelia, Arnold–Chiari malformation, hydromyelia, or a tethered spinal cord.

Meningomyelocele

> - Open sac extending through posterior bone defect. Neural tissue, meninges, and CSF exposed
> - Initial MMC diagnosis with obstetrical ultrasound

- Fetal MR: eligibility for fetal surgery
- Antenatal diagnosis
- Look for open neural arch, MMC sac, and Chiari II findings.
- Rule out associated anomalies: hydrocephalus, diastematomyelia, Chiari II, hydromyelia, or a tethered spinal cord. Important: (1) Diastematomyelia can occur at a higher level than the MMC! (2) Syringohydromyelia may develop and produce late-onset symptoms!
- Low conus on MR imaging is not always a sign of clinical tethering!
- MRI: postoperative clinical deterioration requires craniospinal reevaluation.
- Important: re-tethering of the spinal cord with adhesions to the dura is always present; therefore, it is of questionable diagnostic significance.

Meningomyelocele is the most common form of OSD. It involves the spinal cord and meninges and may be covered by a thin layer of skin or by a membranous sac. Clinically, these patients present with limb paralysis, bladder and bowel incontinence, or dislocations of the hip. Other potential associated abnormalities are hydromyelia, split cord with or without diastematomyelia (Figs. 9.6b and 9.18c), hydrocephalus, Arnold–Chiari malformations (Fig. 9.11) or scoliosis, kyphosis, or lordosis. Congenital scoliosis and kyphosis are found in approximately 30 % of the patients with MMC and are due to associated anomalies, such as hemivertebrae (Fig. 9.10), bony spurs, and unilateral fusions. Developmental scoliosis and kyphosis are present in 30 % of the patients resulting from muscular imbalance.

Sometimes, as a result of the neural tube not closing properly, the spinal cord is exposed, also called myeloschisis. This is the most severe type of spina bifida, and it bears the risk of severe infection. The nervous structures remain as a placode; its ventral surface is lined by pia-arachnoid. The nerve roots arise directly from the ventral surface (Fig. 9.19c). Dorsally the neural placode is freely exposed. Leaking of the cerebrospinal fluid (CSF) is common because of rupture of the thin subarachnoidal membranes.

Advances in prenatal ultrasound and MRI have significantly improved the diagnosis and therapy of spinal dysraphism prenatally. Screening should be performed with ultrasound. In addition, fetal MRI has significantly improved in the recent years and is an excellent tool in the complementary evaluation of the spinal malformation and associated CNS anomalies. Both methods contributed to the evaluation of the malformation, determining the need for in utero surgery. It appears that surgery covering the exposed spinal cord in utero preserves the distal neurological function, due to the reduced chemical irritation caused by amniotic fluid exposure. In addition, in cases treated prenatally, there was a reduction of hindbrain herniation with decreased need for ventricular shunting in some of the cases. Therefore, MRI plays a significant role in confirming the ultrasound findings, making the correct diagnosis, and ruling out additional anomalies and to decide about the eligibility for fetal surgery in case of MMC.

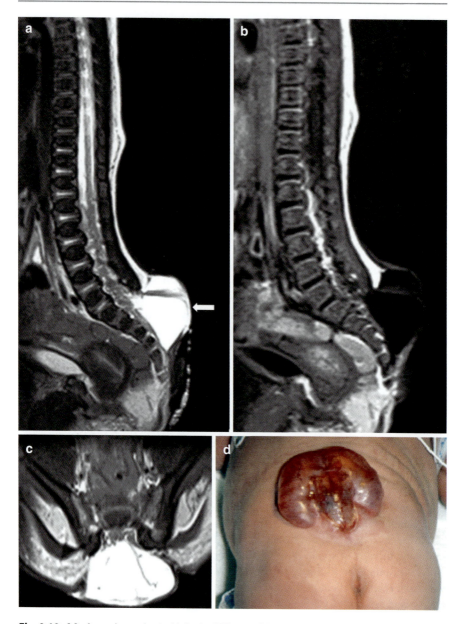

Fig. 9.19 Myelomeningocele. (**a, b**) Sagittal T2-w and T1-w images show, respectively, an unrepaired sacral myelomeningocele with open spinal dysraphism, CSF-filled myelomeningocele sac, and dorsal placode (*white arrow*). (**c**) The axial T2-w image confirms the dysraphism. The nervous structures remain as a placode with the nerve roots arising directly from its ventral surface. (**d**) Another patient. Note that the neural placode is freely exposed with leaking of CSF. The closure has to be performed during the first 48 h to prevent infection

9 Malformations of the Spine

Fig. 9.20 Myelomeningocele after repair. Normal aspect with re-tethering of the cord, scar, and adhesions to the dura. Note the new development of syringohydromyelia, which explains neurological deterioration in this patient

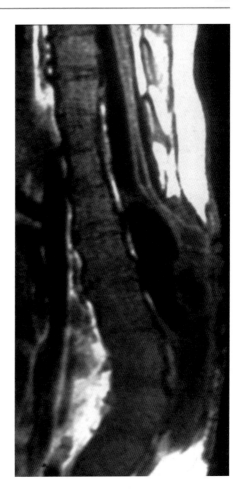

After birth, the diagnosis of OSD is clinically easy (Fig. 9.19d), and imaging untreated MMC is questionable. If indicated, the aim of MRI is to evaluate the malformation in detail and to rule out associated anomalies prior to corrective surgery. Associated anomalies, such as diastematomyelia at a higher level than the MMC, indicate that a more extensive surgery will be necessary.

The best possible outcome in these patients is a stable postoperative deficit. Patients with MMC, who after surgery or later in life show clinical neurological deterioration, should be reevaluated with MRI. The aim is to detect postoperative complications (e.g., constriction secondary to dural ring by scar), concomitant unrecognized abnormality (e.g., split cord with or without diastematomyelia) or changes in the malformation. For example, syringohydromyelia (Fig. 9.20) may develop (29–77 %) and give late symptoms. Other possible postoperative complications are arachnoid cysts, dermoids or inclusion tumors, or cord ischemia. Re-tethering of the spinal cord with adhesions to the dura (Fig. 9.19) is always present and, therefore, is of questionable diagnostic significance.

9.4 Miscellaneous Malformations of the Spine

9.4.1 Tethered Cord and Fibrolipomas of the Filum Terminale

- Thickened filum terminale: >2 mm at L5–S1 level.
- Tethered cord: conus tip below the level of the L2 vertebral body + tethered by thickened filum.
  Usually, patients present with combination of both the above. However, tethered cord may occur without thickened filum, or the filum is thickened, but the conus lies in its normal position. In these cases, it is helpful to evaluate the position of the conus medullaris: it lies dorsal (even in prone position) in tethered cord.
  Important: *tethered cord is a clinical diagnosis*. It can be present regardless of normal conus position and normal thickness of the filum.
- Low-lying conus can present as a normal variant without symptoms.
- Lipomas: incidental findings in 4–6 % of exams.
  MRI: sagittal images alone should not be used to diagnose tethering.
  Look for CSD, hydromyelia, myelomalacia, lumbosacral hypogenesis, and VACTERL syndrome.

The filum terminale is a long and thin (under 2 mm at L5–S1 level) filament. The thickened filum terminale is defined as an enlargement of the filum to a diameter of 2 mm or more at the L5–S1 level. Tethered cord is described as the conus tip below the level of the L2 vertebral body associated with thickened filum terminale und dorsal position of the conus medullaris (even in prone position).

Tethered cord results from an incomplete regressive differentiation with failure of the terminal cord involution or failure of filum terminale to lengthen. The conus should be in the adult normal position (at or above the level of the L2 vertebral body) at the latest by 2 months of age. Lipoma of the filum (Fig. 9.20) can result from minor alteration in the canalization and regression. Note though that lipomas are found as incidental findings in 4–6 % of normal spinal exams.

Patients usually present with a combination of tethered cord and thickened filum terminale. However, tethered cord may occur without thickened filum or the other way around (the filum is thickened, but the conus lies in its normal position). A significant number of patients present with clinical symptoms of tethered cord but on MRI show normal filum diameter and normal conus position. This does not preclude the diagnosis of tethered cord. Conversely, low-lying conus can be present as a normal variant without symptoms. In these patients, prophylactic surgery is controversial. Physiologically, the tethering impairs the oxidative metabolism of conus and nerve roots with secondary abnormal lumbosacral function.

9 Malformations of the Spine

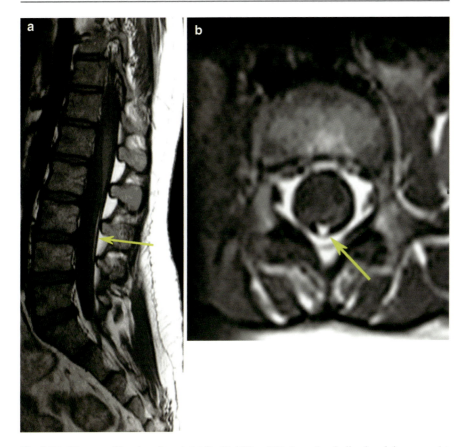

Fig. 9.21 Lipoma with tethered cord. (**a**) Sagittal T1-w MR shows borderline low-lying conus (at the inferior L2 vertebral level). The filum (*yellow arrow*) contains fat. (**b**) Axial T1-w MR confirms the presence of fat in filum terminale (*yellow arrow*)

However, while the filum is usually thickened by fibrosis (55 % of abnormal cases), in ca. 20 % of the cases, a thin lipoma is found (Fig. 9.20) or rarely a filar cyst. Tethered cord is commonly associated with cutaneous stigmata, CSD (33–100 % depending on the references), hydromyelia, myelomalacia, and scoliosis. Clinically, it typically becomes symptomatic during adolescent growth, but symptom onset has been described as early as 3 years of age and as late as 76 years of age.

Imaging

Neurosonography can be used in the diagnosis if the child is less than 6 months old; the findings need to be confirmed with MRI. On MRI, the dural sac is usually widened with dorsal positioning of the conus (even when the patient is scanned in a prone position), and the thickened filum is attached to the dorsal dura. Filum lipoma appears as high signal on T1-w images. When the filum is thickened by dense fibrosis, it has a signal appearance similar to the nerve roots (Fig. 9.21b). It is important to emphasize that sagittal MR images alone should not be used to diagnosis tethering. The exact location of the conus should be determined on axial scans, in which the filum appears as a low signal structure within high signal CSF. If evaluated on the sagittal images, the cauda equina may lead to an ambiguous evaluation of the conus tip.

After surgery, the recurrence of symptoms is rare; if present, a new MRI evaluation is required to rule out re-tethering.

9.4.2 Caudal Regression Syndrome

Abnormal distal spinal cord associated with lumbosacral dysgenesis/agenesis. It can be divided into:
- Group one: severe sacral osseous anomalies and dilated central spinal canal. Abrupt termination of the cord above L1
- Group two: the cord is tapered, low lying, and elongated with tethering, and a spinal lipoma may be present.

Differential diagnosis: tethered spinal cord, no caudal dysgenesis
Rule out tethered cord in all patients with caudal dysgenesis, even in the mild case of an absent coccyx.
Look for genitourinary and anorectal malformations in patients with CRS.

Caudal regression syndrome (CRS) is characterized by sacral dysgenesis (Fig. 9.22) associated with genitourinary and gastrointestinal malformations. Sacral agenesis/dysgenesis is a rare congenital anomaly of the spine, and the incidence is 1/7500 births, mostly milder forms of dysgenesis. In 15–20 % of the cases, the mother has diabetes, but most cases are sporadic. The embryogenesis of this syndrome is still controversial. Patients with a deranged caudal development of the spine, which includes canalization and regression, will show tethered cord with or without dysgenesis of the cord associated with caudal vertebral agenesis. The second group with disruption prior to the fourth gestational week presents with agenesis of parts of the end of the spinal cord, spinal ganglia, and spine. This suggests that the primary neurulation is involved with abnormal neural tube and notochord development (Fig. 9.23).

Morphologically, it presents as a spectrum varying from a mild form with an absent coccyx to a severe form and complete lumbosacral agenesis. It can also present as a unilateral sacral agenesis/dysgenesis with oblique lumbosacral joint, pelvic tilt, and scoliosis. In the case of a bilateral lumbosacral agenesis, the vertebral column terminates at the level of the thoracic spine, and the lowest vertebra articulates with the ilia. Alternatively, the ilia are fused below the lowest vertebrae.

The MR findings in CRS can be divided into two groups. The first is characterized by distal spinal cord hypoplasia; the distal spinal cord typically terminates abruptly in a "wedge-shaped" form. In this case, the dorsal portion of the cord extends more caudally than the ventral portion (Fig. 9.22). Usually, the caudal roots extend downward vertically; it looks like a distal focal "diastematomyelia" is present arising from

Fig. 9.22 A 8 years old boy with typical tethered cord. (**a**) Sagittal T2-w reveals a low-lying hydromyelic tethered cord with fibrolipoma (*curved white arrow*) inserting into a terminal lipoma. Marked signal loss at S1/S2 level compatible with lipoma. (**b**) Sagittal T1-w MRI shows an elongated low-lying hydromyelic spinal cord extending to the S1 level, ending in a small terminal lipoma (*block white arrow*). Notice above the level of the lipoma, the subcutaneous fat extending through the dorsal dysraphism (*straight white arrow*)

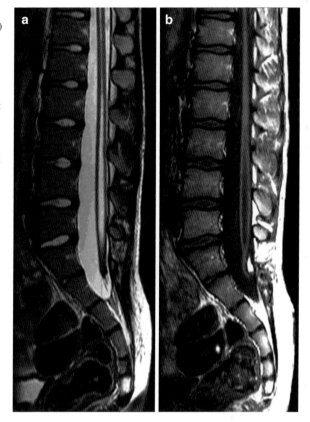

the dysplastic conus with a gap between the anterior and posterior roots. This group of patients usually present with severe sacral osseous anomalies and dilated central spinal canal. In the second group of patients, the cord is tapered, low lying, and elongated with tethering, and a spinal lipoma may be present. The main differential diagnosis is tethered spinal cord, in which patients present no caudal dysgenesis.

There is an association with VACTERL (10 %), which is a nonrandom association of birth defects (V, vertebral; A, anal; C, cardiac; TE, trachea/esophagus; R, renal; and L, limbs). Cardiac anomalies may be present in 24 % of these patients. The lower extremities are often affected; the extreme case with fusion of the lower extremities is called sirenomelia. The peritoneal and gluteal muscles are hypoplastic with fat infiltration. An imperforated anus or anal atresia is frequent. MRI may show not only the anorectal anomalies but also the genitourinary (24 %; such as renal agenesis, ectopia, hydronephrosis, bladder malformations) anomalies and can analyze the pelvic musculature.

A tethered cord is present in all patients with CRS, in whom the conus terminates below L1. Other spinal anomalies may include vertebral anomalies (22 %), lipo- and myelomeningocele (10–50 %), hydromyelia (10 %), diastematomyelia, terminal myelocystocele (15 %), and anterior sacral meningocele.

Fig. 9.23 Caudal regression syndrome with sacral agenesis and multiple vertebral segmentation anomalies. Sagittal T2-w image shows that the dorsal portion of the cord extends more caudally than the ventral portion

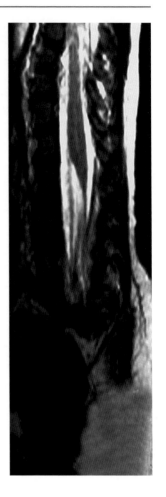

Further Reading

1. Bulas D (2010) Fetal evaluation of spine dysraphism. Pediatr Radiol 40:1029–1037
2. Chen YF, Liu HM (2009) Imaging of craniovertebral junction. Neuroimaging Clin N Am 19:483–510
3. DeLaPaz RL (1993) Congenital anomalies of the lumbosacral spine. Neuroimaging Clin N Am 3:425–442
4. Ghanem I, El Hage S, Rachkidi R, Kharrat K, Dagher F, Kreichati G (2008) Pediatric cervical spine instability. J Child Orthop 2:71–84
5. Lustrin ES, Karakas SP, Ortiz AO, Cinnamon J, Castillo M, Vaheesan K, Brown JH, Diamond AS, Black K, Singh S (2003) Pediatric cervical spine: normal anatomy, variants, and trauma. Radiographics 23:539–560
6. Smoker WR (1994) Craniovertebral junction: normal anatomy, craniometry, and congenital anomalies. Radiographics 14:255–277

Part IV
Diseases of Extramedullary Origin

Diseases of Extramedullary Origin: Degenerative Diseases

10

Stefan Weidauer, Michael Nichtweiß, Werner Wichmann, and Elke Hattingen

Contents

10.1	Back Pain	160
	10.1.1 Local Pain	160
	10.1.2 Radicular Pain	161
	10.1.3 Referred Pain	163
	10.1.4 Pain Caused by Muscle Spasm	167
10.2	Radicular Compression Syndromes	167
	10.2.1 Pathophysiological and Clinical Aspects	167
	10.2.2 Imaging: General Considerations	169
	10.2.3 Intervertebral Disc Degeneration	172
	10.2.4 Degenerative Vertebral Endplate Changes	174
	10.2.5 Disc Herniation	174
	10.2.6 Foraminal Stenosis	179
	10.2.7 Acquired Lumbal Canal Stenosis	182
10.3	Myelon Compression Syndromes	188
	10.3.1 Pathophysiological and Clinical Aspects	188
	10.3.2 Cervical Disc Herniation	192
	10.3.3 Cervical Spondylosis	193
References		200

S. Weidauer (✉)
Department of Neurology, Sankt Katharinen Hospital,
Seckbacher Landstr. 65, D-60389 Frankfurt, Germany
e-mail: stefan.weidauer@sankt-katharinen-ffm.de

M. Nichtweiß
Department of Neurology, Hanse Klinikum Wismar; Wellengang 21, D-23968 Wismar, Germany
e-mail: michael.nichtweiss@gmail.com

W. Wichmann
Department of Neuroradiology, University of Zürich, Rämistr. 100, CH-8091 Zürich, Switzerland
e-mail: werner.wichmann@usz.ch

E. Hattingen
Institute for Neuroradiology, Goethe-University,
Schleusenweg 2-16, D-60528 Frankfurt, Germany
e-mail: elke.hattingen@kgu.de

Abbreviations

ATR   Achilles tendon reflex
BTR   Biceps tendon reflex
PTR   Patellar tendon reflex
TPR   Tibialis posterior reflex
TTR   Tibialis tendon reflex

10.1 Back Pain

The vertebral and paravertebral structures are innervated by meningeal branches (syn.: recurrent meningeal nerves or sinuvertebral nerves) originating from the dorsal rami of the spinal nerves shortly after the dorsal nerve root ganglion (spinal ganglion). The sinuvertebral nerves run recurrently through the intervertebral foramen back into the spinal canal and supply pain fibres to the periosteum of the vertebra, the capsule of the articular facets, the outer layers of the anulus fibrosus and the intraspinal ligaments, e.g. yellow ligament and posterior longitudinal ligament at the segmental level and also in parts at the neighbouring levels. The sinuvertebral nerve also contains fibres from the neighbouring sympathetic ganglion via grey ramus or directly from a thoracic sympathetic ganglion. In general, there are four types of lower back pain [1, 2]:

Local pain. Caused by circumscribed pathological processes in structures containing sensory receptors.

Radicular pain. With projection into a dermatome because of mechanical (i.e. nerve root compression), inflammatory or metabolic aetiologies with consecutive irritation of the nerve root.

Referred pain or reflective pain. One can distinguish two types of referred pain: the first type projects pain from the (lower) spine within lumbar regions and sacral dermatomes and the second projects from visceral structures into the surface of the body [2].

Pain caused by muscular spasm. May be caused by local pain with reflex muscle contraction.

10.1.1 Local Pain

This type of pain has widespread aetiologies including vertebral tumours, fractures, degeneration of vertebral body-disc complex, articular facets and ligamentous structures, inflammatory processes including autoimmune associated diseases (e.g. ankylosing spondylitis, see Fig. 10.1) and bacterial infections (e.g. epidural abscess, spondylitis or spondylodiscitis; see Figs. 10.2, 10.3 and 10.4 and Chap. 13). In addition, orthopaedic diseases and congenital anomalies including spondylolysis (see Fig. 10.19) may cause local back pain. However, detailed description is beyond the scope of this chapter.

10 Diseases of Extramedullary Origin: Degenerative Diseases

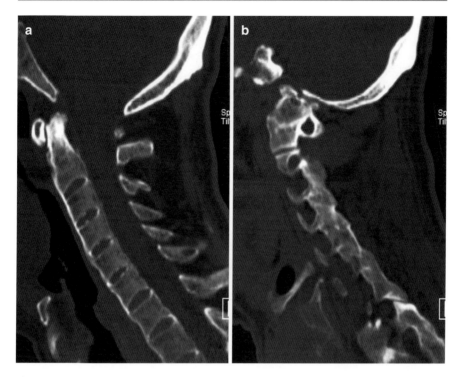

Fig. 10.1 Sag. CT (**a**, **b**): ankylosing spondylitis with "bamboo spine" and fusion of joints

10.1.2 Radicular Pain

Result from mechanical (i.e. compression or stretching), inflammatory or metabolic irritation of the nerve root within the spinal canal or the region of the intervertebral foramen (Fig. 10.5). The pain has a sharp character and radiates into the dermatome including the peripheral parts accordingly to the segmental innervation of the nerve root. When mechanical aetiology is present, e.g. intervertebral disc herniation or stenosis of intervertebral foramen, coughing, sneezing and jugular vein compression (Valsalva manoeuvre) could evoke or increase radicular pain caused by nerve root shifting.

Clinical examination using "straight leg raising" (Lasègue manoeuvre) shows pain exacerbation, when there is L4, L5 or S1 nerve root entrapment caused by nerve stretching. "Straight leg raising" is often restricted to between 20 and 30° in severe sciatica. Inverse Lasègue manoeuvre in a prone position with thigh extension is positive in L3 nerve root entrapment. A crossed positive Lasègue manoeuvre with pain radiation into the contralateral leg is indicative of a ruptured disc prolapse with sequestration (Fig. 10.6). Additional neurological findings may be segmental sensory and motor failures and lowered or extinct muscle jerks. Lateral foraminal or extraforaminal disc herniation in particular often also show a vegetative pain component with a deep gnawing and burning character caused by additional affection of the spinal nerve ganglion (syn.: dorsal root ganglion).

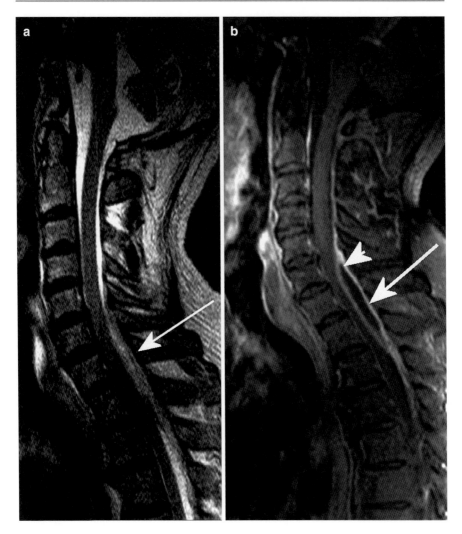

Fig. 10.2 Epidural abscess dorsal accentuated C5/6 to Th2. Sag. T2 WI (**a**) and T1 WI pc (**b**) exhibiting epidural liquid lesion (*arrow*) with marginal enhancement (**b**, *arrowhead*). The 67-year-old man suffered from severe neck pain for 4 days and dysaesthsia in both hands; C reactive protein elevated, leucocytosis; orthopaedic outdoor examination was stated normal 2 days before

In cervical disc herniation, downward pressure on the head in the hyperextended position of the cervical spine as well as bending to the affected side could increase radicular pain.

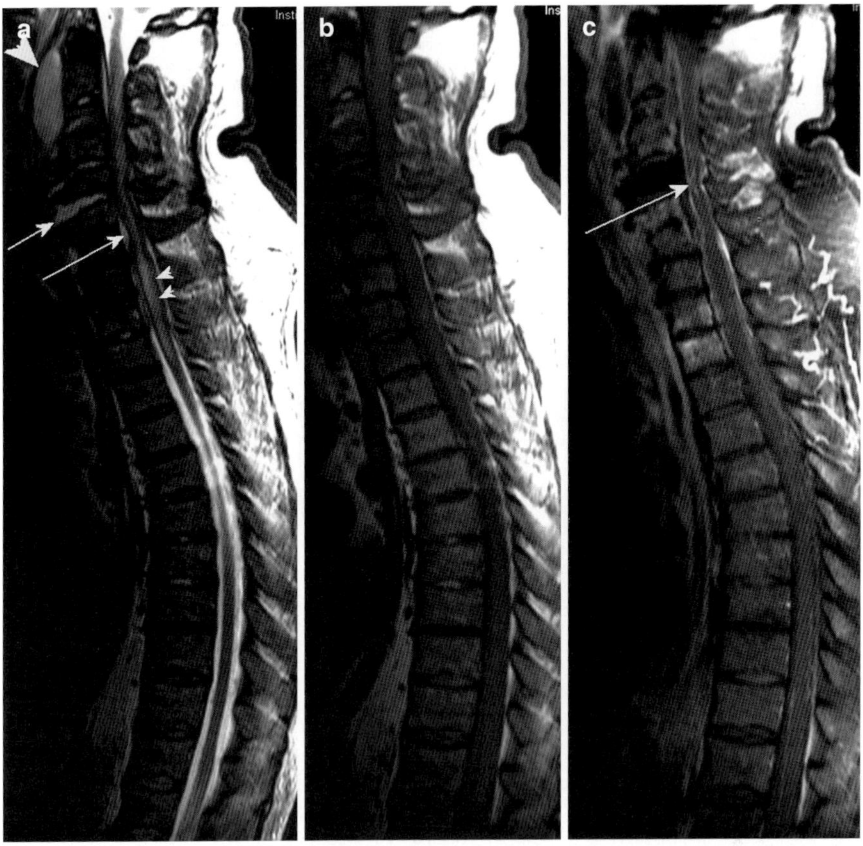

Fig. 10.3 Sag. T2 WI (**a**), T1 WI (**b**) and T1 WI fat sat pc (**c**) showing severe multisegmental spondylodiscitis (**a**, *short arrow*) with epidural abscess/empyema (**a**, *long arrow* and severe myelomalacia with intramedullary signal conversion (**a**, *small arrow heads*), caused by prevertebral abscess (**a**, *large arrow head*). Wallpaper-like pial and epidural enhancement, partially intramedullary (**c**, *arrow*), also enhancement of vertebral structures

10.1.3 Referred Pain

Referred pain from the lower back (*syn: pseudoradicular pain*) originates from the above-mentioned spinal structures (i.e. the periosteum of the vertebra, the capsule of the articular facets, the outer layers of the anulus fibrosus and the intraspinal ligaments, e.g. yellow ligament and posterior longitudinal ligament) at a particular level and, in contrast to the radicular (nerve root) affection, this pain does not

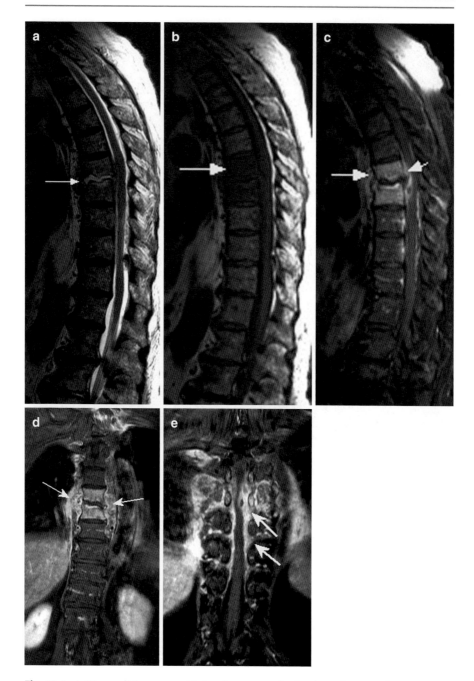

Fig. 10.4 A 91-year-old woman suffering from severe back pain and progressive paraparesis caused by spondylodiscitis at the level T6/7 with epidural abscess. Sagittal T2 WI (**a**) showing hyperintense signal changes of the intervertebral disc (*arrow*); sag. T1 WI (**b**) with signal decrease of the vertebral bodies Th6 and Th7 (**b**, *arrow*) and homogeneous enhancement (**c**, *arrow*; pc T1 WI); note additional enhancing masses preavertebral and epidural (**c**, *short arrow*). (**d, e**) (pc T1 WI coronal) exhibiting extended paravertebral inflammatory masses (**d**, *arrows*) with diffuse infiltration of the intervertebral foramina (**e**, *arrows*). (**f**) (T2 WI ax.) and (**g**) (pc T1WI ax.) revealing thickened paravertebral space (*arrow*) and epidural abscess with myelon compression (*short arrow*); note additional pleural fluid collection

10 Diseases of Extramedullary Origin: Degenerative Diseases

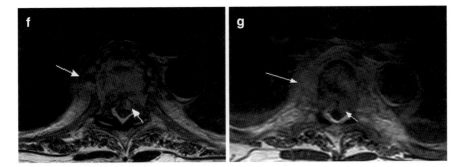

Fig. 10.4 (continued)

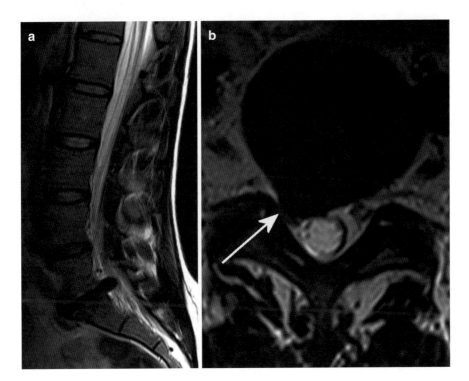

Fig. 10.5 Sag. (**a**) and ax. (**b**) T2 WI showing a mediolateral disc herniation at the level L5/S1 right in a 35-year-old woman suffering from an S1 syndrome right sided. The S1 nerve root is stretched and shifted and in addition there is a nerve root compression against ligamentous and articular structures (*arrow*)

project much below the knees. Pain from the lower spine is often projected into the lower buttocks and posterior thighs. This is because of the activation of the same pool of segmental intraspinal neurons. Therefore, differentiation of the pain origin coming from lower spinal nerves or from the sinuvertebral nerves is sometimes impossible for the patients. However, there are no (segmental) sensory or motor deficits and deep tendon reflexes and the H reflex (e.g. S1 root) are normal. This

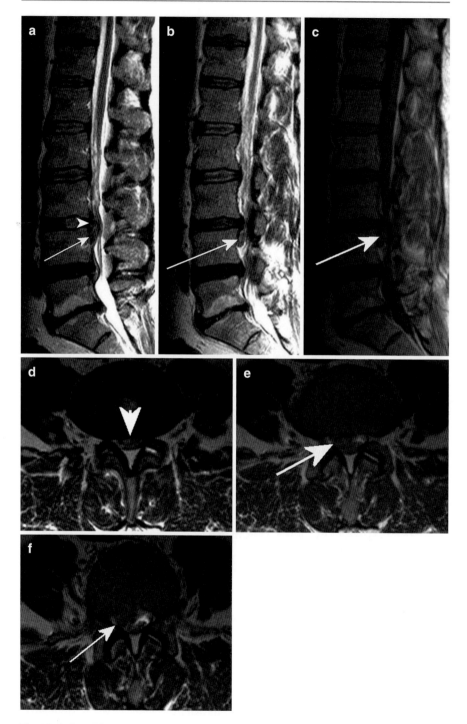

Fig. 10.6 Sag. T2 WI (**a**, **b**) and T1 WI (**c**) revealing a medial and mediolateral disc prolapse (*arrowhead*; **a**, **d**) in L3/4 with a caudal sequestration (*arrow*); (**d–f**) ax. T2 WI showing the sequestrated material within the lateral recessus (*arrow*)

underlines the need for exact neurological assessments including a precise anamnesis of pain evolution and evaluation of triggering manoeuvres. Besides imaging, electrophysiological investigations including nerve conduction studies and electromyography (EMG) can also help to differentiate pseudoradicular from radicular pain.

On the other hand, referred pain from visceral disease may be a challenge. Beside diseases in the pelvic, abdominal and thoracic viscera, including malignant, inflammatory and metabolic aetiologies and retroperitoneal neoplasms, infections and also (dissecting) aortal aneurysm may generate pain localized in the corresponding surface of the body ("Head zones") region because of the above-mentioned convergence of the same intraspinal neuron pool.

10.1.4 Pain Caused by Muscle Spasm

This is often induced by local pain with reflexive muscle contraction attempting to stabilize the affected structure/segment, e.g. facet joint. Medical treatment with muscle relaxants and additional physical therapy to interrupt this circle is therefore an important part of the therapeutic concept.

Besides a wide range of other pain entities including postural back pain and sacroiliac strain, psychiatric diseases should also be considered when careful neurological and radiological investigation rule out an organic origin.

10.2 Radicular Compression Syndromes

10.2.1 Pathophysiological and Clinical Aspects

Segmental anterior and posterior roots run in their intradural sleeve through the lateral recessus and constitute the spinal nerve, which exits through the intervertebral foramen. Whereas the efferent motoric fibres of the spinal nerve derive from the lower motor neurons in the anterior horns of the grey matter of the spinal cord, the sensory afferent fibres derive from the spinal ganglion (dorsal root ganglion) at the level of the intervertebral foramen (see also Chap. 2). Both nerve roots also content visceral autonomic fibres and there are segmental connections to the sympathetic chain and their ganglia via grey and white rami communicantes. After a short distance at the exit of the intervertebral foramen, the extradural spinal nerve divides into a ramus anterior and a ramus posterior.

Radicular compression syndromes are a composition of motoric, sensoric and vegetative segmental disturbances in the corresponding myotome and dermatome. Sometimes even a sclerotome giving irradiation of pain to structures of the pelvis is mentioned. However, because of different myelin sheets, the afferent sensoric fibres are first affected with the clinical phenomena of (segmental) radicular pain and subsequent sensory deficits such as dys- and/or hypaesthesia. In addition, segmental monosynaptic deep tendon reflex via afferent spindle fibres is extenuated or extinct, especially in comparison with the healthy contralateral side. Progressive radicular compression causes additional impairment of the motoric fibres, which have thicker myelin sheets. Partial paresis or, in extremes, paralysis is flaccid and, without radicular decompression, muscle atrophy with permanent lower motor neuron palsy follows.

There is often a typical time course for radicular compression syndromes. Declining radicular pain in the presence of progressive flaccid segmental palsy in the key muscles is a red flag and should initiate emergency diagnostic clarification with a neurological examination and additional spinal imaging on the same day. This course of the disease may represent at least a partial root death and delayed therapy, i.e. neurosurgical decompression often results in partially irreversible radicular deficits. However, *the correlation of clinical symptoms and neuroradiological features with clearly visible nerve root compression is essential for neurosurgical therapy.* If there are any doubts about the mechanical aetiology of radicular symptoms, other causes of radicular diseases such as inflammatory aetiologies (radiculitis, e.g. borreliosis or herpes zoster; see also Chaps. 3 and 15) as well as metabolic disturbances (e.g. diabetic radiculopathy) or peripheral nerve damage (e.g. diabetic mononeuropathy) should be ruled out by additional cerebrospinal fluid (CSF) analysis, nerve conduction studies and electromyographic (EMG) investigations.

Cervical disc herniations most often occur in the segments C5/C6 and C6/C7, and lumbar prolapses in the segments L4/L5 and L5/S1 (Fig. 10.5).

Compression of sacral nerve roots may cause additional bladder dysfunction. Whereas radicular symptoms often caused by mediolateral, lateral foraminal or extraforaminal disc herniations (Figs. 10.5 and 10.6) and/or stenosis of the intervertebral foramen, medial (or central) lumbar/lumbosacral prolapse (Figs. 10.7 and 10.8) may cause a *cauda equine syndrome*. Lesions of the cauda equine may cause with bilateral possibly asymmetric flaccid paresis of the legs, lowered or extinct deep tendon reflexes, sphincteric disorders with disturbance of bladder and bowel function as well as polyradicular sensory loss. With lower motor neuron lesion and intact corticospinal tract, the Babinski sign is negative. Hypaesthesia or anaesthesia in the sacral dermatomes cause so-called "breeches anaesthesia". Equivalent to acute transverse spinal cord syndromes, the acute cauda equine syndrome is an emergency case and immediately diagnostic investigation is necessary, in which initial spinal magnetic resonance imaging (MRI) is the method of choice.

Comparable to isolated radicular syndromes, differential diagnosis includes inflammatory aetiologies, i.e. polyradiculitis, which may be autoimmune associated (Guillain–Barré syndrome; see also Chap. 13) or caused by viral or bacterial (e.g. borreliosis) infections see Chap. 15). Although lesions of the conus medullaris with affection of the lower sacral segments of the spinal cord could be distinguished from the neurological point of view, in daily clinical practice it is sometimes difficult to separate these two entities. Because of lesions at the S3 to S5 level in the spinal cord, in patients with a conus medullaris syndrome paresis of the legs is absent. Table 10.1 summarizes relevant radicular syndromes.

10 Diseases of Extramedullary Origin: Degenerative Diseases

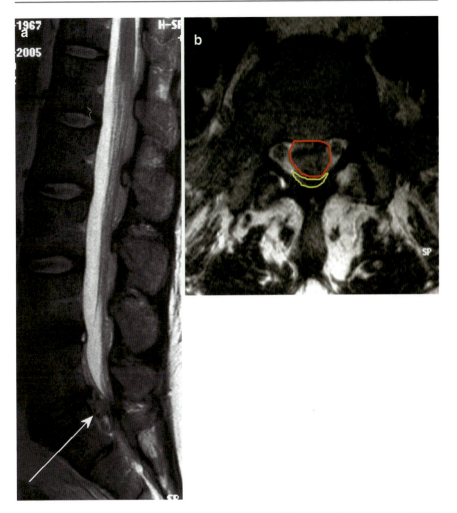

Fig. 10.7 Sag. (**a**) and ax. (**b**) T2 WI demonstrating of a medial mass prolapse at the level L5/S1 (**a**, *arrow*) in a 38-year-old woman with incomplete cauda equine syndrome; (**b**) *red* area show the mass prolapse and *yellow* small sickle-like formation represent the compressed and dorsal shifted thecal sac enclosing the cauda equine

10.2.2 Imaging: General Considerations

10.2.2.1 MRI

For spinal MRI sagittal and axial planes are mandatory. Sagittal T1-w TSE (turbo spin echo) sequences best depict the bone marrow and the cortical rims, especially regarding the endplates. The epidural fat should be considered as an anatomical landmark (spinal canal and intervertebral foramen). Anatomical details, e.g. in spondylolysis and other spine diseases, are also well detectable. One problem can

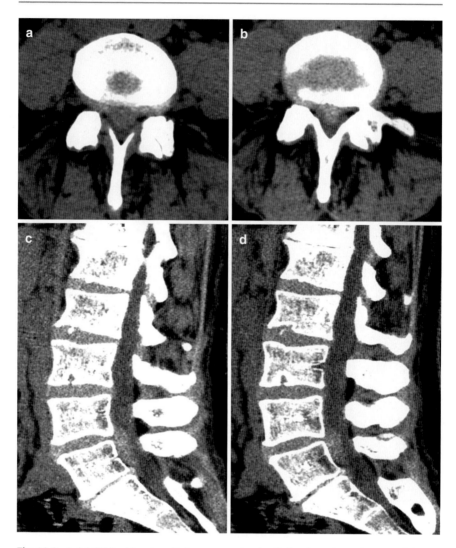

Fig. 10.8 Axial CT (**a**, **b**) and sagittal reconstruction (**c**, **d**) showing a hyperdense medial mass prolapse in L4/L5 with suspected caudal sequestration. Despite the extensive prolapsed material the 46-year-old woman showed only a slight sensomotoric L5 syndrome on the right; bladder function as well as deep sacral dermatomas were unremarkable

be higher field strengths (3 T), because fat is less bright due to longer T1-relaxation times. However, T1-w FLAIR (fluid attenuated inversion recovery) sequence may resolve this problem.

Sagittal T2-w TSE sequences exhibit the best depiction of disc degeneration because of signal decrease of hyperintense nucleus pulposus (see above), best depiction of disc herniation and best depiction of synovial cysts and widening of the facet joints with intraarticular hyperintense signal changes of the joint cavity.

10 Diseases of Extramedullary Origin: Degenerative Diseases

Table 10.1 Radicular syndromes and neurological deficits

Radicular syndrome	Lowered/extinct deep tendon reflex	Paresis	Sensory deficits
C4	–	Diaphragm muscle	Ventral shoulder
C5	(BTR)	M. deltoideus M. biceps	Lateral shoulder Proximal arm
C6	BTR	M. biceps M. brachioradialis	Distal arm radial, Thumb, index finger
C7	TTR	M. triceps	Distal arm, dorsal, finger II – IV
C8	Trömner reflex TTR	M. abductor minimi Mm. lumbricales Mm. interossei	Distal arm, ulnar, finger IV and V
L4	PTR	M. quadriceps	Lateral proximal and medial distal leg
L5	TPR	M. extensor hallucis longus, M. extensor dig. brevis	Lateral proximal and lateral distal leg; medial foot
S1	ATR	M. triceps surae M. glutaeus max.	Dorsolat. proximal and dorsal distal leg, lat. foot
Cauda equine syndrome	Level dependency of cauda compression (PTR, TPR, ATR)	Bilateral possible asymmetric flaccid paresis (level) Gait disturbance up to immobility	Sensation deficits in the legs, "Breeches anaesthesia", bladder and bowel disfunction
Conus medullaris syndrome	–	Paresis of the leg absent	"Breeches anaesthesia", bladder and bowel dysfunction

Abbreviations see above

Sagittal T1-w contrast-enhanced sequences may yield inflammatory reaction of adjacent soft tissue caused by degenerative processes, e.g. posterior longitudinal ligament enhancement in disc herniation, facet joints and endplates. In addition, enlarged epidural space adjacent to disc herniation caused by congestion of epidural veins and reactive fibrotic reaction shows enhancement (Fig. 10.9).

However, in suspected inflammatory diseases autoimmune associated or caused by bacterial infections (e.g. spondylitis, spondylodiscitis; Figs. 10.2, 10.3 and 10.4 and Chap. 13), T1 WI post contrast are also mandatory. The sagittal "Short-Tau Inversion Recovery" (STIR) sequence is sensitive to increased water content of structures, because of, for example, inflammatory processes showing hyperintense signal changes. Edema in the bone marrow and inflammatory reactions of vertebral structures caused by rheumatic and other autoimmune mediated diseases are especially detectable.

Axial planes on T1-w and T2-w sequences are helpful in classifying disc herniation. Images should depict the herniation completely and small stacks covering only the centre of the disc should be avoided. Delineation of the lateral recessus, the facet joint and the adjacent soft tissue, e.g. ligamentum flavum and synovial structures, is well feasible using axial images.

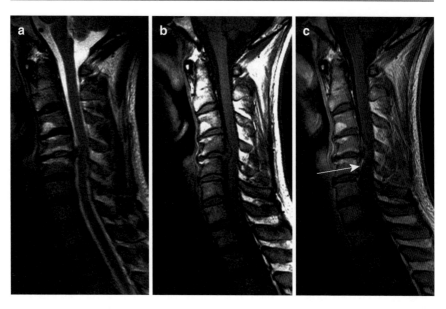

Fig. 10.9 Medial disc herniation at the level C4/5 with exhaustion of the ventral and dorsal subarachnoid space and moderate spinal cord compression. Sag. T2 WI (**a**) without intramedullary signal conversion; (**b, c**) sag. T1 WI pc (**c**) disclosing epidural enhancement near the disc prolapse and partially tended epidural plexus (*arrow*). Vertebral endplate degeneration at C 4/5 Modic type I, at level C3/4 Modic type II

Coronal planes are optional and should be performed as STIR or T2-w SPIR, e.g. for assessment of paravertebral structures in inflammatory (abscess) and neoplastic diseases (lymphoma). In particular, the psoas muscle is of interest in bacterial infections. Further indications may be sacroiliitis, scoliosis and extraforaminal neurofibroma. The latter sometimes resemble a difficult differential diagnosis in regard to extraforaminal disc herniations, especially when post-contrast images are not performed.

Acquisition of dynamic imaging of the spine during flexion–extension may helpful in assessing instability with pathological movement of the vertebra (Fig. 10.10) and in assessing – with axial loading – load-dependent nerve compression. CT distinguishes soft tissue from bony elements and gas and is especially helpful when analysing bony structures.

10.2.3 Intervertebral Disc Degeneration

In childhood the gelatinous matrix of the nucleus pulposus show high signals on T2 WI caused by hydration. In adulthood there is a decrease in water-binding capacity and T2 WI shows lowered signal intensity of the nucleus pulposus with increasing collagen content and indistinct boundaries to the anulus fibrosus. Especially in the

10 Diseases of Extramedullary Origin: Degenerative Diseases

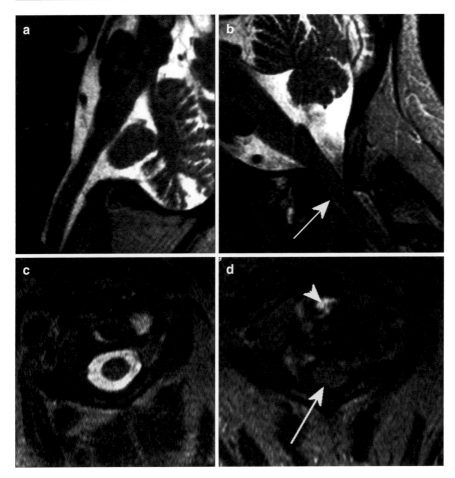

Fig. 10.10 Dynamic imaging of the spine. Pathological mobility at the level C1/2 in a woman suffering from rheumatoid arthritis with severe narrowing of the spinal canal (*arrow*) in anteflexion on T2 WI (**b**, **d**; **a**, **c**: retroflexion/extension); *arrowhead*: inflammatory partially hyperintense reactions around the dens axis

lower lumbar spine, the discs are often comparatively hypointense on T2 WI reflecting decreasing disc hydration and consecutive smaller intervertebral space because of "flat" discs (Figs. 10.5 and 10.6). However, decreasing signal intensity on T2 WI, dehydration, increasing collagen content and lowered disc height are normal features in aging (see also Chap. 2).

Disc degeneration and thinned disc space induce osteophytosis. Osteophytes originate near the discovertebral junctions or the facet joints caused by traction on Sharpey fibres. The osteophytes extend first in a horizontal and then in a vertical direction.

Advanced disc degeneration may also disclose gas inclusions in the intervertebral disc space (vacuum phenomena; Fig. 10.22).

10.2.4 Degenerative Vertebral Endplate Changes

Parallel, and in relation to the intervertebral disc degeneration, additional endplate changes occur. After Modic MT et al. [5] the signal abnormalities in the vertebral body and endplates on MR imaging are classified in three categories in correlation to histopathological findings.

Modic type I: this aggressive type of endplate change often goes ahead with acute disc degeneration and occurs most often in the lower lumbar spine. MRI shows signal increase on T2 WI and signal decrease on T1 WI with partially prominent enhancement on T1 WI pc (Fig. 10.11). Histopathology discloses vascularized fibrous tissue with fibrovascular bone marrow replacement and new bone production (activated osteochondrosis). Important differential diagnoses are spondylitis and spondylodiscitis. However, in contrast to infectious diseases of the disc space and the neighbouring vertebral structures, there is a lack of paravertebral soft tissue masses and bony destruction (Figs. 10.2, 10.3 and 10.4). In addition, infectious diseases of the disc space show, especially in the beginning, hyperintense signal changes of the intervertebral disc on T2 WI (Figs. 10.3 and 10.4). The involvement of epidural structures in the inflammatory process, i.e. epidural abscess, is an important complication of spondylitis and spondylodiscitis and should not be overlooked. Besides a small local epidural reaction often showing central hyperintense signal changes on T2 WI and profound contrast enhancement of the abscess wall on pc T1 WI (Figs. 10.2 and 10.4) at the level of spondylodiscitis, epidural inflammation may also involve numerous segments with longitudinal extended abscesses (Fig. 10.3). Myelon compression caused by epidural mass effect is a likely consequence (Fig. 10.2), but intradural inflammatory complications resulting in meningomyeloradiculitis may also occur (Fig. 10.3 and Chap. 13). Neurological worsening may result in irreversible para- or tetraparesis within a few hours. *Therefore, the combination of progressive back pain and inflammatory constellation on laboratory blood (or CSF) analysis (especially CRP, C reactive protein) represents a "red flag" and spondylitis or spondylodiscitis should be included in the differential diagnosis.*

Beside infectious processes, metastatic and autoimmune associated diseases should also be considered in differential diagnosis.

In *Modic type II*, degenerative endplate changes show a fatty replacement of normal bone marrow with signal elevation on T1 WI and a nearly isointense signal on T2 WI (Fig. 10.9). Finally, in *Modic Type III*, signal of the vertebral body and endplates are lowered both on T1-w and T2-w sequences because of replacement of bone marrow structures by bony sclerosis. Table 10.2 summarizes imaging findings in endplate degeneration.

10.2.5 Disc Herniation

Fissures in the anular fibres and dissection from the vertebral body causes *anular tears* located in the posterior and posterolateral circumference of the anulus fibrosus with a size often smaller than 3 mm and a hyperintense signal on T2 WI within the

10 Diseases of Extramedullary Origin: Degenerative Diseases

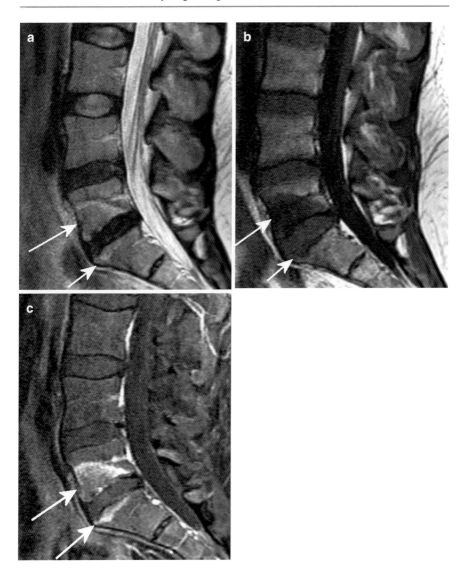

Fig. 10.11 Degenerative endplates changes, type I (Modic). Sag. T2 WI (**a**) showing signal increase at the L5/S1 segment (*arrow*), T1 WI signal decrease (**b**) and T1 WI fat sat. pc. (**c**) inhomogeneous enhancement with sparing the intervertebral disc

Table 10.2 Endplate degeneration and signal changes

Modic type	Histopathological findings	Signal T2 WI	Signal T1 WI	T1 WI pc
I	Fibrovascular bone marrow replacement	↑	↓	(Prominent) enhancement
II	Fatty replacement	~	↑	–
III	Bony sclerosis	↓	↓	–

hypointense fibres (Fig. 10.12). *Herniation* of an intervertebral disc is defined by dislocation of disc material over the margins of the intervertebral disc space. Focal herniation describes a herniation smaller than 25 % of the disc circumference; 25–50 % of the disc circumference is a broad-based herniation. In contrast to a disc herniation, in a *disc bulge* the amount of involved circumference is over 50 %, and the tissue extending over the margins of the adjacent apophyses is smaller than 3 mm. A *protrusion* is a herniation where the distance of the dislocated material is smaller than the distance between the neighbouring apophyses (disc height, base). In contrast, a *disc extrusion* shows a larger distance of dislocated material into the spinal canal than the distance between the neighbouring apophyses. *Sequestration* of a disc herniation means a free fragment of prolapsed material (sequester) without connection to the intervertebral disc (Fig. 10.6). The terminology of the different disc degenerations is summarized in Table 10.3 [3].

From the neuroradiological and clinical points of view, differentiation should be made between medial (central/paracentral), mediolateral (subarticular) and lateral (foraminal and extraforaminal) disc herniations.

> *Classification of disc herniation based on their anatomical boundaries:*
> 1. Medial (central/paracentral)
> 2. Mediolateral (subarticular; lateral recessus)
> 3. Lateral/foraminal
> 4. Lateral/extraforaminal
> 5. Free fragment: sequestration

10.2.5.1 Mediolateral (Subarticular) Disc Herniations

In Fig. 10.5 the typical imaging findings of a mediolateral disc herniation are shown. The prolapsed disc material restricts the lateral recessus with consecutive dorsal shifting of the nerve root and compression. Mediolateral herniations may cause ipsilateral radicular syndromes of the nerve root running through the lateral recessus. If the prolapse is greater and has more medial aspects, as well as the segmental nerve root the next lower nerve root is also affected. Figure 10.6 illustrates a mediolateral disc herniation with caudal sequestration.

10.2.5.2 Medial (Central/Paracentral) Disc Herniations

In the lumbar spine, medial intervertebral disc prolapse may compress the cauda equina with the resulting neurological features mentioned above (Table 10.1), especially in the case of mass prolapse (Figs. 10.7, 10.8 and 10.13). In a smaller prolapse, clinical examination often shows no neurological disorders, although the patient may have distinct back pain. However, because of the relatively soft disc tissue in younger patients, medial mass prolapse may cause only slight sensation deficits or no neurological disturbances and, in the first place, conservative therapy is the method of choice. With dehydration, over time the prolapse becomes smaller with declining pain. Post contrast (pc) T1 WI often shows enhancement around the

10 Diseases of Extramedullary Origin: Degenerative Diseases

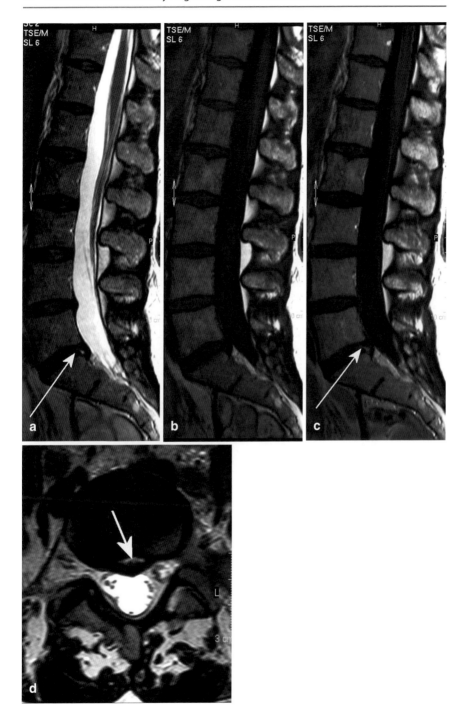

Fig. 10.12 Sag. (**a**) and ax. (**d**) T2WI disclosing a focal hyperintense lesion (*arrow* **a, d**) within the posterior medial anulus fibrosus representing an anular tear. T1 WI sag. (**b, c**) exhibiting slight contrast enhancement in this area (**c**, pc, *arrow*)

Table 10.3 Classifications of disc degeneration

Anular tear	<3 mm, hyperintense signal ((T2 WI) within the anulus fibrosus
Bulge	>50 % circumference, distance <3 mm
Herniation	Circumscribed dislocation of disc material beyond the margins of the intervertebral disc space; Focal: <25 % of disc circumference Broad based: 25–50 % of disc circumference
Protrusion	Distance < height of intervertebral disc space; base of the protruded disc broader than any other diameter of the displaced disc material
Extrusion	Distance > height of intervertebral disc space; base of the protruded disc smaller than any other diameter of the displaced disc material
Sequester	Disconnection of herniated material from the parent disc (fragment)

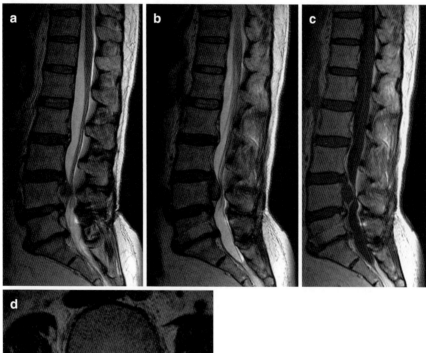

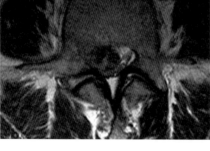

Fig. 10.13 Paracentral right sided mass prolapse in L3/4 in a 58-year-old woman suffering from acute sensomotoric L4 syndrome right sided. Sag. (**a**, **b**) and ax. (**d**) T2 WI disclosing a large disc herniation causing nearly complete constriction of the lateral recessus and impressive shifting of the thecal sac. Sag. T1WI pc show (**c**) removed enhancing epidural space

10 Diseases of Extramedullary Origin: Degenerative Diseases

herniation of the nucleus pulposus caused by epidural structures with partially dilated veins and surrounding reactive fibrosis in the epidural space (Figs. 10.9 and 10.13). There may also be a circumscribed enhancement in the posterior disc margin and the herniation itself because of the repair mechanism with granulation tissue and new micro-vascularization (Fig. 10.12).

10.2.5.3 Lateral Foraminal and Extraforaminal Disc Herniations

Lateral disc herniation compresses the nerve root intraforaminal and often also affects the dorsal root (spinal) ganglion. Because of the intraspinal course of the nerve root running downwards and laterally through the lateral recessus lumbar foraminal disc herniations, e.g. at the level L2/3 compromise the L2 nerve root in the intervertebral foramen L2 (Figs. 10.14 and 10.15). In contrast, a mediolateral (subarticular) disc herniation at the level L2/3 causes an L3 syndrome due to nerve root compression during the course through the lateral recessus. Analysis of sagittal images covering the whole vertebra and the foramen may be helpful in detecting intraforaminal disc tissue.

10.2.6 Foraminal Stenosis

Foraminal stenosis is an important cause of back pain and radicular symptoms, especially in the elderly. The aetiology of narrowed intervertebral foramen is multifactorial and caused by:
1. Degeneration of the intervertebral disc with bulging or herniation and reduced disc height
2. Degeneration of the facet joint with osteophytes
3. Spondylolisthesis with pathological mobility

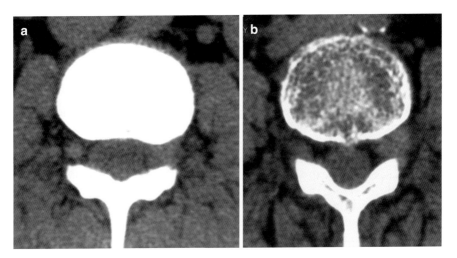

Fig. 10.14 Axial CT demonstrating left sided lateral foraminal (**a**) and lateral partially extraforaminal (**b**) lumbal hyperdense soft tissue, i.e. disc herniation, respectively

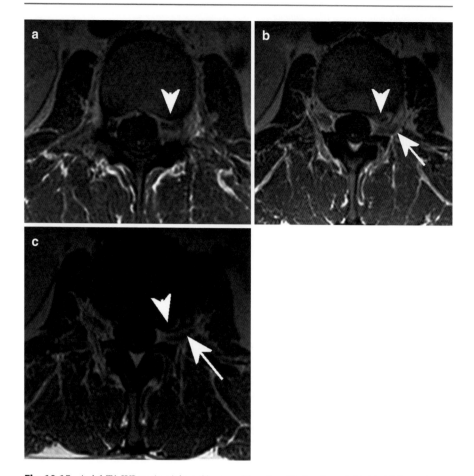

Fig. 10.15 Axial T1 WI pc (**a–c**) in a 41-year-old male suffering from left sided L2 syndrome, disclosing an intraforaminal disc herniation (*arrowhead*) at the level L2/3 with compression of the nerve root L2 (*arrow*) and the dorsal root (spinal) ganglion (see also normal nerval configuration on the right side). Note hyperintense filum terminale (also visible on T1 WI before Gd. application, i.e. fat, not shown)

Description of the anatomical form of disc herniation in axial and vertical orientations and the foraminal epidural fat are important to assess affection of the radicular structures during their course through the lateral recessus and the intervertebral foramen and possible surgical approach. Classification of the foraminal epidural fat differentiates between:
1. Normal
2. Deformed, but completely surrounding the spinal nerve
3. Deformed, only partly surrounding the spinal nerve
4. Obliteration of the epidural fat

In addition, *facet joint degeneration* is an important cause of back pain because of rich innervation of the synovia and capsule by the sinuvertebral nerve (see above) and radicular symptoms are caused by narrowing of the lateral recess and/or intervertebral foramina. It mostly occurs in the lumbar spine (i.e. L 4/5 and L5/S1). A weak point of the facet joint is the ventral aspect, which has no fibrous capsule. In this region *juxtaarticular cysts* filled with clear or mucinous fluid or gas are in contact with the joint and cause (additional) narrowing of the lateral recessus and sometimes of the spinal canal (Figs. 10.16 and 10.17). Haemorrhage into the cysts may also occur with acute aggravation of pain and radicular symptoms. For clinical and neuroradiological assessment, additional functional investigations during ante- and retroflexion as well as axial loading (upright and horizontal positions) may be necessary, especially to analyse the impact of pathological mobility with consecutive foraminal or spinal canal stenosis (see below).

In *spondylolisthesis* based on widened facet joints, especially axial, T2 WI may show increased intraarticular fluid or even gas (Figs. 10.17 and 10.18). Besides normal aging of the spine, a wide differential diagnostic spectrum, especially regarding autoimmune associated (rheumatic) diseases, may affect the facet joints. Red flags are, for example, additional sacroiliitis, and ankolytic disorders (see below and Fig. 10.1). However, description of detailed differential diagnosis of inflammatory and congenital spine diseases is beyond the scope of this chapter.

Spondylolysis (Fig. 10.19) with open clefts in the pars interarticularis may also cause foraminal and spinal canal stenosis because of pathological mobility with displacement of the vertebra, best visible in sagittal projection, classified after Meyerding, grades I to V. Grade I describes a displacement below 25 % of the vertebra amplitude, grades II–IV 25–50 %, 50–75 % and <75 %, and, finally, grade V a spondyloptosis. Bilateral lucent clefts in the pars interarticularis at different

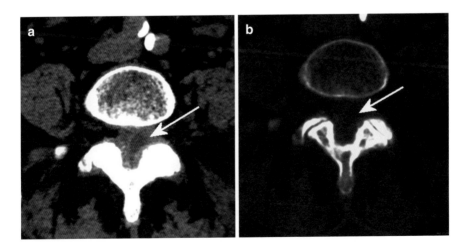

Fig. 10.16 Axial (**a**, **b**) CT and sagittal (**c**, **d**) reconstruction showing a juxtaarticular cyst in L4/5 left (*arrow*) with hyperdense rim and impressive constriction of the thecal sac

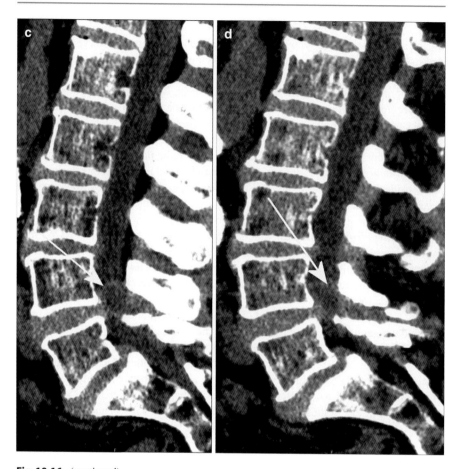

Fig. 10.16 (continued)

locations are best visible on axial CT and sagittal reconstructions (bone window), in which angulation along the vertebral arch are often helpful. A widened spinal canal may be indicative of spondylolysis (Fig. 10.19).

10.2.7 Acquired Lumbal Canal Stenosis

Comparable to foraminal stenosis, spinal canal stenosis is also a multifactorial process secondary to degenerative changes and most often located in the lower lumbar spine (L4/5 or L5/S1) (Figs. 10.18 and 10.20) [6, 7]. Beside the above-mentioned *disc degeneration* with narrowing of the spinal canal from ventral direction, *altered facet joints* with widened joint space, *osteophytic appositions,* and *degenerative changes of the yellow* ligament are present (Figs. 10.21 and 10.22). Ligamentum flavum degeneration with laxity and thickening (hypertrophy) narrows the spinal canal

10 Diseases of Extramedullary Origin: Degenerative Diseases

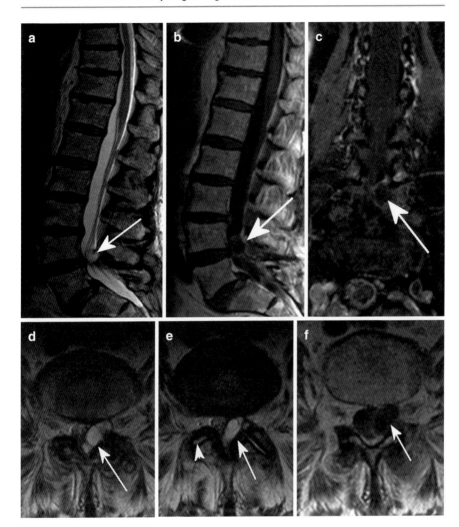

Fig. 10.17 Same Pat. as shown in Fig. 10.16. Juxtaarticular cyst in L4/5 (*arrow*) with slight contrast enhancement of the cyst wall on T1 WI pc (**b, c, f**; sag., cor., ax.); T2 WI (**a, d, e**) showing hyperintense signal inside the cyst; note also hyperintense intraarticular signal caused by widened facet joints (*arrowhead*)

and the recessus from dorsolateral and *pathological mobility* accentuate stenosis (Figs. 10.20 and 10.21). Midsagittal diameter of the spinal canal <12 mm reflects relative stenosis, whereas a diameter <10 mm is defined as an absolute stenosis (Fig. 10.22). However, beside acquired degenerative alterations, congenital anatomical variations, e.g. "short pedicule syndrome" or chondrodysplasia (Fig. 10.23) may also accentuate clinical symptoms in the elderly.

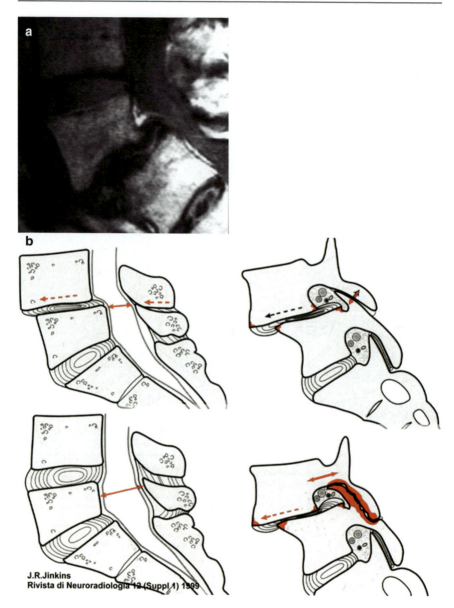

Fig. 10.18 Spondylolisthesis with pathological mobility at segment L4/5 (**a**: T1 WI sag.); (**b**) schematic illustration. (From: Jinkins RJ (1999) Riv Neurorad 12: suppl1; Centauro, Bologna, Italy, with permission). *Red double headed arrows* demonstrating narrowing of the thecal sac (above) and segmental widened spinal canal (*lower row*) due to altered facet joints with consecutive pathological movement (*dotted arrows*).

10 Diseases of Extramedullary Origin: Degenerative Diseases

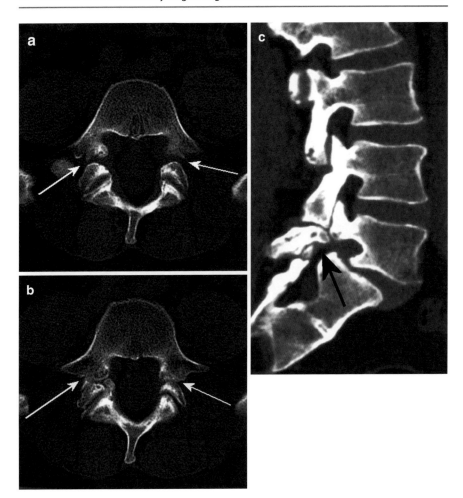

Fig. 10.19 Spondylolysis with lucent clefts bilateral (**a, b**, *arrows*), widened spinal canal and vertebral displacement according Meyerding II° (**c**, *arrow*)

Clinical examination in acquired spinal canal stenosis shows a wide range of symptoms. Neurological symptoms beside local and pseudoradicular (referred) pain may be radicular pain, the latter often accentuated in an upright position and walking (claudicatio radicularis), possibly with neurological failures (Fig. 10.24; also Fig. 8.1a, b, e and f in Chap. 8). Claudicatio spinalis involves at least two (bilateral) nerve roots and a cauda equine syndrome (see above) represents the worst

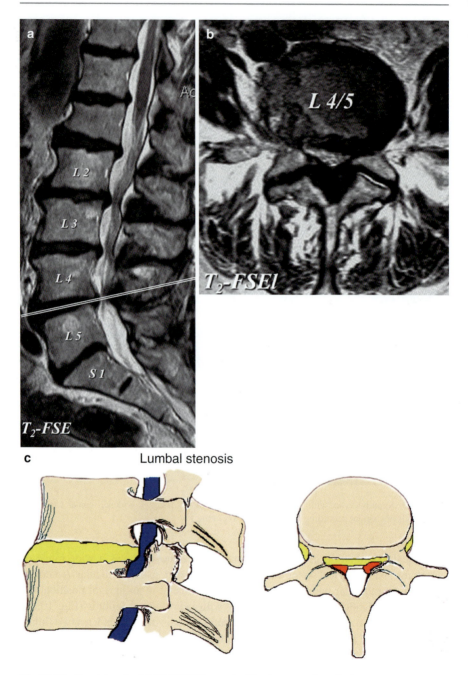

Fig. 10.20 Sag. (**a**) and axial (**b**) T2 WI in acquired lumbar stenosis at the level L4/5 with ventral and dorsolateral narrowing (**c**; after [6, 7]) caused by degeneration of disc, facet joints, thickened yellow ligamentum and osteophytes (FSE: fast spin echo; L1: vertebral body L1)

10 Diseases of Extramedullary Origin: Degenerative Diseases

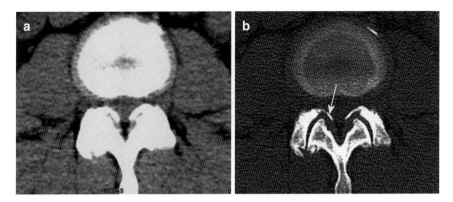

Fig. 10.21 Axial CT (**a**, **b**) showing facet joint degeneration with additional partial sclerosis of the articular capsule and the yellow ligamentum (**b**, *arrow*)

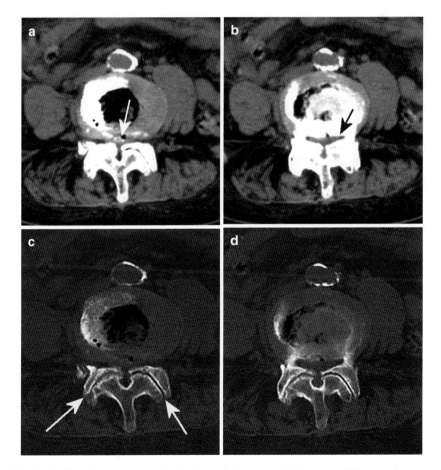

Fig. 10.22 Combined stenosis of the lumbar spinal canal at L4/5 in a hale 93-year-old woman suffering from claudicatio spinalis with accentuation of the L5 nerve roots. Axial CT disclosing medial disc herniation (**a**, *arrow*), degeneration of the facet joints (**c**, **d**; *arrows*) and impressive narrowing of the lateral recessus; typical "bicycle saddle" configuration (**b**, *arrow*), in addition, there are short pedicles; vacuum phenomena with intradiscal gas caused by advanced disc degeneration. In anteflexion the pat. had no pain

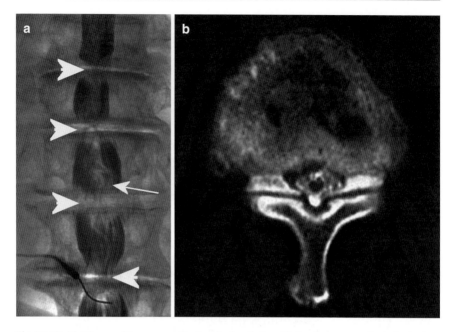

Fig. 10.23 A 68-year-old woman with chondrodysplasia suffering from paraesthesia in the legs during Valsava manoeuvre. Myelography (**a**) exhibiting multisegmental severe stenosis (*arrowheads*) with tortuous nerve roots (*arrow*); (**b**) postmyelo CT

case, which is an emergency situation requiring rapid neurosurgical decompression. Sagittal T2 WI and myelography may exhibit dilated veins and elongated nerve roots with a meander-like tortuous intrathecal course above and below the hourglass appearance of the canal stenosis (Figs. 10.20 and 10.23) caused by ventral and dorsolateral narrowing ("nipper pliers"). Increased epidural fat (e.g. Morbus Madelung) may accentuate compression of the thecal sac. However, differential diagnosis of thickened nerve roots should include inflammatory (e.g. borreliosis) and neoplastic aetiologies (e.g. meningeosis carcinomatosa, lymphoma). Uncommon diseases are sarcoidosis or multiple nerve root tumours (e.g. neurofibromatosis, often multinodular) (see also Chap. 13).

10.3 Myelon Compression Syndromes

10.3.1 Pathophysiological and Clinical Aspects

Spinal cord compression caused by extradural or intradural/extramedullary lesions shows a wide range of clinical syndromes. Extent and composition of neurological failures depend on the:

10 Diseases of Extramedullary Origin: Degenerative Diseases

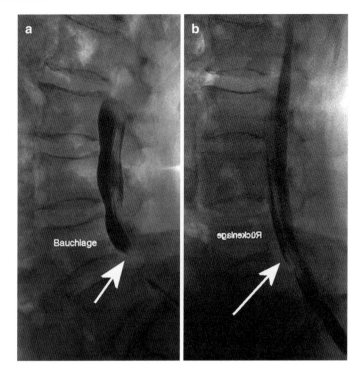

Fig. 10.24 Functional myelography: position depending stenosis at the level L4/5 (*arrow*), ventral accentuated especially caused by disc bulging and pathological mobility in retroflexion (**a**: ventral position; **b**: dorsal position; see also Fig. 8.1 in Chap. 8)

1. Time course of compression
2. Degree of spinal cord compression
3. Location
4. Additional pathophysiological components, e.g. vascular disorders, inflammation, and others

10.3.1.1 Time Course of Spinal Cord Compression

Spinal trauma is the most frequent cause of *acute complete transverse spinal cord syndrome* with a *spinal shock* or areflexia. At the time of injury the spinal neural structures below the lesion are inoperative. Depending on the topography, neurological examination can disclose complete loss of motor function with flaccid tetraplegia caused by lesions of the upper cervical spinal cord and flaccid paraplegia caused by lesions in the thoracic spinal cord. In addition, there is complete loss of sensation (at and) below the level of spinal cord injury, atonic paralysis of the bladder with urinary retention, bowel and gastric atony and also loss of sexual, vegetative and autonomic functions. The duration of the spinal shock with areflexia varies from 1 to 6 weeks in the majority of patients. After this period, a different degree of reflex activity appears. Beside genital, bowel and bladder reflexes, heightened reflex activity of the motor systems also develops. Neurological examination discloses to a different degree progressive spasticity of the muscles and the plantar responses are extensor, i.e. positive Babinski sign with dorsiflexion of the big toe. Deep tendon reflexes of the extremities are exaggerated. Improvement of initial para- or tetraplegia within the first week after spinal cord injury may result in partial remission; otherwise, prognosis of neurological failures is unfavourable with irreversible severe transverse spinal cord syndrome.

Beside spinal traumata, further aetiologies of acute spinal cord syndromes are vascular disorders, e.g. spinal cord infarction or intramedullary haemorrhage, epidural haemorrhage, inflammatory lesions (fulminant myelitis), epidural inflammation (abscess) or rapidly progressive spinal cord compression in case of spontaneous or malignant vertebral fractures.

In contrast to spinal shock, in chronic incomplete or complete transverse spinal cord syndromes, neurological examinations exhibit spastic tetraparesis (tetraplegia) or paraparesis (paraplegia). Because of reflex bladder dysfunction, urine retention is incomplete and reflex micturition occurs. Muscle tonus is spastic elevated, deep tendon reflexes are exaggerated and plantar responses are extensor, i.e. the Babinski sign is positive. There are different degrees of gait disturbance up to immobility. In relation to the extent and location of myelon compression, sensation deficits below the level of the damaged spinal cord show different characteristics.

In the case of marginal compression increase over a long time, e.g. several years, initial spinal cord symptoms especially could be discrete and misdiagnosed. The patients report slight gait disturbances and onset of sensation deficits in the feet- and possible bladder dysfunctions, only mentioned when asked about. Typical aetiologies for such neurological constellations are spinal meningeoma and cervical spondylosis in the elderly. Often they are misdiagnosed as a "polyneuropathy syndrome" or "multifactorial gait disturbance". Therefore it isn't surprising that spinal imaging exhibits, for example, extensive thoracic meningeoma causing advanced spinal cord compression and intramedullar hyperintense signal changes on T2 WI as an imaging finding for myelopathy could be absent (see Chap. 8, Fig. 8.3). *However, it must be noted that imaging features alone in degenerative diseases should never indicate surgery.* This is always a clinical decision and neurological disturbances and radiological findings should be conclusive.

10.3.1.2 Location of Spinal Cord Compression

Because of the topographic distribution of the spinal segments within the different fibre tracts, extradural as well as intradural-extramedullar spinal cord compression result in ascending transverse spinal cord syndromes. Regarding, for example, the spinothalamic tract, the fibre bundles originating from the lower spinal segments, i.e. lumbar and sacral segments, are located onionskin-like in the outer edge of the tract, whereas the fibre bundles from the segments above are attached interiorly. Extramedullar compression compromises first the outer layers in the tracts and therefore neurological disturbances ascent over time. Beside segmental neurological disturbances, e.g. radicular pain, cervical spinal cord compression first causes spastic paraparesis and sensation deficits in the legs, and, in addition, possibly bladder and vegetative dysfunctions (see also Chap. 14; pathophysiological regards on diagnostically important white matter tracts).

Therefore, very often the neurological level of sensation deficits is below the level of the spinal cord lesion. It should be mentioned that the vegetative fibres, e.g. bladder and sexual function, are sensitive to mechanical compression and may be the first neurological disorders in (acute) spinal trauma. Interestingly, this is not valid for cervical stenosis and disc prolapse. In contrast, intramedullary tumours, e.g. gliomas, may cause descending spinal cord symptoms with sparing sacral segments. Furthermore, the experienced neurologist differentiates several types of transverse spinal cord syndromes, but detailed description is beyond the scope of this section. However, dissociate sensation deficits as well as Brown-Séquard syndrome should be mentioned.

Brown-Séquard described in 1851 for the first time a hemi-spinal cord syndrome with ipsilateral paresis and hypaesthesia (epicritic sensation) and contralateral disturbance of pain and temperature sense (protopatic sensation), i.e. dissociated sensation deficit below the lesion. Segmental crossing of the spinothalamic tract cause contralateral dysfunction of temperature and pain sense (see Chap. 14, Fig. 14.1).

The extent of neurological disorders caused by spinal cord compression may be accentuated by chronic or acute additional (segmental) vascular disorders. Beside disturbance of spinal cord microcirculation, syndromes of the anterior spinal artery (ASA) or posterior/posterolateral spinal arteries (PSA, PLSA) may also occur and should be considered in acute deterioration (see below and Chap. 20) [4].

In addition, inflammatory diseases, e.g. autoimmune associated myelitis, may emphasize initial spinal cord syndromes. As an example, in late onset multiple sclerosis with additional cervical spondylosis it could be difficult to correlate clinical symptoms to one of the diseases (see below). Table 10.4 summarizes clinical signs of transverse spinal cord syndromes.

Table 10.4 Transverse spinal cord syndromes

1. Spinal shock (acute complete transverse spinal cord syndrome)
   Flaccid para- or tetraparesis
   Atony of the muscles
   Sensory loss (at and) below the level of spinal cord lesion
   Atonic paralysis of the bladder with urinary retention, bowel and gastric atony and also loss of sexual, vegetative and autonomic functions
   Areflexia
   Plantar responses are extensor, i.e. positive Babinski sign (however, in the first hours after spinal cord injury Babinski sign could be negative)
2. Subacute/chronic (complete/incomplete) transverse spinal cord syndrome
   Spastic para- or tetraparesis, para- or tetraplegia
   Spasticity (elevated muscle tonus)
   Sensory disturbances (often) below the level of spinal cord lesion
   Ascending disturbances in progressive myelocompression
   Possible dissociated sensation deficits
   Exaggerated deep tendon reflexes
   Plantar responses are extensor, i.e. positive Babinski sign
   Bladder and bowel dysfunction
   Spastic ataxic gait disturbance (up to immobility)

(See also Table 15.1, Chap. 15)

10.3.2 Cervical Disc Herniation

In an emergency setting with acute spinal cord symptoms, MRI is the method of choice for differential diagnosis. Especially in space-occupying lesions, immediate diagnosis with consecutive neurosurgical treatment option is essential for a good clinical outcome with remission of neurological disturbances. However, in chronic myelopathy syndromes, e.g. cervical spondylosis, the aim of neurosurgical intervention is primarily to stop symptom progression.

Medial and mediolateral cervical disc herniation may cause acute and subacute transverse spinal cord syndromes caused by cord compression with consecutive myelopathy. T2 WI images disclose a depleted ventral and dorsal subarachnoid space and ventral spinal cord compression. In the acute phase hyperintense signal changes are often caused by edema, whereas in the subacute and chronic phase intramedullary hyperintense lesions may resemble (irreversible) gliosis (Fig. 10.25, see also Chap. 14, Fig. 14.10). However, there is no direct correlation between T2 spinal cord signal changes and clinical symptoms. Edema with extinct signal conversion (Fig. 10.25) may be accompanied by only slight neurological disturbances, whereas, in patients suffering from cord compression without detectable T2 myelopathy, obvious disturbances of the spinal tracts are present (Fig. 10.26).

However, the extent of cord compression caused by medial disc herniation depends on the diameter of the spinal canal. Therefore, *congenital spinal canal stenosis* with a central canal diameter anterior-posterior (ap.) smaller than 14 mm may aggravate the space-occupying effect of the herniated disc. In sagittal projection the Torg ratio (ap. diameter of the spinal canal/ap. diameter of the vertebral body) in congenital stenosis of the cervical spine is <0.8. Additional imaging findings are short pedicles ("short pedicle syndrome"). On conventional imaging on lateral projection, the articular pillar takes up the entire ap. canal diameter. T2* sequences may overestimate narrowing because of blooming artefact, and therefore ap. measurement should be performed on T1 WI or CT, whereas postmyelo CT provides the most exact method.

Differential diagnosis should include inherited spinal canal stenosis, e.g. caused by achondroplasia, mucopolysaccharidosis and ossification of the posterior longitudinal ligament (OPLL). Superimposed slight disc degenerations and *cervical spondylosis* (see below) may also cause spinal cord symptoms in younger patients because of limited reserve capacity of the small subarachnoid space (Fig. 10.27).

On the other hand, intramedullary signal conversion should have a clear spatial relationship to the stenotic segment. Intramedullary longitudinal extension of the mechanically-induced myelopathy is most often smaller than half of the vertebra height in the cranial and caudal directions. *A red flag will be missed clear spatial relationship of intramedullary hyperintense signal changes on T2 WI to the narrowed canal and/or cord compression is not visible* (Fig. 10.28). In such a constellation, inflammatory aetiology, e.g. autoimmune associated or even neoplastic diseases, must be discussed, which require detailed differential diagnostic considerations including

Fig. 10.25 Sag. T2 WI disclosing intramedullary hyperintense signal changes at level C6/7 (*arrow*), initial frequently representing edema, because of acute medial disc herniation (painless!) with spinal cord compression; note also posterolateral degenerative changes

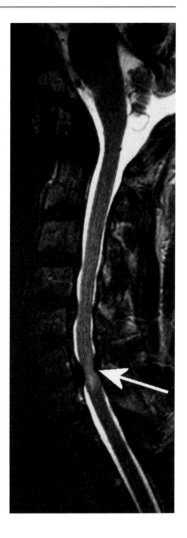

laboratory and CSF analysis, total spine imaging and cranial MRI. In rare cases, additional vascular complications might extend primary mechanical induced myelopathy (Fig. 10.29) [4], and sometimes only follow-up examinations are decisive.

10.3.3 Cervical Spondylosis

Comparable to acquired lumbar spinal canal stenosis, cervical spondylosis (syn.: acquired cervical spinal canal stenosis) contain multifactorial degenerative changes with consecutive narrowing of intervertebral foramina and/or the cervical spinal canal. In addition, congenital features such as short pedicles (see above) may

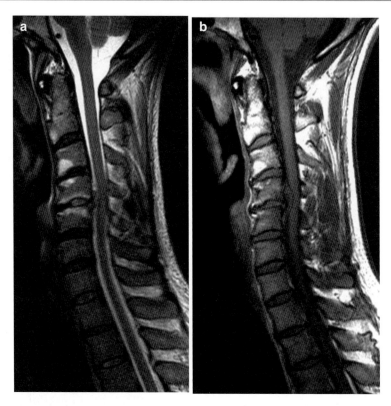

Fig. 10.26 (Same pat. as in Fig. 10.9). The 39-year-old woman suffered from paraesthesia in both hands and feet and deep tendon reflexes were exaggerated on the left. Anteflexion aggravate sensation deficits (Lhermitte sign). Sag. T2 WI (**a**) and T1 WI (**b**) demonstrating cervical medial mass prolapse and cord compression at C4/5 without intramedullary signal changes

accentuate the narrowing. Sagittal diameter is smaller than 13 mm and sagittal T2 WI shows typical "washboard spine" (or "nipper pliers phenomena", when accompanied by hypertrophic changes of ligaments posterior to the dural tube) (Figs. 10.30 and 10.31). Besides disc degeneration and ventral osteophytes, facet joint and uncovertebral joints are also altered with narrowing of the intervertebral foramina. From a clinical point of view, cervical myelopathy with hyperintense signal changes on T2 WI in cervical spondylosis often show a more chronic course with slight progression of spinal cord symptoms (see above) in comparison to medial disc herniation. However, mild whiplash injuries with cervical hyperextension and hyperflexion during drops especially in the elderly may also cause acute aggravation of spinal cord symptoms (contusio spinalis).

10 Diseases of Extramedullary Origin: Degenerative Diseases

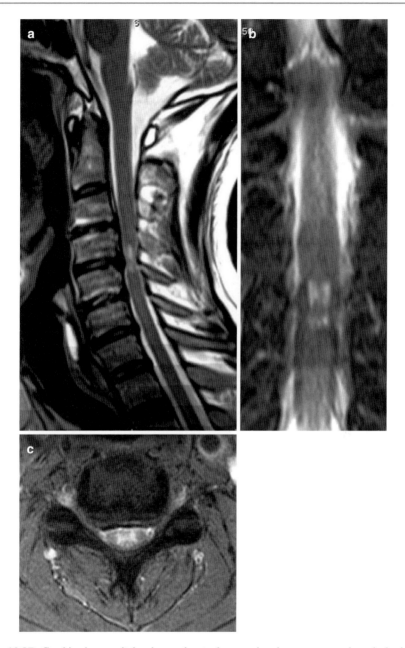

Fig. 10.27 Combined congenital and secondary to degenerative changes narrowed cervical spinal canal at C4/5 with intramedullary hyperintense signal changes in a 50-year-old man (**a–c**, T2 WI; sag., cor., ax.); exaggerated reflexes at the upper extremities, no gait disturbance and spasticity

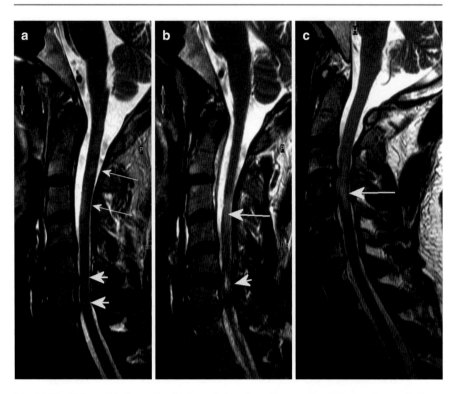

Fig. 10.28 Differential diagnosis of intramedullary hyperintense signal changes in acquired cervical spinal stenosis, sag. T2 WI (**a–c**). (**a**) Moderate cervical stenosis at C5/6 and C6/7 without intramedullary signal conversion (*arrowhead*), but several spinal lesions caused by multiple sclerosis (*arrows*); (**b**) cervical spondylosis with myelopathy at C5/6 (*arrow head*) and additional inflammatory spinal cord lesions (*arrow*); (**c**) astrocytoma at level C4 (*arrow*) beside degenerative changes. (With courtesy Prof. H. Lanfermann, Hannover)

10 Diseases of Extramedullary Origin: Degenerative Diseases

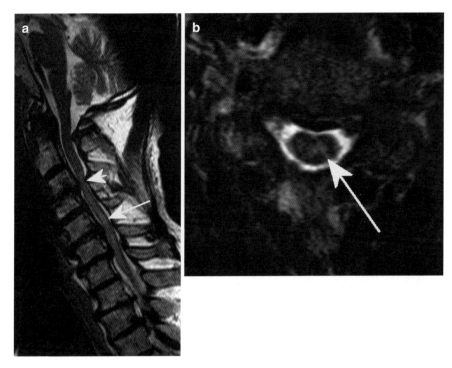

Fig. 10.29 An 81-year-old man suffering from acute onset of ataxic gait disturbance, hypaesthesia and paresis in both distal arms. Sag. T2 WI (**a**) demonstrating severe cervical multisegmental spondylosis, p.m. at level C3/4 with additional spondylolisthesis (*arrowhead*). Longitudinal extended myelopathy C4–C7 (**a**, **b**; *arrow*) suggesting spinal cord ischemia, possibly induced by compression of the anterior spinal artery

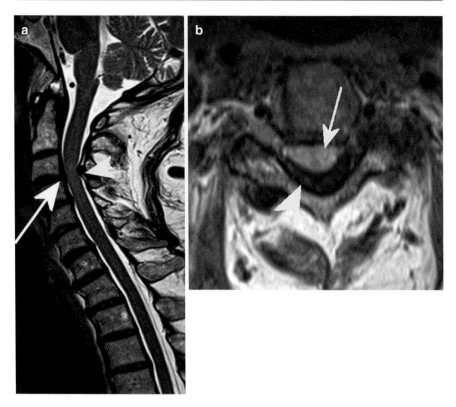

Fig. 10.30 Sag. (**a**) and ax. (**b**) T 2 WI demonstrating myelopathy with intramedullary hyperintense signal changes (*arrow*) at C3/4 in a 55-year-old man suffering from progressive ataxic gait disturbance; main component of narrowed spinal canal derive from dorsolateral degenerative changes (*arrowhead*)

10 Diseases of Extramedullary Origin: Degenerative Diseases

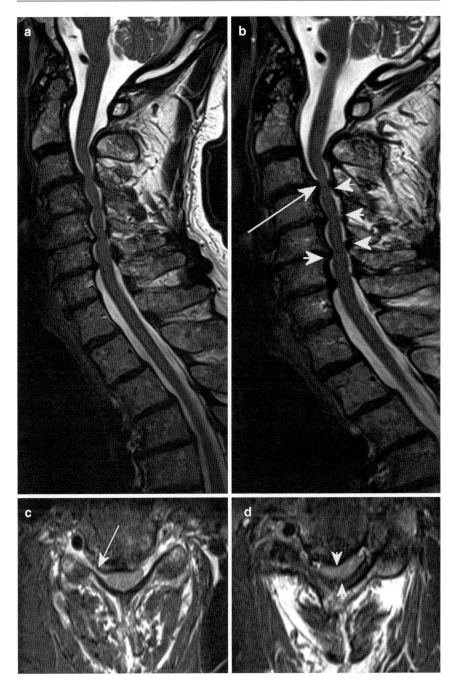

Fig. 10.31 Cervical spondylosis. T2 WI sag. (**a**, **b**) and ax. (**c–e**) demonstrating multisegmental degenerative narrowed cervical spinal canal from C3/4 to C6/7, punctum maximum at level C3/4 with intramedullary hyperintense signal conversion (**b**, *arrow*). Note "washboard spine" (or: nipper pliers sign) caused by complex narrowed canal caused by disc degeneration and osteophytic fittings (**b**, **d**; *arrowheads*), additional stenotic intervertebral foramen (**c**, *short arrow*). A 77-year-old man with progressive sensory deficits in all extremities and gait disturbance

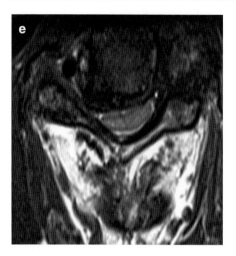

Fig. 10.31 (continued)

References

1. Adams RD, Victor M (1989) Principles of neurology, 4th edn. McGraw-Hill, New York
2. Duus P (1988) Neurologcial topical diagnostic, 4th edn. Thieme, Stuttgart
3. Ross JS, Moore KR, Shah LM, Borg B, Crim J (2010) Diagnostic imaging – spine, 2nd edn. Amirsys, Salt Lake City, Utah
4. Thron A (ed) (1989) Vascularisation of the spinal cord. Springer, Wien/New York
5. Modic MT et al (1988) Degenerative disk disease: assessment of changes in the vertebral body marrow with MR imaging. Radiology 166:193–199
6. Benini A (1986) Sciatica without disc prolaps: The stenosis of the lumbar spinal canal (Ischias ohne Bandscheibenvorfall: Die Stenose des lumbalen Spinalkanals). 2nd edn. Publisher Hans Hubert, Bonn Stuttgart Toronto
7. Benini A (1991) The lumbar disc damage. Instability, disc herniation, spinal canal stenosis. A clinical compendium (Der lumbale Bandscheibenschaden. Instabilität, Diskushernie, Wirbelkanalstenose. Ein klinischer Leitfaden). W. Kohlhammer, Stuttgart Berlin Ulm

Extramedullary Space-Occupying Pathologies: Epidural and Intradural Extramedullary Disorders

11

Stefan Dützmann and Matthias Setzer

Contents

11.1	Introduction to Extradural Extramedullary Pathologies	202
11.2	Epidural Tumours	203
	11.2.1 Primary Benign and Malignant Epidural Tumours	203
	11.2.2 Vertebral Hemangioma	205
	11.2.3 Aneurysmal Bone Cyst	207
	11.2.4 Osteoid Osteoma/Osteoblastoma	207
	11.2.5 Osteochondroma	207
	11.2.6 Chordoma	207
	11.2.7 Chondrosarcoma	209
	11.2.8 Giant Cell Tumour	209
	11.2.9 Brown Tumour	209
	11.2.10 Fibrous Dysplasia	209
	11.2.11 Langerhans Cell Histiocytosis/Eosinophilic Granuloma	210
	11.2.12 Solitary Plasmacytoma/Multiple Myeloma	210
	11.2.13 Lymphoma	211
	11.2.14 Osteosarcoma	212
	11.2.15 Ewing Sarcoma	215
	11.2.16 Fibrosarcoma	215
	11.2.17 Malignant Fibrous Histiocytoma	216
	11.2.18 Sacrococcygeal Teratoma	216
11.3	Secondary Malignant Epidural Tumours	218
	11.3.1 Metastases	218
11.4	Epidural Empyema	223
	11.4.1 Aetiology	223
	11.4.2 Prevalence	225
	11.4.3 Neurological Symptoms	225

S. Dützmann • M. Setzer (✉)
Department of Neurosurgery, Goethe-University,
Schleusenweg 2-16, D-60528 Frankfurt, Germany
e-mail: matthias.setzer@kgu.de

		11.4.4	Important Diagnostic Findings	225
		11.4.5	Differential Diagnosis	226
		11.4.6	Therapy	227
		11.4.7	Outcome	227
	11.5	Epidural Hemorrhage		227
		11.5.1	Aetiology	227
		11.5.2	Prevalence	229
		11.5.3	Neurological Symptoms	230
		11.5.4	Important Diagnostic Findings	230
		11.5.5	Differential Diagnosis	230
		11.5.6	Therapy	230
		11.5.7	Outcome	230
	11.6	Introduction to Intradural Extramedullary Pathologies		231
	11.7	Intradural Extramedullary Benign Tumours		231
		11.7.1	Meningiomas	231
		11.7.2	Schwannomas	234
		11.7.3	Neurofibromas	236
		11.7.4	Paragangliomas	237
		11.7.5	Ganglioneuromas	237
		11.7.6	Ependymomas	237
	11.8	Intradural Extramedullary Malignant Tumours		238
		11.8.1	Malignant Peripheral Nerve Sheath Tumour	238
		11.8.2	Hemangiopericytoma	238
		11.8.3	Leptomeningeal Metastases	239
Further Reading				241

11.1 Introduction to Extradural Extramedullary Pathologies

This chapter summarizes concisely the pathologic anatomy of the epidural space and its most relevant tumorous, inflammatory and hemorrhagic diseases. The aim is to demonstrate case illustrations for the aforementioned diseases. After studying this chapter the reader should be able to explain the clinical features and the standard treatment of these diseases.

The epidural space is the anatomical space between the dura and the bony and ligamentous limits of the spinal canal which are ventrally the vertebral bodies and the intervertebral discs. Dorsally and dorso-laterally, the epidural space is restricted by the spinal laminae and the yellow ligaments. The epidural space is usually filled with fat and veins adjacent to the dura which are especially prominent around the axilla of the nerve roots and ventral to the thecal sac. These veins communicate with the veins of the vertebral body, both forming the internal vertebral venous plexus. This plexus is connected over a network of valveless veins (Batson plexus) with pelvic and thoracic veins and accounts for the spreading route of cancers and infections of pelvic organs to the spine. Furthermore, the epidural veins are prone to congestion in the case of narrowing epidural space. Then they are vulnerable and can be the origin of brisk intraoperative bleedings. The epidural fat serves as a sliding contact bearing, since the thecal sac is usually not attached to the spinal canal. Under normal conditions the thecal sac can slide up to several centimetres with flexion/extension movements of the spine.

Since the introduction of myelography in clinical practice, spinal tumours have been traditionally classified according to their relation to the dura and spinal cord in (1) epidural tumours, (2) intradural extramedullary tumours and (3) intradural intramedullary tumours. Epidural and intradural extramedullary tumours are addressed in this chapter and intradural intramedullary tumours are addressed in Chap. 18.

In spondylodiscitis and spondylitis, infections affect the intervertebral discs or/ and the adjacent vertebral bodies and, in approximately half of the patients, they also extend to the epidural space.

11.2 Epidural Tumours

11.2.1 Primary Benign and Malignant Epidural Tumours

11.2.1.1 Aetiology

According to their site of origin, spine tumours can also be classified as primary spinal tumours arising from cells of the vertebral body, pedicle and laminae such as osteocytes, osteoblasts, chondrocytes, fibroblasts and hematopoietic cells and secondary spine tumours, usually metastases, which originate from distant tumours in the body and spread on a hemotogeneous route to the spine.

11.2.1.2 Prevalence

Primary spinal tumours are rare lesions and amount to only about 0.4–0.5 % of all spinal neoplasms. Because of their rarity, larger surgical series are lacking. The peak age for benign primary spinal tumours is between 20 and 30 years, whereas malignant primary and secondary spine tumours predominantly occur in patients older than 40 years. Further detailed information about the prevalence of the specific tumour entities, if available, follows in the description of these tumour entities.

11.2.1.3 Symptoms

Symptoms of spinal tumours are not specific for single tumour entities and largely depend on the velocity of tumour growth and the extent of destruction of spinal structures. Progressive destabilization of the spine leads to mechanical back pain which is usually a severe and localized pain which is exacerbated by movement. Patients with mechanical back pain show tenderness to percussion at the site of the tumour. Biological pain is the second type of pain in spinal tumours. It is characterized by a dull pain which is independent of movement, increases during the night and is thought to be caused by periosteal stretching. Tumours which extend beyond the bony structures into the spinal canal can cause compression of the spinal cord and spinal nerve roots, depending on location. Spinal cord compression is characterized by motor, sensory or vegetative deficits (paraparesis, tetraparesis, sensory level, bladder and bowel dysfunction). Nerve root compression usually causes radicular pain, which is the third type of pain in spine tumours and/or radicular motor and sensory deficits. Benign primary spine tumours usually cause only pain. Because of their slow growth the spinal cord can compensate even high grade compression before neurological deficits occur as a late symptom. With malignant primary spine tumours, pain is found in the majority of patients and neurological deficits are much more frequently found than in patients with secondary spine tumours. Children with primary spine tumours can additionally present with a deformity with or without pain.

11.2.1.4 Diagnosis

For diagnostic work up of primary spinal tumours, both CT and MRI should be used. CT scans demonstrate the bone matrix and the osteolytic destruction and are therefore valuable for evaluation of instability. MRI is superior to CT in depicting the spinal cord and the nerve roots. Often CT and MRI provide first hints for differential diagnosis. If the tumour appears to be highly vascularized, a spinal angiography should be performed to obtain information about the tumour feeders and, if necessary, a preoperative embolization should be performed. Furthermore, a spinal angiography demonstrates the radiculomedullary arteries if the surgical procedures require sacrificing several nerve roots. If there suspicion of a primary spinal tumour, a biopsy should be performed to obtain the histological diagnosis and to plan further therapy. The biopsy should be planned carefully to prevent a spreading of the tumour. It is very important not to contaminate the epidural space. Usually the biopsy tract should be excised during the definitive surgery. Therefore the biopsy should be carried out in a spine centre where the definitive surgical tumour resection takes place.

11.2.1.5 Therapy

In contrast to secondary spine tumours, where the therapeutic concept is usually palliative, the surgical therapy in primary spine tumours is often curative. Therefore an exact oncological and surgical staging is mandatory. For the oncological staging the Enneking system, initially developed for the long bones, has also gained widespread acceptance in the treatment of spine tumours. This system defines the necessary extent of tumour resection on the basis of tumour dignity, growths characteristics and morphology. However, the unique anatomy of the spine with the spinal canal and its contents, the spinal cord and the nerve roots, required the development of spine-specific staging systems. The WBB surgical staging system was developed by Weinstein, Boriani and Biagini for surgery planning. It allows spine surgeons to plan the extent and type of tumour resection and whether a radical "En bloc" procedure is feasible at all. The WBB surgical staging system was validated for benign as well as malignant tumours. Figure 11.1 gives a detailed overview of the WBB system and its zones.

11.2.1.6 Outcome

The outcome of primary spinal tumours largely depends on the histology and the extent of tumour resection. Incomplete resection of primary tumours or violation of tumour margins carries a high risk for local tumour recurrence and determines ultimately the survival of the patients. Survival of patients with primary spine tumours decreases dramatically in the case of a tumour recurrence. The best results are obtained with "en bloc resection techniques" with tumour-free margins. Therefore a complete en bloc resection of the tumour should be carried out whenever technically feasible.

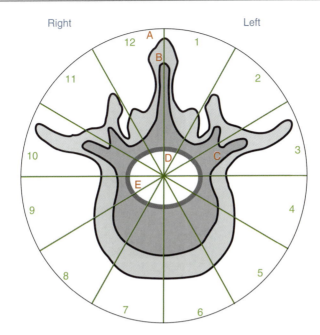

Fig. 11.1 Surgical staging system for primary spinal tumours according to Weinstein, Boriani and Biagini (WBB). The spinal column and its surrounding soft tissue, the spinal canal with the thecal sac and its contents are divided into 12 zones and 5 lettered compartments from outside the spine to the spinal canal: extraosseous paraspinal soft tissue compartment (*A*), superficial intraosseous compartment (*B*), deep intraosseous compartment (*C*), epidural compartment (*D*), intradural compartment (*E*)

11.2.2 Vertebral Hemangioma

Vertebral hemangiomas are the most common benign tumours of the spine and account for approximately 2–3 % of all spine tumours. From larger autopsy studies the incidence is reported to be 10–12 %; however vertebral hemangiomas are usually asymptomatic and usually diagnosed incidentally. The peak incidence is the fourth to sixth decade. Vertebral hemangiomas are extremely vascularized slowly growing tumours histologically composed of irregular vascular space collections surrounded by endothelial cells. On MRI, vertebral hemangiomas appear as T1 and T2 hyperintense lesions within the vertebral body. Symptomatic vertebral hemangiomas are usually treated conservatively. Further treatment options are vertebroplasty and embolization. In very rare cases vertebral hemangiomas cause instability and spinal cord compression (Fig. 11.2a–f). In these cases, open surgical decompression and spine stabilization is indicated. However it should be kept in mind the these highly vascularized lesions can lead to significant blood loss during open surgery. A preoperative embolization should be strongly considered. En bloc resection techniques without violation of the hemangioma can also reduce blood loss.

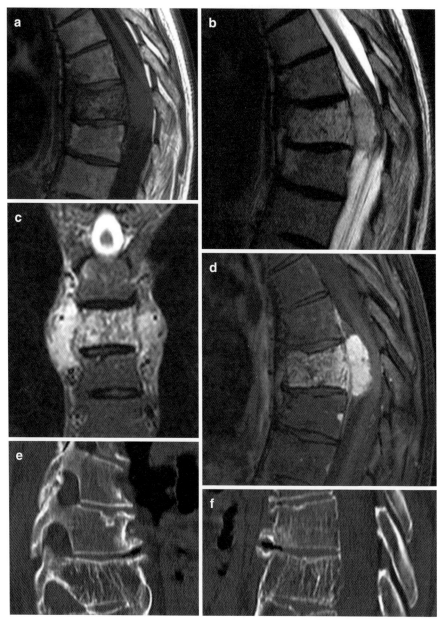

Fig. 11.2 Typical hemangioma shows a hyperintense signals on T1- and T2-weighted images reflecting adipose tissue within the stroma. Aggressive hemangiomas (**a–f**) however show atypical MRI features with hypointense signals on T1- (**a**) and hyperintense signals on T2-weighted images and on STIR sequences (**b**, **c**). Because of the vascularised stroma within an osseous matrix of bone erosion with interspersed thickened vertical trabeculae, hemangiomas show a high gadolinium uptake (**d**) and on CT a "honeycomb" appearance

11.2.3 Aneurysmal Bone Cyst

Aneurysmal bone cysts are cystic lesions with differently sized cavities filled with fluid and clotted blood separated by fibrous septa and do not have an endothelial lining. However, even if the histological pattern is benign with absence of atypical mitoses, aneurysmal bone cysts sometimes show rapidly progressive growth with destruction of the bone. They can affect every bone in the body and arise de novo as primary aneurysmal bone cysts or complicate other bone tumours as secondary aneurysmal bone cysts. Therapy of choice is surgical intralesional curettage/resection. If the cyst is large and needs extensive surgery, preoperative embolization should be considered.

11.2.4 Osteoid Osteoma/Osteoblastoma

These tumour are most common in adolescents and young adults. Osteoid osteomas and benign osteoblastomas belong to the same tumour entity and are only differentiated by size. Osteoid osteomas larger than 1.5 cm^2 are referred to as osteoblastomas. Osteoid osteomas are typically found in long bones whereas osteoblastomas are more frequent in the spine. Histologically they do have a nidus consisting of bony trabeculae with intervening vascular tissue and are preponderantly slowly growing benign tumours; however, very rarely, osteoblastomas show a more aggressive behaviour and histological appearance. Patients with osteoid osteomas almost always present with pain as the major symptom which is promptly relieved by Non steroidal antiinflammatory drugs NSAIDs, especially by aspirin. Pain from osteoblastomas, in contrast, is usually not influenced by NSAIDs. Therapy of choice is surgical resection. In osteoid osteomas it is sufficient to do an intralesional resection whereas marginal en bloc resection is the best option for osteoblastomas.

11.2.5 Osteochondroma

Osteochondromas are the most common benign bone tumours usually found in long bones and rarely in the spine (4 % of the solitary osteochondromas). Osteochondromas are benign low grade lesions which consist of columnar cartilage and maturing bone surrounded by a fibrous capsule. Therapy of choice is surgical en bloc resection.

11.2.6 Chordoma

Chordomas derive from remnants of the notochord. They are usually found in midline structures of the skull base which is the most common region of origin. Within the spine, chordomas develop most often in the sacrum (~50 %) followed by the cervical spine. Chordomas are composed of cells arranged in small clusters or cords

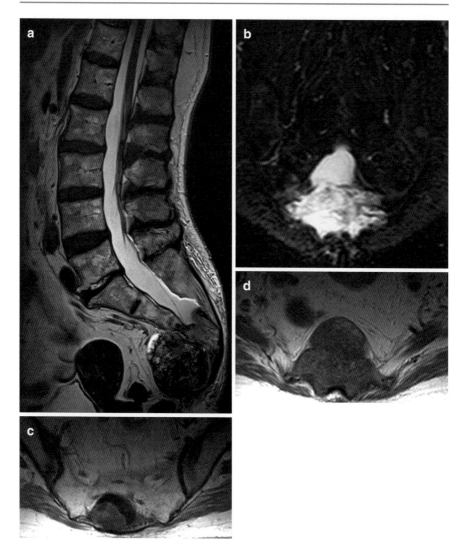

Fig. 11.3 Chordomas are midline tumours with destructive growth patterns (**a–d**). On T2WI they are hypo- to hyperintense depending on the fibrous tissue component (**a, b**). Sacral chordomas usually have a large presacral tumour component (**a**). On T1WI chordomas are hypo-/isointense (**d**) and show a heterogeneous enhancement

within a myxoid matrix. CT scans show soft tissue mass and usually osteolytic lesions. On T1WI MRI chordomas are hypo-/isointense and on T2WI hyperintense, depending on the fibrous tissue component (Fig. 11.3a–d). The most important differential diagnosis is chondrosarcoma. Chordomas show a strong keratin and S100 immunoreactivity while chondrosarcomas are only S100 immunopositive. Chordomas are slowly but locally aggressive growing tumours and therefore have to be resected en bloc whenever technically feasible.

11.2.7 Chondrosarcoma

Chondrosarcomas arise from neoplastic chondrocytes. Low grade chondrosarcomas are mild to moderately hypercellular tumours, whereas high grade chondrosarcomas show increasing nuclear atypia, sometimes associated with necrosis. Chondrosarcomas are immunopositive for S100 but not for keratin. They are rare lesions occurring most often in patients between 30 and 50 years of age and are most common in the thoracic spine. The prognosis is always dependent on the possibility of a local recurrence. Intralesional resections of chondrosarcomas are associated with high recurrence rates of up to 100 %. Therefore it should be the aim to do a complete "en-bloc" resection if possible. If a complete "en-bloc" resection is achieved, the local recurrence rate is given as 20 % in the literature. Chondrosarcomas are not sensitive to conventional radiotherapy and chemotherapy.

11.2.8 Giant Cell Tumour

Giant cell tumours are locally aggressive semi-malignant tumours most frequently found in the sacrum. They usually occur in younger patients with immature skeletal system. Histologically they are composed of giant cells resembling osteoclast and spindle- to ovoid-shaped mononuclear stromal cells. These mononuclear stromal cells are thought to be the neoplastic component of these tumours, the osteoclast-like giant cells being considered as non-neoplastic reactive tumour components. Giant cell tumours sometimes spread to the lung. They are usually highly vascularised tumours, and therefore a preoperative embolization should be considered before surgery. "En-bloc" resection is the therapy of choice.

11.2.9 Brown Tumour

Brown tumours are bone lesions associated with hyperactivity of osteoclasts as seen in hyperparathyroidism. Brown tumours are non-neoplastic lesions and typically found in long bones. Spinal involvement is exclusively seen in primary hyperthyroidism. The primary therapy consists of medical treatment of the causal condition. Surgery is only indicated in cases of acute neurological deterioration and instability despite adequate therapy of the causal condition.

11.2.10 Fibrous Dysplasia

Fibrous dysplasia is a non-malignant fibroosseous disorder of the skeletal system significant for the replacement of the normal bone with fibrous tissue and irregular osteoid. Besides the skeletal system, other organs may be involved (McCune Albright syndrome). Fibrous dysplasia usually affects one bone (monostotic form ~ 70–80 %); less frequently, more than one bone is affected (polyostotic form ~ 20–30 %). Spinal involvement is very rare and can be monostotic or polyostotic. Patients with spinal fibrous dysplasia have an increased risk of vertebral body fracture and of the development of a secondary osteosarcoma. Therapy is symptomatic to control pain. Surgery is reserved for complications such as spinal instability or neurological compromise by spinal cord or nerve root compression.

11.2.11 Langerhans Cell Histiocytosis/Eosinophilic Granuloma

Langerhans cell histiocytosis is an abnormal proliferation of histiocytes resulting in focal or multiple granulomatous lesions of the bone. The clinical spectrum reaches from focal bone lesions to multifocal multisystem disease. Langerhans cell histiocytosis can affect every organ. It shows characteristics of both malignant and non-malignant diseases and it is still unclear whether Langerhans cell histiocytosis is a true neoplasm or an inflammatory process. Eosinophilic granuloma is the localized type of the Langerhans cell histiocytosis and shows a localized uni- or multifocal bone involvement being observed in around 70 % of patients with histiocytosis. Hand–Schüller–Christian disease is significant for localized bony involvement, usually the skull, with exophthalmus and diabetes insipidus caused by the involvement of the pituitary stalk. This type of Langerhans cell histiocytosis is seen in about 15–40 % of the cases. Abt–Letterer–Siwe disease refers to the disseminated form of Langerhans cell histiocytosis which occurs in around 10 % of the cases. Although Langerhans cell histiocytosis can occur in every age, it is usually diagnosed in the pediatric population and younger adults. In children the incidence is estimated to be 3–5 per 1,000,000. Around 8–15 % of eosinophilic granulomas affect the spine and can cause pain and instability as well as neurological compromise (Fig. 11.4a–d). Very often eosinophilic granuloma is self limiting and results in spontaneous resolution, and therefore therapy should be conservative and address predominantly the pain symptoms. Surgery is reserved for cases with spinal instability, intractable pain or neurological compromise caused by spinal cord or nerve root compression. In cases with multifocal or multisystem disease, radio- and chemotherapys are treatment options.

11.2.12 Solitary Plasmacytoma/Multiple Myeloma

Plasmacytoma/multiple myeloma is a neoplastic disorder of the antibody producing plasma cells. It belongs to the B-cell non-Hodgkin lymphomas and occur with an incidence of 4–6 per 100,000 per year. The terms plasmacytoma and myeloma are often used synonymously, although, strictly speaking, only one solitary intramedullary or one extramedullary focus are referred to as plasmacytoma without systemic involvement; multiple intramedullary foci are referred to as multiple myeloma. Around 55 % of all solitary plasmacytomas affect the spine. Usually they are located within the vertebral bodies but can cause osteolytic lesions with pathologic vertebral body fractures and extend to the spinal canal with subsequent spinal cord compression (Fig. 11.5a–l). Spinal manifestation per se is not an indication for

11 Extramedullary Space-Occupying Pathologies

surgery, because solitary plasmacytoma/multiple myeloma is sensitive to radio- and chemotherapy. Painful pathologic fractures can be treated successfully with kypho- or vertebroplasty (Fig. 11.6a, b). Open surgery is indicated in patients with high grade spinal instability and progressive neurological deficits.

11.2.13 Lymphoma

Spinal lymphomas arise from the bone marrow of the vertebral body, infiltrate the bone of the vertebral body and extend per continuitatem to the epidural space or metastasize hematogenously from extraspinal sites to the epidural space (Fig. 11.7a–f). Spinal lymphomas are usually non-Hodgkin lymphomas. Therapy of choice is chemo- and radiotherapy. Surgical therapy is reserved for cases with instability and acute

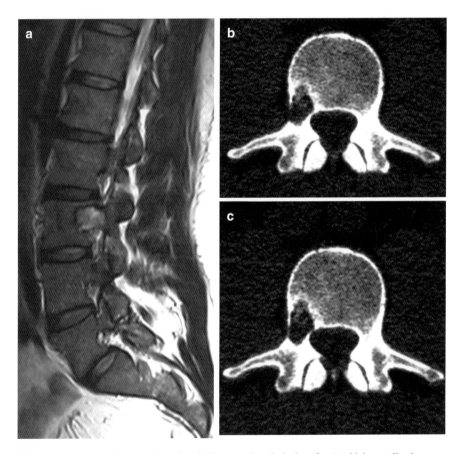

Fig. 11.4 Eosinophilic granuloma is a lytic non-sclerotic lesion (**b, c**) which usually does not enter the disc space, nor the epidural space or the paravertebral region. T2WI show a high signal soft tissue mass (**a, d**)

Fig. 11.4 (continued)

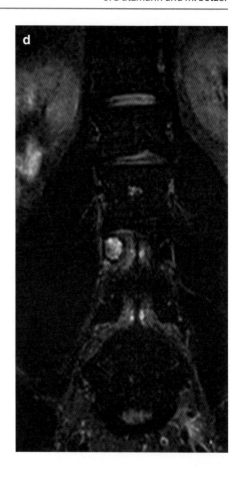

neurological deterioration caused by spinal cord compression. Spinal cord compression without involvement of the vertebral body is amenable to sole decompressive surgery.

11.2.14 Osteosarcoma

Osteosarcoma is a common bone tumour; however, primary spinal osteosarcomas are rare at around 2 % of all osteosarcomas. Histologically they consist of malignant spindle or round cells which form osteoid. Risk factors for the development of an osteosarcoma are preexisting bony pathologies such as Paget's disease or osteoblastomas and radiation therapy. Pain is the most common presenting symptom in patients with spinal osteosarcomas. Treatment consists of a combination of chemotherapy, en bloc resection when technically feasible and postoperative radiation. However, because of the aggressiveness of the tumour, the prognosis is poor.

11 Extramedullary Space-Occupying Pathologies

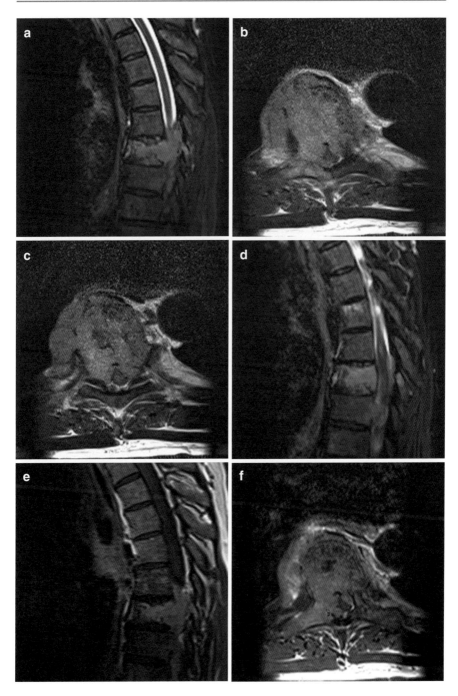

Fig. 11.5 Solitary plasmacytoma shows a lytic tumour with sclerotic margins. (**h, i**) On T1WI it is an iso- or slightly hyperintense tumour mass with homogenous enhancement. (**e–g**) On T2WI it can show a variable hyperintensity. (**a–c**) In this case the tumour has entered the spinal canal with high grade spinal cord compression. (**a–g**) Because of the significant bone destruction with subsequent instability therapy was surgical with vertebrectomy, tumour resection, anterior reconstruction with cage and posterior instrumentation over dorsoventral approach (**j–l**)

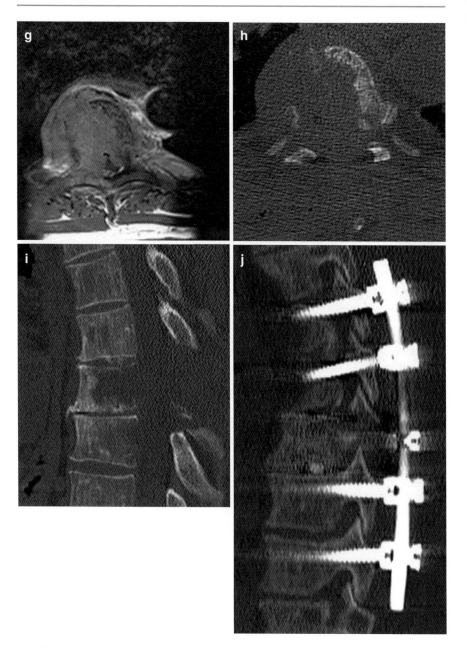

Fig. 11.5 (continued)

11 Extramedullary Space-Occupying Pathologies

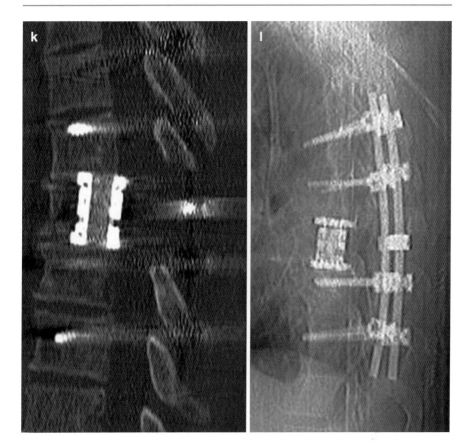

Fig. 11.5 (continued)

11.2.15 Ewing Sarcoma

Ewing sarcoma is the most common malignant bone tumour in children. It usually affects long bones; primary spinal involvement is rare and occurs in less than 10 % of cases. Of the primary spinal Ewing sarcomas, the sacrum is the most common localization. Ewing sarcomas are chemo- and radiosensitive. Therefore surgery is limited to acute neurological deterioration and biomechanical instability.

11.2.16 Fibrosarcoma

Fibrosarcoma is a rare soft tissue tumour which arises typically from the fascia of the deep musculature and the periosteum. It consists of proliferating fibroblasts and anaplastic spindle cells. Known risk factors for fibrosarcomas are conditions such as fibrous dysplasia, radiation therapy and Paget's disease. Fibrosarcomas

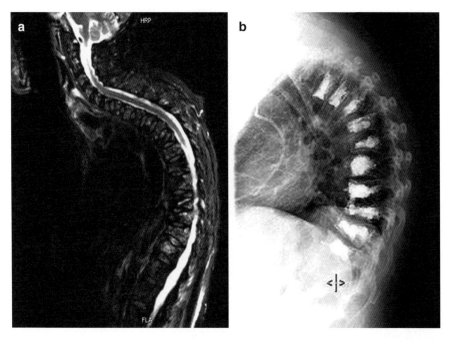

Fig. 11.6 Multiple myeloma with involvement of several vertebral bodies can lead to pathological fractures with significant pain (**a**). Kypho- and vertebroplasty is a minimally invasive therapy option which can usually address pain from multiple pathologic fractures in patients with multiple myeloma (**b**)

usually involve the soft tissue of the extremities and the trunk. The spine is a rare location. In bones, surgical radical resection is the standard therapy for fibrosarcomas. Chemotherapy may be administered neoadjuvantly or adjuvantly. Typically fibrosarcomas are not very radiosensitive.

11.2.17 Malignant Fibrous Histiocytoma

Malignant fibrous histiocytoma is a soft tissue sarcoma which occasionally occurs in bone and very rarely as a primary spine tumour. Treatment consists primarily of radical resection if possible. Sometimes radiation is indicated. The role of chemotherapy in the treatment of fibrous histiocytoma is controversial at the present time.

11.2.18 Sacrococcygeal Teratoma

Sacrococcygeal teratoma is the most common extragonadal germ tumour in children, with an incidence of 1 in 350,000 live births, usually located in front of the sacrum. They consist of entodermal, ectodermal and mesodermal derivatives and have a potential to be malignant. Sacrococcygeal teratoma has been classified into four types according to their extent outside and inside the body. Type 1 tumours are completely outside the body, sometimes connected with a narrow stalk. Type 4 tumours are completely inside the body in a presacral/retrorectal location. Therapy depends on the size of the tumour and the age of manifestation. Beside close observation, complete resection is the favourite treatment option.

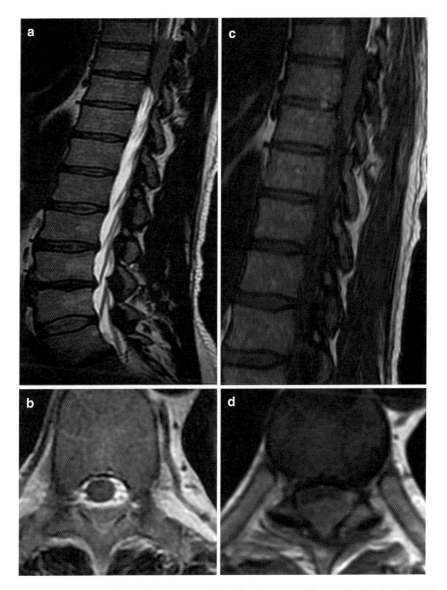

Fig. 11.7 Lymphoma of the epidural space without involvement of the vertebral body. On T2WI lymphomas can have hypo- to isointense signals (**a**, **b**) and usually enhance uniformly (**c–f**)

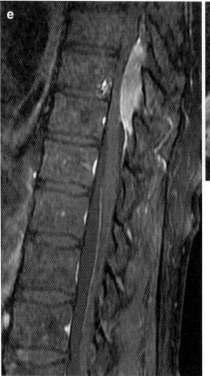
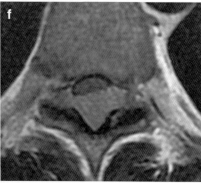

Fig. 11.7 (continued)

11.3 Secondary Malignant Epidural Tumours

11.3.1 Metastases

11.3.1.1 Prevalence

The spinal column is the most frequent site of bone metastasis. Metastatic spinal disease is a significant problem for a large number of patients: spinal metastases develop in 5–10 % of all patients with cancer during the course of their disease. Approximately 40 % of persons dying of cancer have autopsy evidence of spinal metastases. Of these, 10 % experience spinal cord compression with subsequent neurological deficits. The annual incidence of spinal cord compression caused by spinal metastases is estimated to be 20,000 cases. In recent autopsy studies, investigators found metastatic involvement of the spine in 90 % of patients with prostate carcinoma, in 75 % of those with breast carcinoma, in 55 % of those with melanoma, in 45 % of those with lung carcinoma, and in 30 % of those with renal carcinoma. Specific carcinomas cause clinically significant spinal cord compression in a higher percentage of patients. Twenty-two percent of patients with breast cancer, 15 % of those with lung cancer and 10 % of those with prostate carcinomas experience symptomatic spinal cord compression.

11.3.1.2 Symptoms
Symptoms of secondary spine tumours do not differ significantly from malignant primary spine tumours. In most cases spinal metastases present with mechanical back pain because of instability and/or radicular pain. When the metastatic tumour enters the spinal canal and compresses the spinal cord, an acute neurological deterioration with transverse spinal cord syndromes are often seen. Symptoms progress much more rapidly in metastases than in primary malignant extradural tumours.

11.3.1.3 Diagnosis
Metastatic cancer is a systemic disease. Therefore an oncological staging is very important and should answer the question of life expectancy. Preoperative MRI of the whole spine reveals further metastases which may cause instability and may have to be addressed surgically. CT scans are important for exact measurement of the pedicles and the implants and to evaluate the quality of bone. In highly vascularised metastases (renal cell, thyroid) it is recommended to perform a preoperative angiography with embolization, since intralesional resections of these tumours can cause massive blood loss (Fig. 11.8a–h).

11.3.1.4 Therapy
Surgical treatment options are decompression by anterior and posterior approaches as well as minimally invasive treatment with vertebro- or kyphoplasty. Possible non-surgical treatments for metastatic spinal tumours include radiotherapy alone, radiotherapy plus systemic chemotherapy, hormone therapy, surgical decompression followed by radiotherapy, and, more recently, extracranial radiosurgery. Traditionally, spinal metastases have been treated by surgical decompression over a posterior approach with a single or multilevel laminectomy to treat radicular pain and spinal cord compression. However, several studies carried out in the 1980s, including a randomized clinical trial, have shown that the outcome after surgical decompression followed by radiotherapy is not superior to treatment by radiotherapy alone. These studies led to the abandonment of surgical decompression by laminectomy alone and resulted in treatment of spinal metastases by radiotherapy alone. However, with the advent of more sophisticated techniques for complex spine reconstruction, and because of the fact that simple laminectomy and radiotherapy do not address biomechanical instability, a main feature of spinal metastases, spine surgeons started again to treat spinal metastases more aggressively compared to simple laminectomy with subsequent stabilization of the spine. Recent studies have shown that surgical decompression with complex spine reconstruction can successfully improve the neurological status, improve severe pain and restore biomechanical stability. One well designed randomized clinical trial could show that, in a selected patient group with spinal metastases, the neurological outcome and the survival after surgical decompression with subsequent stabilization followed by

radiation is better than with radiation therapy alone. The present generally accepted treatment algorithm embraces that, when a metastatic spinal tumour causes compression of the spinal cord or other neural elements, surgical decompression is often chosen. Based on the extent of spinal column destruction and the resulting biomechanical instability of the spine, fixation may be elected. The goal of both surgery and local radiation therapy in the treatment of spinal metastases in the majority of patients is basically palliation of painful symptoms, prevention of pathological fractures of the vertebral body, and halting or reversing progression of neurological compromise rather than a curative concept (Fig. 11.9a–c). However, in single metastases from slowly growing tumours (renal cell, thyroid cancer) a

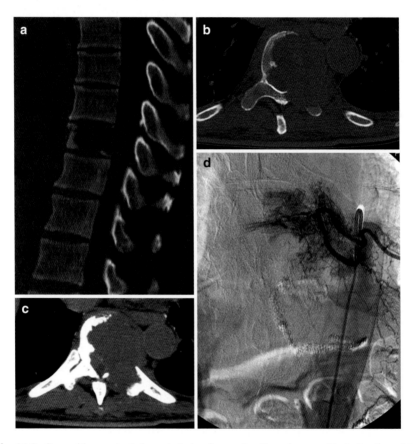

Fig. 11.8 Case with an osteolytic metastasis of a renal cell carcinoma with destruction of the larger part of the vertebral body, the left pedicle and transverse process, the facet joint and the left lamina (**a, b**). The tumour has entered the spinal canal with subsequent spinal cord compression (**c**). Because of the primary renal cell carcinoma, a preoperative angiography was carried out, demonstrating the high vascular supply (**d**). Embolization could significantly reduce the vascularization (**e**) and the patient underwent a single-stage posterolateral transpedicular vertebrectomy with anterior reconstruction with expandable cage and posterior instrumentation with a screw rod system (**f–h**)

11 Extramedullary Space-Occupying Pathologies

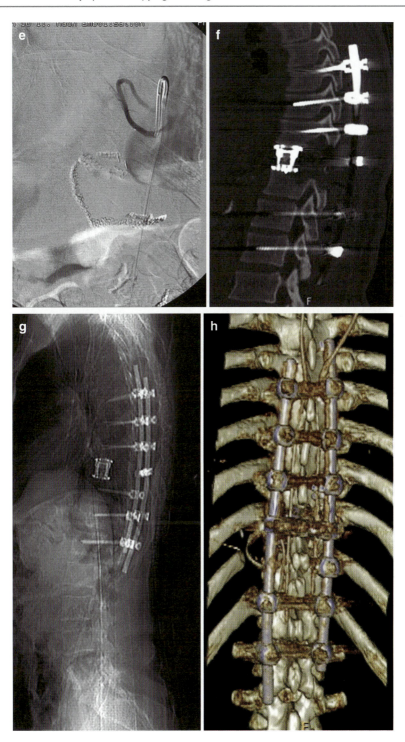

Fig. 11.8 (continued)

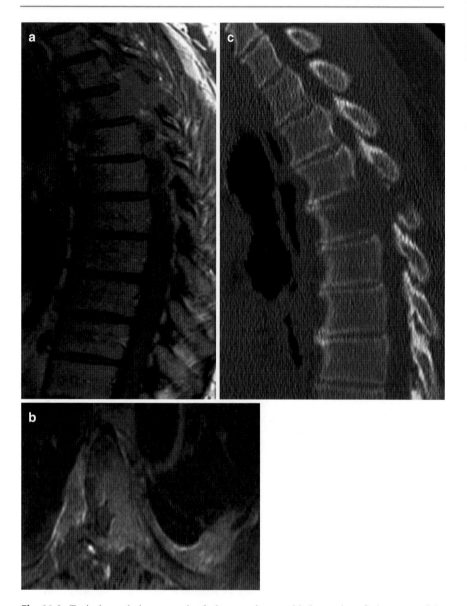

Fig. 11.9 Typical osteolytic metastasis of a lung carcinoma with destruction of a large part of the vertebral body causing instability with the typical mechanical back pain (**c**). MRI shows a slightly hyperintense tumour with a strong contrast enhancement and compression of the spinal cord (**a, b**)

curative therapeutic concept may apply with a radical "en-bloc" resection of the spinal metastasis. The role of radiosurgery has yet to be defined but is likely limited to treatment of focal or recurrent disease or use as a supplement to fractionated radiotherapy.

11.3.1.5 Outcome

Outcome in spinal metastases is largely dependent on the type and treatment response of the primary tumor, the number and site of further metastases and the presence or absence of neurological deficits.

Take Home Message

Because of their high recurrence rates, primary malignant extradural tumours should be treated with "en bloc" resection techniques if technically feasible. Table 11.1 provides an overview of the primary benign and malignant extradural spine tumours and the recommended treatment.

Surgical treatment of spinal metastases is in most cases palliative. Circumferential decompression with stabilization and subsequent radiotherapy is superior to radiotherapy alone. Surgical indications are (pending) instability, intractable pain, deformity and progressive neurological deficits. Spinal metastases are treated best by an interdisciplinary team consisting of spine surgeons, oncologists and radiotherapists.

11.4 Epidural Empyema

11.4.1 Aetiology

Epidural infections are generally of bacterial origin and very rarely fungal. The epidural space consists of fat tissue and venous vessels. It is highly vascularized and therefore under good surveillance of the immune system. Since the epidural compartment is a preformed space, collections of infectious fluid is referred to as empyema consistent with the pathological definition and not as abscess. The term epidural abscess, however, is also found abundantly in medical literature. As the dura, the posterior longitudinal ligament and the periosteum of the vertebral bodies usually lie close together, most abscesses develop lateral or posterior. Depending on the stage of the infection, the abscess itself is usually built up of granulation tissue and pus.

Therefore about half of non-iatrogenic epidural abcesses are either in continuum with a spondylitis or even a spondylodiscitis or are outgrowths of prevertebral infections such as abscesses of the psoas muscle or retroperitoneal space. Pathophysiologically important are the multiple venous channels which form a venous network between the vertebral bodies and the epidural veins. The remaining abscesses are infections in the rest of the body with the most prevalent being those which can easily spread hematogenously like endocarditis. Pneumonias and skin infections such as furuncles are also commonly found as distant sources. Typically the epidural abscess develops with a latency of weeks after the initial infections has subsided.

A significant portion of spinal infections are from iatrogenic sources, such as injections, epidural catheters or instrumentation.

Isolated specimens show predominantly *Staphylococcus aureus*. More rarely found bacteria are *Eschericcia coli*, Streptococcus, coagulase – negative

Table 11.1 Primary spine tumors and their preferred treatment

Tumor	Tissue of origin	Histology	Clinical course	Therapy of choice
Vertebral hemangioma	Blood vessels	Benign	Benign	Vertebroplasty, radiation, embolization
Aneurysmal bone cyst	Blood vessels	Benign	Semimalignant	Intralesional curettage
Osteoid osteoma	Bone	Benign	Benign	Intralesional curettage
Osteoblastoma	Bone	Benign	Benign	Mariginal En bloc resection
Osteochondroma	Cartilage	Benign	Benign	En bloc resection
Chordoma	Notochord	Malignant	Malignant	En bloc resection + radiation
Chondrosarcoma	Cartilage	Malignant	Malignant	En bloc resection
Giant cell tumor	Bone	Benign	semimalignant, osteodestructive, metastases	En bloc resection
Brown tumor	Bone	Benign	Benign	Treatment of hpyerparathyroidism
Fibrous dysplasia	Bone	Benign	Osteodestructive no causal therapy	Symptomatic bisphosphonates
Langerhans cell histiocytosis/ eosinophilic granuloma	Mononuclear phagocyte system	Benign	Benign to malignant	Symptomatic surgery in selected cases
Solitary plasmacytoma	Hämatopoietic system	Malignant	Malignant	Radiation, surgery in selected cases
Multiple myeloma	Hämatopoietic system	Malignant	Malignant	Radiation, chemotherapy
Lymphoma	Hämatopoietic system	Malignant	Malignant	Radiation, chemotherapy
Osteosarcoma	Bone	Malignant	Malignant	Chemotherapy + En bloc resection
Ewing sarcoma	Hämatopoietic system	Malginant	Malignant	Radiation + chemotherapy
Fibrosarcoma	Connective tissue	Malignant	Malignant	En bloc resection
Malignant fibrous histiocytoma	Connective tissue	Malignant	Malignant	En bloc resection
Sacrococcygeal teratoma	Germ cells	Potentially malignant	Potentially malignant	Complete resection

Staphylococcis and Pseudomonas. In i.v. drug abusers an atypically high frequency of anaerobic specimen and Pseudomonas is observed. In immunosuppressed patients, mixed infections including fungal infections often occur.

If these infections occur they can progress to potentially severe life-threatening conditions. In modern medicine, however, mortality has decreased significantly with the advent of modern imaging and diagnostic techniques.

11.4.2 Prevalence

U.S. population data estimated the incidence of epidural abscess between 0.2 and 2 % per 10,000 hospital admissions. The incidence may have a rising tendency, possibly because infections are detected better. There seems to be a female predominance (f:m ratio 2:1). Concerning age, these infections are predominant in the 50- to 70-year-olds, which may also be shifting towards a higher age in the aging Western population.

In the thoracic region about half of the abscesses develop, followed by the lumbar region.

11.4.3 Neurological Symptoms

In general, epidural abscesses can be a challenge to the diagnosing physician since symptoms are highly variable and also depend on underlying medical conditions such as immune suppression.

Clinical features depend highly on location and timing of the infection. Acute infections cause fever usually with systemic infection signs and strong back pain. Depending on the location and size of the infections, neurologic deficits (caused by compression, small vein thrombosis or an associated myelitis/meningitis) may develop acutely. The neurologic deficits may be radicular or may involve the cauda or the spinal cord. Classically, fever, lower back pain and radicular symptoms were seen with epidural abscesses. In the modern MRI era this triad is only seen in a minority of patients with spinal epidural abscesses detected by MRI. Rarely seen today is the sequence of back pain which progresses to a radiculopathy to a cauda syndrome to complete paralysis. These infections can potentially lead to sepsis and systemic shock, but this is mostly prevented by the institution of antibiotic therapy. Chronic infections lead to milder back pain, and often non-ambulating and a reduced pain associated mobility. Often no fever or systemic infection signs are present and the diagnosis is almost entirely based on imaging criteria.

11.4.4 Important Diagnostic Findings

The most important diagnostic tool to diagnose spinal infections is MRI. Prior to these parameters of systemic infections such as elevated WBC, C-reactive protein and elevated ESR support the suspicion and are useful markers for follow up.

Blood cultures are positive in little more than half the cases. A lumbar puncture is contraindicated in patients with suspected spinal epidural abscesses.

MRI with gadolinium may show two basic patterns: a homogenous enhancement of the era caused by granulation tissue with associated microabscesses or the typical ring-type contrast enhancing lesions also seen on brain abscesses (Fig. 11.10a–d).

If MRI is not available, a contrast CT scan is a significantly inferior alternative since it may show a block to the flow of contrast but not the cause of the block.

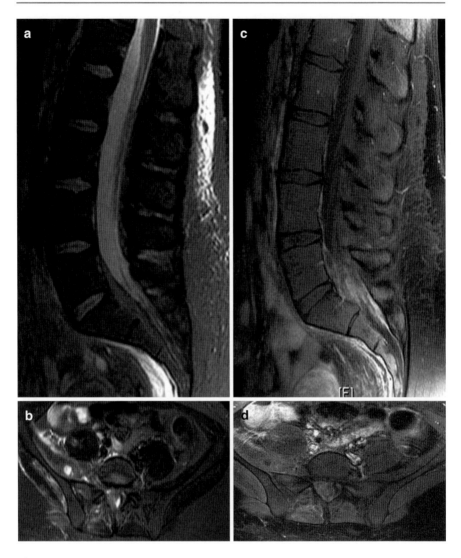

Fig. 11.10 Case of a spinal empyema without concomitant spondylodiscitis (**a**, **b**) caused by multiple analgesic infiltration for lower back pain. After gadolinium a typical marginal enhancement around the empyema is seen (**c**, **d**)

11.4.5 Differential Diagnosis

The differential diagnosis is usually broad since symptoms are highly variable. They include epidural hematoma, spinal cord hemorrhage metastatic diseases, transverse myelitis and multiple sclerosis.

11.4.6 Therapy

Generally supportive measures such as fever control should be instituted immediately. Like many other complex diseases, the management is a team effort. The team in this case consists of infectious disease specialists, spine surgeons and radiologists.

Therapy in general should be operative, especially when associated neurological deficits are present. Thus the cause of the deficits can be eliminated and the microbial origin isolated.

The initiating of antibiotic therapy has to be delayed until a sample of the infection is obtained if possible.

Because the operation is usually done emergently, a posterior approach with a laminotomy abscess drainage and irrigation of the epidural space is employed. This provides quick access and causes low surgical morbidity. If the infection has a wider spread, a (hemi-)laminectomy and even multilevel or a split laminectomy may be employed (Fig. 11.11a–h).

In the case of coexisting spinal instability concomitant spinal instrumentation is indicated. Infection is not a contraindication in modern instrumentation.

In patients with minimal or no neurological deficit having small epidural abscesses, a conservative management might be justified. Microbial sample should still be obtained, i.e. with CT guided needle aspiration.

Antibiotic therapy is given for at least 6 weeks and for up to 12 weeks with underlying osteomyelitis/spondylodiscitis.

11.4.7 Outcome

The outcome of epidural abscesses is highly variable and depends greatly on duration of symptoms, age and comorbid conditions. Prognostically important imaging findings are the length of the abcesses, and underlying core edema.

Take Home Message
The most important diagnostic tool to diagnose spinal infections is MRI. Acute infections usually cause fever with systemic infection signs and strong back pain. Chronic infections lead to milder back pain, and often also non-ambulating and reduced pain-associated mobility. Therapy in general should be operative.

11.5 Epidural Hemorrhage

11.5.1 Aetiology

Epidural hematoma can either occur iatrogenic or spontaneous. The epidural space is highly vascularized predominantly with venous vessels. Most commonly iatrogenic hemorrhage occurs following lumbar puncture, epidural anaesthesia and spinal surgery. Usually a bleeding diathesis through either anticoagulant medication, thrombocytopenia or coagulation abnormality is present.

Spontaneous spinal epidural hematoma is sometimes caused by arteriovenous malformations or vertebral hemangiomas, but usually has no bleeding source and therefore stems from spontaneous bleeding of the above-mentioned venous plexus. This may be caused by intraabdominal or intrathoracic pressure which is transmitted to the epidural plexus.

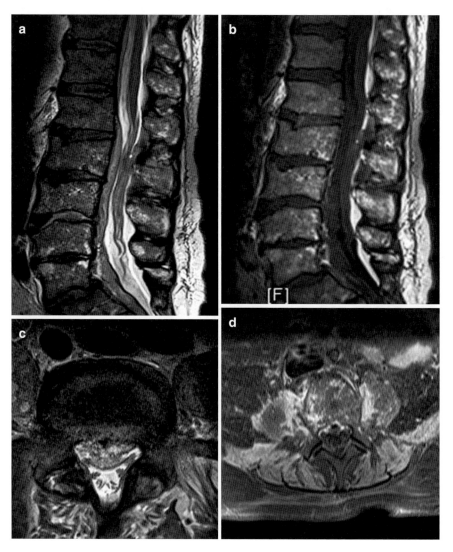

Fig. 11.11 Case of a large spinal epidural empyema extending from L1 to the sacrum (**a**) and compression of the thecal sac (**c, d**) and a weak enhancement after gadolinium injection (**b**). After laminotomy of the segment L5/S1 on the right side the empyema could be drained almost completely (**e–h**)

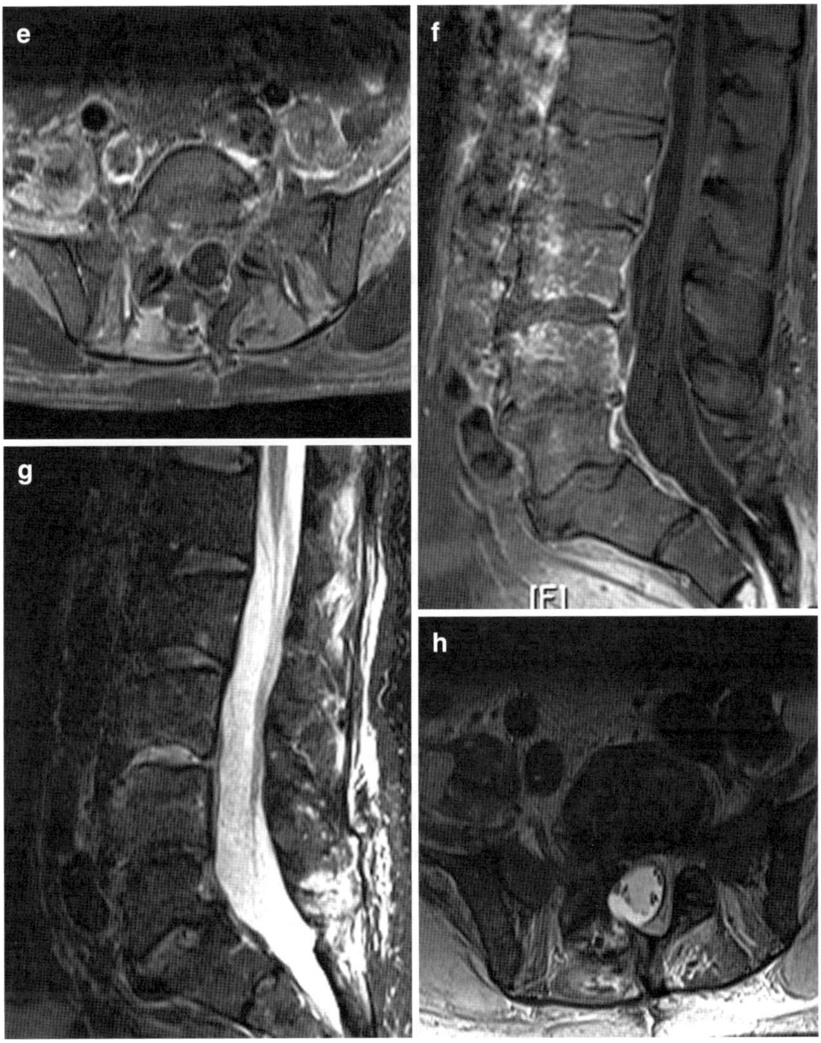

11 Extramedullary Space-Occupying Pathologies

Fig. 11.11 (continued)

11.5.2 Prevalence

Spinal epidural hematoma is very rare. Iatrogenic cases are more common than spontaneous but valid epidemiological data is missing. Counts can be done of reported cases in the international medical literature where even large case series are missing. To date, about 500 cases have been reported since its first description in 1869. The hemorrhage may occur at any level, but the thoracic region is predominant. Intraspinally they are typically located posterior or posterolateral.

rate of tumour growth, and the extent of spinal cord compression. The most common presenting symptom in the reported series was a sensory deficit, followed by gait ataxia and weakness. The least common symptom was pain and sphincter dysfunction.

11.7.1.4 Diagnosis

The current standard diagnostic study for spinal tumours is MR imaging. MRI provides exact information about tumour localization (affected segment, relation to spinal cord and nerve root, and relation of the tumour to the dura), the extent of spinal cord compression, and further information about the spinal cord and the tumour itself (presence of cord edema and intratumoral signal changes such as necrosis, hematoma or calcification). Spinal meningiomas are usually isointense to the spinal cord (T1- and T2-weighted MR images) and show an enhancement after contrast medium (Gd) administration (Fig. 11.12a–d). In limited cases, computed tomography scanning is

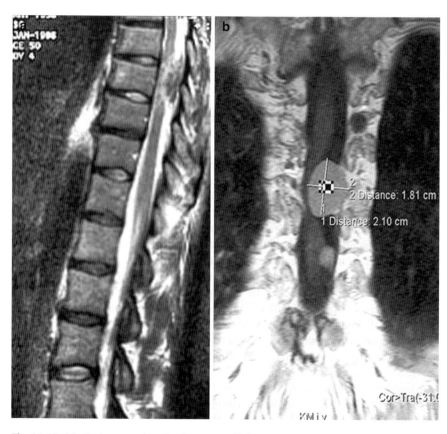

Fig. 11.12 Meningiomas are intradural tumours which are usually isointense to the spinal cord on T2 images. (**a**) After administration of gadolinium they usually show a homogeneous enhancement. (**b**) Since these tumours are slow growing they can cause a massive spinal cord compression until they become symptomatic. (**c**) The image shows a meningioma which almost fills the complete spinal canal and causes a high grade compression of the spinal cord. (**d**) Intraoperative photograph of a spinal meningioma which causes a high grade compression of the spinal cord

Fig. 11.12 (continued)

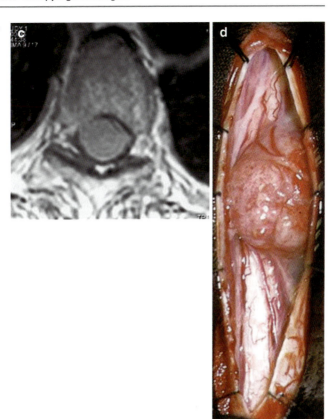

indicated alone or in addition to MR imaging (contraindications for MR imaging or destruction of osseous structures for better depiction of bone or, in the case of a heavy tumour, calcification). The main differential diagnosis of spinal meningiomas includes intradural extramedullary schwannomas. Although there are hints for differentiating spinal meningiomas from schwannomas (dural tail, broad dural contrast of meningioma, regressive changes within the tumour, more lateral position of schwannomas, and relation to the nerve root), a reliable differentiation between spinal meningiomas and schwannomas is not possible with MR or any other imaging techniques. There is no pathognomonic picture of atypical and invasive spinal meningiomas. On MR images these tumours can enhance as solitary or multiple lesions. The tumour can enhance heterogeneously or in a ringlike fashion. Angiography can reveal a tumour blush with pathological vessels or early venous drainage.

11.7.1.5 Therapy

The approach should allow an exposure which is wide enough to survey the tumour and the dural attachment. The most frequent approach has been dorsal; by laminectomy at one level or by hemilaminectomy at one or two levels with lateral extension when necessary (anterior and anterolateral tumours). In the majority of patients with spinal menigniomas it is possible to resect even large tumours safely and without causing spinal instability by using a standard dorsal or dorsolateral laminectomy approach. In patients with calcified ventral or ventrolateral tumours, a partial vertebrectomy and/or a costotransversectomy approach allows safer tumour manipulation and removal. In tumours occurring at the cervicothoracic and/or thoracolumbar junction, dorsal stabilization should be considered to prevent junctional kyphosis.

The primary goal of surgery is complete and safe tumour removal and decompression of the spinal cord. Dorsally placed tumours can be removed totally with or without resection of the dural attachment. Anterior lesions should be debulked before dissection of the tumour capsule, exposure of the plane between the tumour and spinal cord, and finally tumour removal. Intraoperative ultrasonography to localize the tumour is recommended by some authors. In previously reported series, the percentages of total resection ranges from 82 to 99 %. It is usually sufficient to coagulate the dural attachment. Resection of the dural attachment with suturing of a patch graft is in most cases unnecessary. For the majority of spinal meningiomas, the dorsal approach (with partial facetectomy, if necessary) is sufficient to achieve complete tumour resection and prevent spinal instability. However, in rare cases of heavily calcified meningiomas with a ventral or ventrolateral location where internal tumour debulking is not possible via a dorsal approach, it can be safer to perform a partial or complete vertebrectomy for tumour resection along with subsequent instrumentation. Morbidity and mortality rates for spinal meningiomas are low with an average of 6.2 % for morbidity and 2.1 % for mortality. The most frequent complications include CSF leak and wound infection, occurring in 0–4 % and 0–6 %, respectively. Other, less frequent complications are pulmonary embolism, pneumonia, and myocardial infarction. The major cause of death in the previously published studies was pulmonary embolism. Today most of the neurosurgical centres use neurophysiological monitoring on a routine basis in spinal meningioma surgery.

11.7.1.6 Outcome
The prognosis of benign spinal meningioma treated with complete resection is excellent, with low complication rates and a good long-term functional outcome. Recurrence and malignant transformation rates are low.

11.7.2 Schwannomas

Spinal schwannomas are encapsulated tumours which typically arise from Schwann cells of the dorsal sensory root. However, schwannomas may also arise from the motor nerve root. They account for 30 % of all spinal tumours and have approximately the same incidence as spinal meningiomas. The peak incidence of schwannomas is the third to sixth decades of life. Schwannomas are usually solitary lesions; however, they may be associated with genetic syndromes such as neurofibromatosis type 2 (NF2) and in these instances show multiple manifestations. Schwannomas are usually intradural tumours; however they may be completely extradural in up to 15 %. Schwannomas are usually isodense to the spinal cord on CT with low density

11 Extramedullary Space-Occupying Pathologies

cystic changes. Often a remodelling of the adjacent bone can be observed, such as enlargement of the neural foramen or expansion of the spinal canal. Schwannomas may be located completely intraspinally or extraspinally (Fig. 11.13a, b). The sand glass-like growth pattern is typical but rather infrequent. On MRI, schwannomas are iso- or hypointense on T1-weighted images and hyperintense on T2 sequences.

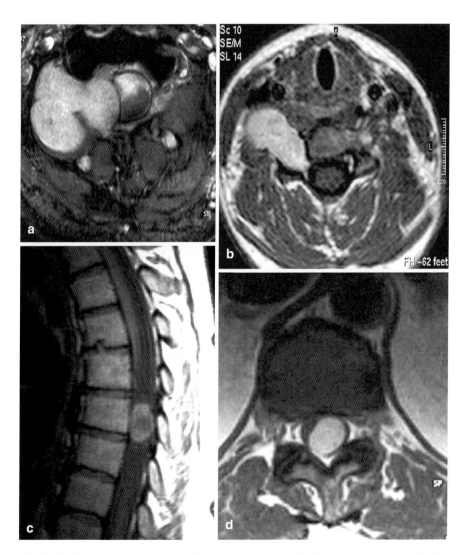

Fig. 11.13 Neurinomas are tumours arising from Schwann cells. The may be located within the neuroforamen with an intra- and extradural growth (**a**) or with a completely extradural growths. (**b**) They may also be located exclusively within the spinal canal and can be confused with meningiomas. (**c, d**) Sometimes they show regressive changes within the tumour which are not typical for meningiomas. *Arrow* in (**e**) indicates vertebral body Th5. (**c, e**) Intraoperative photograph of a neurinoma within the spinal canal which causes a high grade compression of the spinal cord (**f**)

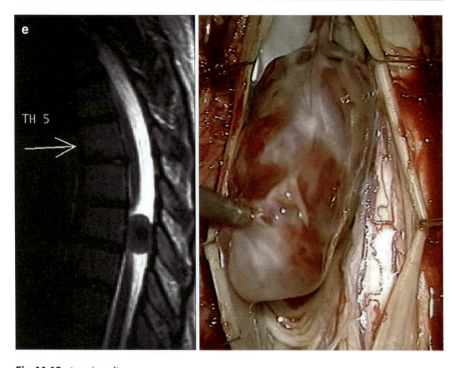

Fig. 11.13 (continued)

Focal areas of regressive (cystic) changes appear hypointense on T1 images and hyperintense on T2 images (Fig. 11.13c–f). These regressive changes and the lack of dural enhancement help to differentiate schwannomas from meningiomas, which is the main differential diagnosis. The therapy of choice for schwannomas is complete surgical resection. In many cases it is possible to separate the involved fascicle and preserve the majority of the nerve root. Electrophysiological monitoring with stimulation of the involved fascicle helps to differentiate sensory from motor nerve roots. Recurrence rates are comparable to spinal meningiomas and are reported to account for 6–12 % with a mean time of 4 years. In the case of neurofibromatosis, recurrence rates are much higher, reaching up to 40 % at 5 years postoperatively in some studies.

11.7.3 Neurofibromas

Spinal neurofibromas may occur sporadically or in the setting of neurofibromatosis. The cell of origin of neurofibromas is not known; however, it is assumed that neurofibromas stem from the mesenchymal line. Neurofibromas are grade I lesions which show a proliferation of all components of the nerve including Schwann cells, perineural cells and collagen. As a result, neurofibromas usually show a fusiform growth pattern. The incidence of spinal neurofibromas is estimated to be as high as the incidence of spinal meningiomas or slightly higher. On CT, neurofibromas are isodense to the spinal cord and sometimes enlargement of the neural foramen is seen. On T1 images the signal of neurofibromas is similar to that of the spinal cord; on T2 images neurofibromas show an isointense or hyperintense signal. After administration of contrast medium, neurofibromas show a moderate to intense enhancement Therapy of choice is the gross total tumour resection. In some cases the involved nerve roots have to be sacrificed. The recurrence rate has been estimated to be around 12 %.

11.7.4 Paragangliomas

Paragangliomas are benign tumours which derive from neural crest cells and most commonly occur in the carotid body or glomus jugulare. In the adrenal medulla these tumours are called phaeochromocytomas and usually secrete catecholamines. In contrast, paragangliomas rarely produce excessive catecholamines. Spinal paragangliomas are uncommon and the incidence has been estimated to be 0.07 per 100,000. Paragangliomas of the spine most commonly occur in the cauda equine. It is supposed that they originate from sympathetic neurons of the lateral horn of the spinal cord and extend over the nerve roots or the filum terminale. There is no pathognomonic MRI feature for paragangliomas; however, they are usually hypervascular with an intense contrast enhancement. Therapy of choice is a complete surgical resection. Recurrence rates are estimated to be 4–10 %. Radiotherapy is an option in the case of incomplete resection or in the case of a recurrence.

11.7.5 Ganglioneuromas

Ganglioneuromas are slowly growing benign tumours which show the features of mature neuronal phenotypes. Ganglioneuromas usually involve the peripheral nervous system and are thought to derive from multipotent neural crest cells and are related to the embryological development of the sympathetic nervous system. Ganglioneuromas of the central nervous system are less common and the histogenesis is not completely understood. Spinal ganglioneuromas show features of both central and peripheral ganglioneuromas. Ganglioneuromas most commonly occur in childhood and adolescence. On MRI they are usually hypointense on T1-weighted images and heterogeneously hyperintense on T2-weighted images. After administration of contrast medium they show an intense enhancement, sometimes with foci of lower signal. Surgical therapy with a complete removal is indicated whenever feasible to obtain histology. Because of their benign character, additional therapies are usually not indicated.

11.7.6 Ependymomas

Intradural extramedullary ependymomas comprise ependymomas arising from the filum terminale. Filum terminale ependymomas are common and comprise approximately 50 % of all spinal ependymomas. They originate from ependymal cells covering the filum terminale. The most common histological type is the myxopapillary type; however, papillary and cellular ependymomas also occur. Myxopapillary ependymomas of the filum terminale grow slowly and are usually considered as benign tumours. On MRI these tumours are iso- or hypointense in T1-weighted images and hyperintense on T2-weighted images. They show an intense contrast enhancement. Therapy of choice for these lesions is surgical with the goal of a complete resection. However, because these tumours are sometimes adherent to the nerve roots, in some cases remnants have to be left in situ, which may be the origin of local recurrences. The recurrence rate after "complete" resection is therefore reported in the literature to be up to 19 %. Radiotherapy is reserved for patients with an incomplete tumour removal or for recurrent tumours.

11.8 Intradural Extramedullary Malignant Tumours

11.8.1 Malignant Peripheral Nerve Sheath Tumour

Malignant peripheral nerve sheath tumours (MPNST) are very aggressive tumours of neural origin. They are regarded as derivatives of Schwann cells. Other terms for MPNST are malignant schwannoma, neurogenic sarcoma or neurofibrosarcoma, which are also found frequently in the literature. Although the majority of MPNST arise de novo from normal peripheral nerves or from malignant transformation of neurofibromas, a smaller proportion develops from benign schwannomas and from sympathetic ganglion tumours. The most common sites for MPNST are the sciatic nerve, brachial plexus and the larger nerves of the upper arm. Neurofibromatosis type 1 predisposes for the development of MPNST. MPNST are confined to the cells intrinsic to the peripheral nerves including perineurium and endoneurium. They are generally considered as Schwann cell derivatives. Histologically, MPNST are hypercellular with spinal cell proliferation. On CT scans MPNST may show calcifications as benign tumours. Therefore calcification is not a reliable sign of a benign dignity. On T1-weighted MRI, with MPNST the signal is isointense to muscle and hyperintense on T2-weighted images, usually with a heavy contrast enhancement which is often inhomogeneous (Fig. 11.14a–e). MPNST are very aggressive tumours which need to be excised in an en bloc fashion or with exarticulation. In the spine this is usually not feasible so radio- or chemotherapeutic options need to be considered. The overall prognosis of MPNST is dismal.

11.8.2 Hemangiopericytoma

Hemangiopericytomas are thought to arise from pericytes, modified smooth muscle cells which surround reticulary sheath capillaries and postcapillary venules. The spinal column is a rather rare location for hemangiopericytomas. Intradural hemangiopericytomas are exceedingly rare. On T1-weighted images hemangiopericytoma show an intermediate signal and a hyperintense signal on T2-weighted images. After administration of contrast medium they show a diffuse enhancement. Hemangiopericytomas are aggressive tumours which should be excised en bloc whenever feasible, followed by radiotherapy. The local recurrence rates are above 60 and 20% of hemangiopericytoma patients develop metastases.

11.8.3 Leptomeningeal Metastases

The majority of metastases are localized in the extradural compartment and are addressed in Chap. 15. Only 5 % of metastatic lesions involve the intradural

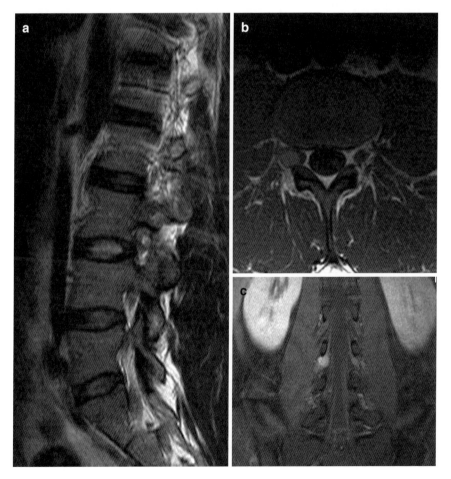

Fig. 11.14 Small Gd enhancing MPNST within the right neuroforamen L3/4. (**a–c**) After 6 months the patient developed an osteolytic metastasis within the vertebral body of Th 11 (**d, e**)

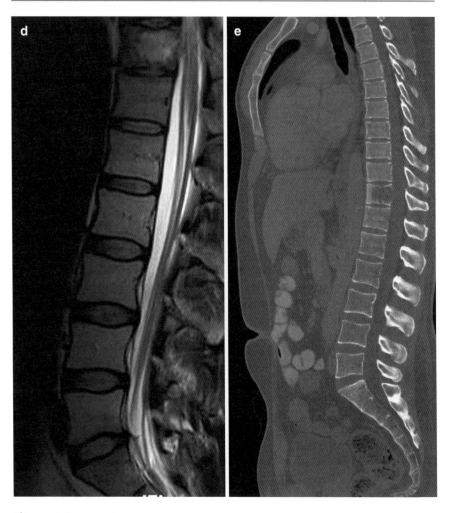

Fig. 11.14 (continued)

compartment and are usually seen in leptomeningeal carcinomatosis, which is caused by dissemination of malignant cells by the CSF. Leptomeningeal carcinomatosis is a devastating complication of systemic cancer in an advanced stage of the disease. It is reported to occur in about 3–8 % of all cancer patients. The primary cancer types which commonly cause leptomeningeal carcinomatosis are breast and lung cancer as well as melanoma. However, leptomeningeal spread is also seen in primary brain tumours (gliosarcoma, glioblastoma) as well as lymphoreticular tumours (leukaemia and lymphoma). In MRI, leptomeningeal carcinomatosis shows a smooth or nodular dural enhancement along the spinal cord and the nerve roots (Fig. 11.15a, b). Treatment is basically non-surgical and the option of intrathecal chemotherapy has to be considered.

11 Extramedullary Space-Occupying Pathologies

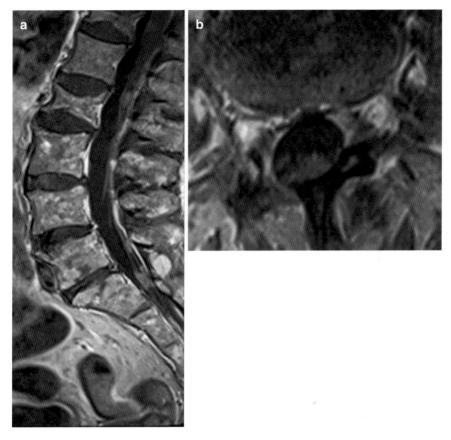

Fig. 11.15 Leptomeningeal carcinomatosis shows a smooth or nodular dural enhancement along the spinal cord and the nerve roots, sometimes with a focal compression of the spinal cord (**a, b**)

Further Reading

1. Boriani S, Weinstein JN, Biagini R (1997) Primary bone tumors of the spine. Terminology and surgical staging. Spine (Phila Pa 1976) 22:1036–1044
2. Dickman CA, Fehlings MG, Gokaslan ZL (eds) (2006) Spinal cord and spinal column tumors. Principles and practice. Thieme, Stuttgart/New York
3. Enneking WF (1983) Musculoskeletal tumor surgery. Churchill Linvingstone, New York
4. Enneking WF, Spanier SS, Goodman MA (1980) A system for the surgical staging of musculoskeletal sarcoma. Clin Orthop Relat Res 153:106–120
5. Kim DH, Chang UK, Kim SH, Bilsky MH (eds) (2008) Tumors of the spine. Saunders Elsevier, Philadelphia
6. Patchell RA, Tibbs PA, Regine WF, Payne R, Saris S, Kryscio RJ, Mohiuddin M, Young B (2005) Direct decompressive surgical resection in the treatment of spinal cord compression caused by metastatic cancer: a randomised trial. Lancet 366:643–648
7. Quiñones-Hinojosa A, Jun P, Jacobs R, Rosenberg WS, Weinstein PR (2004) General principles in the medical and surgical management of spinal infections: a multidisciplinary approach. Neurosurg Focus 17(6):E1

8. Rigamonti D, Liem L, Sampath P, Knoller N, Namaguchi Y, Schreibman DL, Sloan MA, Wolf A, Zeidman S (1999) Spinal epidural abscess: contemporary trends in etiology, evaluation, and management. Surg Neurol 52:189–197
9. Setzer M, Vatter H, Marquardt G, Seifert V, Vrionis FD (2007) Management of spinal meningiomas: surgical results and a review of the literature. Neurosurg Focus 23(4):E14
10. Tomita K, Toribatake Y, Kawahara N, Ohnari H, Kose H (1994) Total en bloc spondylectomy and circumspinal decompression for solitary spinal metastasis. Paraplegia 32(1):36–46
11. Wiley AM, Trueta J (1959) The vascular anatomy of the spine and its relationship to pyogenic vertebral osteomyelitis. J Bone Joint Surg Br 41-B:796–809

Spinal Trauma

12

Matthias Setzer

Contents

12.1	Cervical Spine	244
12.1.1	Aetiology and Prevalence	244
12.1.2	Symptoms	244
12.1.3	Diagnosis	244
12.1.4	Therapy and Outcome	245
12.2	Craniocervical Junction	245
12.2.1	Occipital Condyle Fractures	245
12.2.2	Atlantoccipital Dislocation (AOD)	247
12.3	Upper Cervical Spine	249
12.3.1	Atlas Fractures	249
12.3.2	Traumatic Atlantoaxial Dislocations	252
12.3.3	Fractures of the Axis	254
12.3.4	Odontoid Fractures	255
12.3.5	Atypical Fractures of the Body of the Axis	258
12.4	Subaxial Cervical Spine	259
12.4.1	Type A Fractures of the Cervical Spine	259
12.4.2	Type B Fractures of the Cervical Spine	262
12.4.3	Type C Fractures of the Cervical Spine	263
12.5	Sacral Fractures	264
12.5.1	Aetiology	264
12.5.2	Classification	264
12.5.3	Prevalence	266
12.5.4	Symptoms	266
12.5.5	Diagnosis	266
12.5.6	Therapy	266
12.5.7	Outcome	267
12.6	Traumatic Spinal Cord Injury	267
12.6.1	Aetiology	267
12.6.2	Prevalence	267

M. Setzer
Department of Neurosurgery, Goethe-University,
Schleusenweg 2-16, D-60528 Frankfurt, Germany
e-mail: matthias.setzer@kgu.de

12.6.3 Symptoms	267
12.6.4 Diagnosis	269
12.6.5 Therapy	269
12.6.6 Outcome	269
References	270
Further Reading	270

12.1 Cervical Spine

12.1.1 Aetiology and Prevalence

Because of its high flexibility, the cervical spine is prone to injury during accidents. The most common injury mechanisms are traffic accidents, falls and strangulations. The injuries may be mere soft tissue injuries, ligamentous or osseous or a combination of all. The prognosis of cervical spine injuries is determined by concomitant spinal cord injuries or by injuries of the nerve roots. The incidence in adults is estimated between 3 and 4.5% and in children below 1 %. The incidence of injuries without spinal cord injury (SCI) is about 3 %. SCI without concomitant fractures are found in about 0.7 %. The incidence of cervical spine injuries in polytraumatized patients is estimated to be about 6 %. Mortality is about 15 % and morbidity about 45–60 %. The most common cause for cervical spine injuries are traffic accidents in modern industrial nations. While the frequency of traffic accidents decreases, the frequency of cervical spine injuries in older people increases.

12.1.2 Symptoms

General symptoms such as spasms of the neck muscles and headaches are common even in mild forms of cervical spine trauma. Mechanical neck pain (increases in motion, decreases in rest) and fixed subluxation positions or deformity are indicative of a luxation or fracture. If neurological injury is present it largely depends on the localization (nerve root vs spinal cord lesion) and the level of injury.

12.1.3 Diagnosis

Every radiological examination of the cervical spine has to be preceded by a clinical examination. Radiological examination can be avoided if the patient is awake and alert and is not under the influence of drugs, denies neck pain and does not have tenderness to palpation, does not show any neurological symptoms and does not have any other severe injuries. If history or clinical examination supports the suspicion of a cervical spine injury it has to be ruled out thoroughly. Standard cervical AP, lateral and odontoid views have been reported to reach a sensitivity of 92 % in adults and 94 % in children. Although in recent years the increased use of CT has been able to detect more injuries plain radiograms remain an important tool if they are adequately carried out. CT scans are indicated in the case of pathological plain films if an area cannot clearly be seen in standard radiographs (craniocervical or cervicothoracic area). For special questions an additional MRI is indicated (ligamenteous or avulsion injuries, differentiation between acute and old fractures). For evaluation for vascular injury, especially injury of the vertebral artery, CT or MRI angiography has largely replaced the conventional angiography. The incidence of injury to the vertebral artery is estimated to range between 17 and 44 % in patients with cervical spine injury and is therefore not an uncommon finding. Therefore a CTA (CT angiography) should be added to a normal CT scan in the case of C1 and C2 injuries and in cases with fractures which involve the foramen of the vertebral artery to rule out a traumatic dissection. Furthermore, a CTA provides valuable information about the normal anatomy (unilateral dominant vertebral artery).

For the classification and documentation of the neurological status the American Spinal Injury Association and the International Medical Society of Paraplegia developed a scheme for a standardized documentation of neurological status which has gained wide acceptance. In cases of spinal cord injury this ASIA Impairment Scale (AIS) should be used for documentation of initial status at admission and for follow-up evaluations.

12.1.4 Therapy and Outcome

Therapeutic options and outcome are described in the sections on the special fracture types below.

12.2 Craniocervical Junction

The craniocervical junction is the transitional zone between the skull base and the upper cervical spine and is prone to injuries such as fractures and luxations. Although injuries of the craniocervical junction are rarely seen in clinical practise, some of them are potentially life threatening and the diagnosis may be difficult. They are frequently seen in combination with a traumatic brain injury or in polytrauma patients.

12.2.1 Occipital Condyle Fractures

Occipital condyle fractures are classified according to Anderson and Montesano into three types or, according to Jeanneret, four types.
Type I (Jeanneret) = Type II (Anderson and Montesano). This fracture is part of a transverse fracture of the petrosal part of the temporal bone. It may affect the foramen of the hypoglossal nerve and a hypoglossal palsy is the most frequent cranial nerve palsy in this type (Fig. 12.1a).

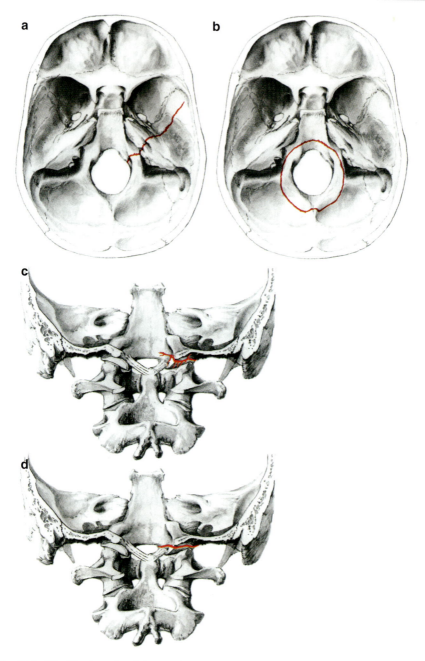

Fig. 12.1 Classification of occipital condyle fractures according to Jeanneret and Anderson and Montesano: (**a**) *Jeanneret type I* (*Anderson and Montesano type II*) fracture is part of a transverse fracture of the petrosal part of the temporal bone. (**b**) *Jeanneret type II* is a ring fracture of the cranial base. (**c**) *Jeanneret type III* (*Anderson and Montesano type I*) is a compression fracture of the occipital condyle. (**d**) *Jeanneret type IV* (*Anderson and Montesano type III*) is an avulsion fracture of the alar ligament and is frequently combined with an atlantooccipital dislocation (AOD). Reprinted with permission from Tscherne and Blauth [3]

Type II (Jeanneret). A ring fracture of the cranial base which has only been observed in victims killed in traffic accidents (Fig. 12.1b).

Type III (Jeanneret)=Type I (Anderson and Montesano). This type is a compression fracture of the occipital condyle and usually does not cause a neurological deficit (Fig. 12.1c).

Type IV (Jeanneret)=Type III (Anderson and Montesano). An avulsion fracture of the alar ligament which is frequently (25 % of the cases) combined with an atlantooccipital dislocation (AOD) (Fig. 12.1d).

Therapy. Type I is usually treated with a soft cervical collar until improvement of the symptoms. Types II and III without AOD are treated with a soft cervical collar for 6 weeks. Types II and III with AOD has to be treated surgically with a craniocervical fixation. If a dislocation of the fracture is seen it might also be treated in a halo fixateur.

12.2.2 Atlantoccipital Dislocation (AOD)

AOD is a severe injury which usually results in death at the scene caused by brain stem or upper spinal cord injury or injuries of the carotid or vertebral arteries. Sometimes surviving patients show cranial nerve deficits. AOD is caused by a disruption of the ligaments between the skull base and C1 (alar ligaments, tectorial membrane, anterior and posterior atlanto-occipital membrane). The extent of the ligamentous injury determines the grade of instability. The direction of dislocation of the skull in relation to the atlas determines the type of AOD (according to Harris [5]; Traynelis et al. [6]).

Type I. The skull is dislocated anteriorly. The ventral dislocation is the most common type of AOD with instability in the sagittal plane alone or combined with axial instability (Fig. 12.2a)

Type II (Traynelis)=Type III (Harris). The skull is dislocated axially. This is the most unstable form of AOD and is equivalent to a complete separation of the skull from the spine (Fig. 12.2b). There is a high risk of stretch injury of vessels and spinal cord.

AOD is usually diagnosed in a trauma scan. If the patient is stable an MRI of the spine and the skull should be performed to evaluate the brainstem and the brain for infarctions and to give further hints for the prognosis.

Type III (Traynelis)=Type II (Harris). The skull is dislocated posteriorly. Type II is a rare form of AOD (Fig. 12.2c).

Type IV. A lateral dislocation of the skull which was described by Collato and Jevtich.

AOD is usually diagnosed in a trauma scan. If the patient is stable an MRI of the spine and the skull should be performed to evaluate the brainstem and the brain for infarctions and to give further hints for the prognosis.

Therapy. AOD in adults is managed by surgical occipitocervical instrumentation with fusion. In children AOD can alternatively be managed with immobilization in a halo fixateur if a good closed reposition can be achieved. Another treatment possibility in children is a temporary occipitocervical instrumentation without bony fusion. Extension is absolutely contraindicated.

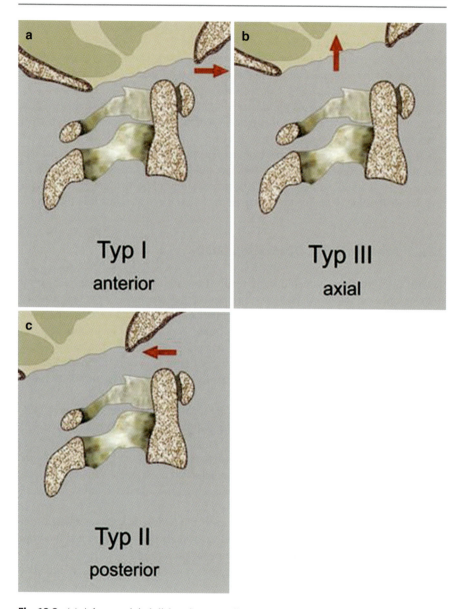

Fig. 12.2 (a) Atlantooccipital dislocation according to Traynelis and Harris. Type I: the skull is dislocated anteriorly (*red arrow*). (b) Type II (Traynelis), type III (Harris): the skull is dislocated axially (*red arrow*) – this is the most unstable form of AOD. (c) Type III (Traynelis), type II (Harris): the skull is dislocated posteriorly (*red arrow*). Reprinted with permission from Kandziora et al. [1].

12.3 Upper Cervical Spine

12.3.1 Atlas Fractures

Fractures of the atlas are common injuries with a percentage of up to 13 % of all cervical injuries. The most common classification is that of Gehweiler et al. who differentiated between five types of atlas fractures.

Type 1 is an isolated fracture of the anterior arch of the atlas. The frequency of this type in the literature is given with around 2 % of all atlas fracture. This fracture type is caused by an abrupt contraction of the longus colli muscle in hyperextension injuries. It is generally considered as stable (Fig. 12.3a).

Type II is an isolated fracture of the posterior arch occurring always bilaterally at the thinnest portion of the posterior arch which is usually the sulcus of the vertebral artery (Fig. 12.3b). Unilateral fractures are combined with anterior arch fractures and are classified as type III. The mechanism of injury is a hyperextension combined with an axial compression. Type II atlas fractures are frequently combined with additional injuries or fractures of the cervical spine (e.g. fractures of the dens axis). Involvement of the sulcus of the vertebral artery needs further evaluation (CT angiography, MR angiography) of the vertebral artery to rule out traumatic arterial dissection.

Type III is a combined fracture of the anterior and posterior arch of the atlas. This is the classical atlas ring burst fracture which was first described by Jefferson. The fracture lines can be uni- or bilateral, and therefore two-, three- and four-part fractures are possible (Fig. 12.3c–e). The stability of this fracture form is largely determined by the integrity of the transverse ligament. *Type IIIa* are stable fractures where the transverse ligament is intact (Fig. 12.3f) and type *IIIb* are unstable fractures where the transverse ligament is not intact (Fig. 12.3g). Disruption or bony avulsion of the transverse ligament leads to a lateral shifting of the lateral masses which may be seen in plain radiograms and in CT scans (Fig. 12.3h). If the sum of shifting distances on both sides exceeds 7 mm, a lesion of the transverse ligament must be assumed (*Spence rule*) (Fig. 12.3i). *Gehweiler type IIIb* can be further subclassified according to *Dickman*. *Dickman type I* encompasses the injuries with an interligamentous rupture. In *type Ia* the rupture is located centrally while in type *Ib* the rupture site is more lateral near the massa lateralis (Fig. 12.3j, k). *Dickman type II* injuries are injuries disconnecting the tubercle for insertion of the transverse ligament from the C1 lateral mass involving a comminuted C1 lateral mass (*type IIa*) or avulsing the tubercle from an intact lateral mass (*type IIb*) (Fig. 12.3l, m). *Type IIa* lesions also belong to the group of the *Gehweiler type IV* fractures (Fig. 12.3n). This type describes an isolated lateral mass. If there is no lesion of the transverse ligament, *Gehweiler type IV* fractures are stable.

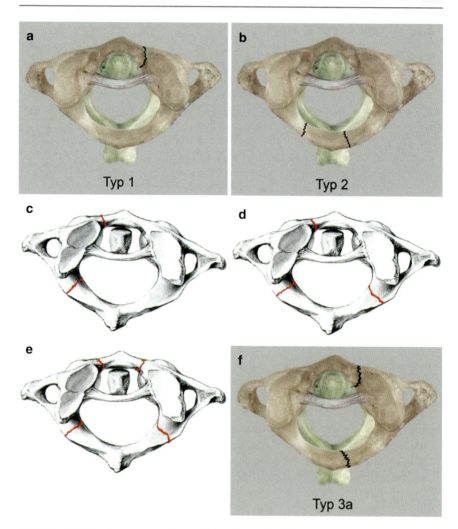

Fig. 12.3 (a) Atlas fractures according to Gehweiler et al. and ruptures of the transverse ligament according to Dickman et al. Type 1 is an isolated fracture of the anterior arch of the atlas, which is stable. (b) Type II is an isolated fracture of the posterior arch occurring always bilaterally. (c–e) Type III is a combined fracture of the anterior and posterior arch of the atlas. (f) Type III a are stable fractures where the transverse ligament is intact. (g) Type IIIb are unstable fractures where the transverse ligament is not intact. (h) Disruption or bony avulsion of the transverse ligament leads to a lateral shifting of the lateral masses (*single arrows*) which may be seen in plain radiographs and in CT scans. (i) If the sum of shifting distances on both sides exceeds 7 mm (*double arrows*) a lesion of the transverse ligament must be assumed (Spence rule). (j, k) Dickman type I encompasses the injuries with an interligamentous rupture. In type Ia the rupture is located centrally in type Ib the rupture site is more laterally near the massa lateralis. (l, m) Dickman type II injuries injuries disconnect the tubercle for insertion of the transverse ligament from the C1 lateral mass involving a comminuted C1 lateral mass (type IIa) or avulsing the tubercle from an intact lateral mass (type II b). (n) Type IIa lesions also belong to the group of the Gehweiler type IV fractures. (o) This type describes an isolated lateral mass fracture. Gehweiler type V fractures are isolated fractures of the transverse process. (p) Besides the indirect signs (Spence rule, ADI, PADI), MRI of the craniocervical junction might be helpful to directly assess the transverse ligament, with a pathological signal in the vicinity of the transverse ligament. Reprinted with permission from Kandziora et al. [2], Tscherne and Blauth [3]

12 Spinal Trauma

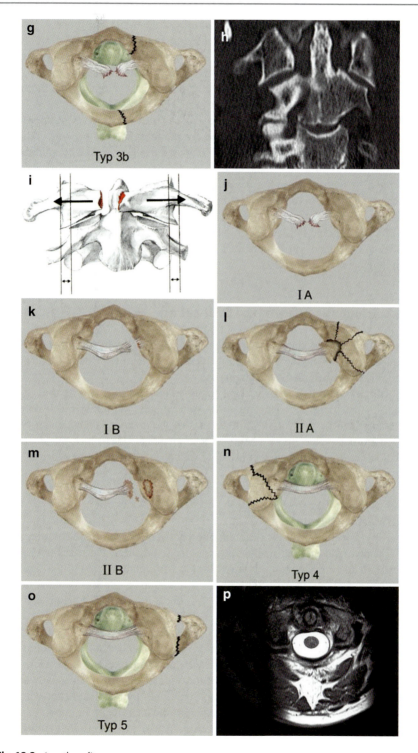

Fig. 12.3 (continued)

Gehweiler type V fractures are isolated fractures of the transverse process. This is a rare fracture type which is typically caused by punches (Fig. 12.3o). In *type III Gehweiler* fractures it is of paramount importance to estimate the stability of the transverse ligament. Besides the indirect signs (Spence rule, ADI, PADI), MRI of the craniocervical junction might be helpful to assess directly the transverse ligament (Fig. 12.3p).

Therapy. Stable *Gehweiler fractures types I, II, IIIa, V and type IV fractures* with minimal or no dislocation can be treated by immobilization in a soft collar for 8 weeks. Type IV fractures with a marked dislocation can be treated by immobilization for 12 weeks in a halo fixateur if a good reposition is achieved and can be maintained. If reposition cannot be achieved or maintained in a halo immobilization, a surgical fixation (either C1/C2 fixation or atlas-osteosynthesis) is indicated. Unstable type IIIb fractures with an interligamentous rupture of the transverse ligament (Dickmann type I) need to be stabilized by C1/C2 fixation. Dickman type 2 injuries can be treated with a mere atlas osteosynthesis or a C1/C2 fixation depending on the degree of dislocation.

12.3.2 Traumatic Atlantoaxial Dislocations

Ligamenteous atlantoaxial dislocations can basically be classified into three groups: translatory, rotatory and axial. Osteoligamentous instabilities such as transdental luxation fractures belong to a different entity.

Translatory atlantoaxial dislocation occurs as consequence of a rupture or bony avulsion of the transverse ligament. As a general rule, the transverse ligament is more stable than the dens axis. On the basis of the anterior atlantodental interval (AADI) (normal value up to 3 mm in adults) which determines the degree of translation Caffinière classified translatory atlantoaxial instabilities fall into three types:
Type I: AADI 4–5 mm (Fig. 12.4a)
Type II: AADI 6–10 mm (Fig. 12.4b)
Type III: AADI > 11 mm (Fig. 12.4c)

Therapy. For treatment, the differentiation between bony avulsions of the transverse ligament and an interligamentous rupture is important. In cases with minor dislocation and contact, a conservative therapy with immobilization in a rigid collar can be carried out. In cases with severe dislocation or interligamentous rupture which have a very low healing tendency, a surgical atlantoaxial fixation has to be carried out.

Traumatic rotatory atlantoaxial dislocation is caused by rupture of the alar ligaments and additional rupture of the capsules of the lateral atlantoaxial joints, and occurs in children and adults after a sufficiently dramatic trauma. However, there is also a non-traumatic form of rotatory atlantoaxial dislocation which usually occurs in children spontaneously without trauma. Sometimes the medical history of these patients is significant for a surgical procedure of the pharynx or an infection of the upper respiratory tract. The degree of dislocation varies and the etiology of the non-traumatic atlantoaxial dislocation remains unclear.

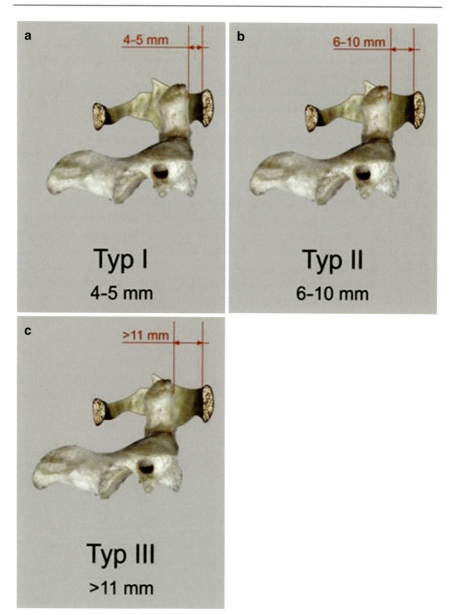

Fig. 12.4 (a) Translatory atalantoaxial dislocations. On the basis of the anterior atlantodental interval (AADI) Caffinière classified translatory atlantoaxial instabilities in three types: *Type I*: AADI 4–5 mm, (**b**) *Type II*: AADI 6–10 mm, (**c**) *Type III*: AADI >11 mm. Reprinted with permission from Kandziora et al. [1]

Fieldings and Hawkins differentiated four types of atantoaxial dislocation:

Type I. Rotatory dislocation without anterior translation of the atlas. The center of rotation is the dens axis, the transverse ligament is intact and the AADI is normal (Fig. 12.5a).

Type II. Rotatory dislocation with anterior translation of the atlas. The sliding distance ranges from 3 to 5 mm. The transverse ligament may be insufficient. One lateral mass of the atlas is dislocated and the contralateral acts as the center of rotation (Fig. 12.5b).

Type III. Rotatory dislocation with anterior translation of the atlas of more than 5 mm. Besides an insufficiency of the transverse ligament, further ligaments and capsules are ruptured (Fig. 12.5c).

Type IV. Rotatory dislocation with posterior translation of the atlas. This type of dislocation is only possible if an additional instability of the dens is present (Fig. 12.5d).

Therapy. Atlantoaxial dislocations with rupture of the transverse ligament usually have to be treated with an atlantoaxial or occipitoatlantoaxial fixation. In cases with intact transverse ligament, a conservative treatment with immobilization in a rigid collar after repositioning is the therapy of choice. In cases with a tendency of relaxation, a halo should be used for immobilization.

Axial (cranial) atlantoaxial dislocations are very rare, unstable injuries with only a few reported cases in the literature. Partial dislocations with high grade instability are differentiated from complete dislocation (Fig. 12.5e, f).

12.3.3 Fractures of the Axis

Fractures of the axis can be assigned to three principal fracture types: (1) fractures of the odontoid, (2) atypical vertebral body fractures of the axis and (3) traumatic spondylolisthesis with fractures of the pars interarticularis.

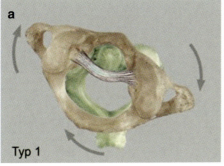 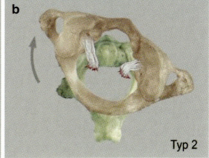

Fig. 12.5 (**a**) Traumatic rotatory atlantoaxial: *Type I*: rotatory dislocation without anterior translation of the atlas. The center of rotation is the dens axis, the transverse ligament is intact and the AADI is normal. (**b**) *Type II*: rotatory dislocation with anterior translation of the atlas. The sliding distance ranges from 3 to 5 mm. (**c**) *Type III*: rotatory dislocation with anterior translation of the atlas of more than 5 mm. (**d**) *Type IV*: rotatory dislocation with posterior translation of the atlas (*arrows* in **a**–**d** indicate the direction of rotation). (**e**) (Axial (cranial) atlantoaxial dislocations are very rare. (**f**) Partial dislocations are differentiated from complete forms. Reprinted with permission from Kandziora et al. [1]

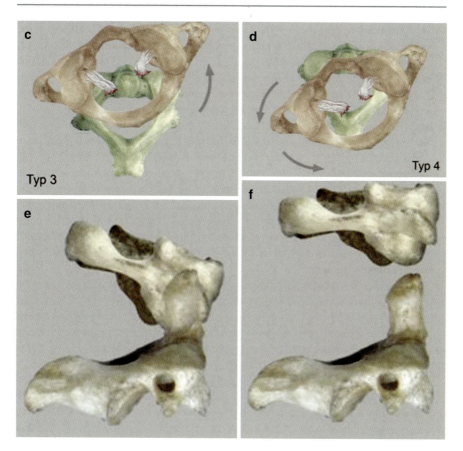

Fig.12.5 (continued)

12.3.4 Odontoid Fractures

Odontoid fractures are a very common fracture type with a reported incidence of 10–20 % of all spine injuries and 17–27 % of cervical spine injuries. Although odontoid fractures occur predominantly in older adults, they may occur at any age. Odontoid fractures are serious injuries with a potential for instability and spinal cord damage. The most commonly used classification was initially described by Anderson and D'Alonzo.

Type 1. Fractures of the tip of the odontoid which are extremely rare and are thought to be avulsion injuries of the apical ligament. They are considered to be stable fractures although they are commonly associated with an atlantooccipital dislocation (Fig. 12.6a).

Type 2. The fracture runs through the base (junction of odontoid and C2 body) of the odontoid (Fig. 12.6b). Based on the orientation of the fracture, type 2 fractures can be subclassified into anterior oblique (Fig. 12.6c), posterior oblique (Fig. 12.6d) and horizontal (Fig. 12.6e). This subclassification has implications for the surgical management. Type 2 odontoid fracture is the most common odontoid fracture and also the most common cervical spine injury.

Type 3. The fracture starts at one cortical surface of the odontoid and runs down into the vertebral body. Usually the fracture line runs in a U-like fashion into the body and separates the dens from the body of the axis (Fig. 12.6f).

Treatment and outcome. Type 1 and 3 fractures and type 2 fractures which are not dislocated and do not show any instability in flexion extension films can be treated with immobilization in a rigid cervical collar for 6–12 weeks. Some spine surgeons prefer an immobilization in a halo vest since this allows for the least motion in flexion extension. However, the halo immobilization is an uncomfortable procedure for the patient and carries a significant risk of morbidity and mortality, especially in older patients.

Dislocated or unstable type 2 fractures need to be surgically stabilized since the fusion rate of this fracture type with external immobilization is low. There are a couple of factors which have been identified as risk factors for a non-union such as patient age, amount of fracture gap, amount of fracture displacement, direction of fracture displacement, redislocation and fracture comminution. Of these factors, patient age is most likely the strongest factor affecting the outcome of type II odontoid fractures.

The overall reported fusion rate of type II odontoid fractures treated with external immobilization in a halo vest is around 70 %. However, this rate decreases with increasing age, with older patients having a significantly increased risk of a fracture non-union after halo vest immobilization. Fracture displacement is another

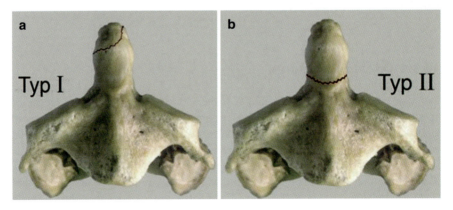

Fig. 12.6 (a) Odontoid fractures. The most commonly used classification was initially described by Anderson and D'Alonzo. *Type 1*: fracture of the tip of the odontoid. (b) *Type 2*: the fracture runs through the base of the odontoid. Based on the orientation of the fracture type 2 fractures can be subclassified into anterior oblique (c), posterior oblique (d) and horizontal (e). This subclassification has implications for the surgical management. (f) *Type 3*: The fracture starts at one cortical surface of the odontoid and runs down into the vertebral body. (g, h) The surgical procedure depends from the orientation of the fracture line. Reprinted with permission from Kandziora et al. 2

12 Spinal Trauma

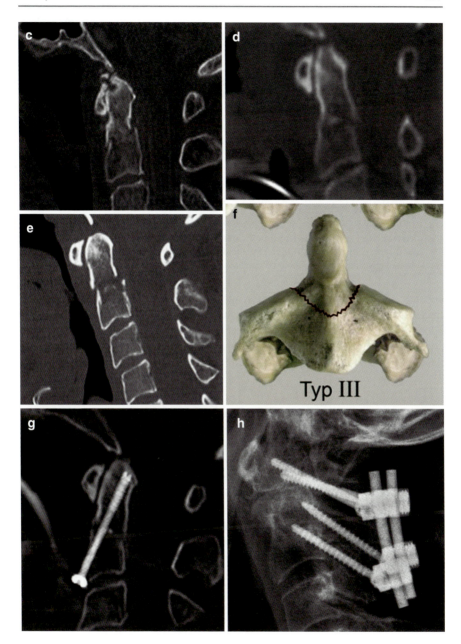

Fig. 12.6 (continued)

significant risk for a non-union with non-union rates of up to 88 % in fracture displacement of more than 4 mm. Therefore primary surgical fixation is the treatment of choice in older patients and fractures with displacement. The surgical procedure

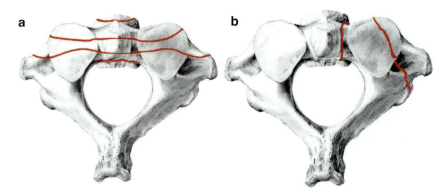

Fig. 12.7 (**a**) Atypical fractures of the vertebral body of the axis are very rare. They have been classified by Benzel et al. in *type 1* fractures with a predominantly coronal orientation of the fracture line, (**b**) *type 2* fractures with sagittal fracture line orientation and *type 3* fractures with a horizontal fracture orientation. Reprinted with permission from Tscherne and Blauth [3]

depends on the orientation of the fracture line. Posterior oblique and horizontal fractures as well as shallow type III fractures should be stabilized with a ventral odontoid screw fixation (Fig. 12.6g). Anterior oblique fractures, dislocated fractures as well as fractures older than 6 months should be treated by a posterior atlantoaxial fixation (Fig. 12.6h).

12.3.5 Atypical Fractures of the Body of the Axis

Atypical fractures of the vertebral body of the axis are very rare and usually occur in combination with other cervical spine injuries. They have been classified by Benzel et al. as *type 1* fractures with a predominantly coronal orientation of the fracture line (Fig. 12.7a), *type 2* fractures with sagittal fracture line orientation and *type 3* fractures with a horizontal fracture orientation (Fig. 12.7b).

Treatment. Types 1 and 2 fractures are usually stable and are treated with immobilization in a soft cervical collar. In dislocated fractures an immobilization in a halo vest or an atlantoaxial stabilization should be considered. In type 3 fractures with instability in functional radiograms, an atlantoaxial fixation should be considered.

12.3.5.1 Traumatic Spondylolisthesis of the Axis

Traumatic spondylolisthesis of the axis, also known as hangman fracture, is a rare injury of the axis which is caused by a hyperextension distraction or hyperextension compression mechanism. The first injury mechanism is seen in judicial hanging which causes a transaction of the spinal cord at the level of C2 and C3. The second mechanism is seen in traffic accidents with impact of the head in hyperextension.

Traumatic spondylolisthesis has initially been classified by Effendi et al. into three types:

Type 1. Fractures with minimal anterior displacement and angulation.

Type 2. Fractures with obvious forward listhesis or angulation in either flexed or extended position.

Type 3. Fractures with anterior displacement with bilateral dislocated and locked facets.

The Effendi classification has been modified by Levine and Edwards:

Type 1. Fractures through the pars interarticularis with displacement of < than 1 mm and no angulation as a result of a hyperextension and axial load (Fig. 12.8a).

Type 1a. Fractures with oblique fracture line often extending into the body on one side as a result of hyperextension and lateral bending.

Type 2. Fractures with displacement of > than 1 mm and significant ventral angulation as a result of hyperextension, axial load and rebound hyperflexion. The C2/C3 disc is disrupted, the anterior longitudinal ligament is intact (Fig. 12.8b, c).

Type 2a. Fractures with displacement of < than 3 mm and significant dorsal angulation (extension) as a result of hyperflexion and distraction. The C2/C3 disc and the anterior longitudinal ligament are disrupted (Fig. 12.8d).

Type 3. Fracture with bilateral locked C2-C3 facet dislocation with ventral angulation (flexion) and displacement as a result of hyperflexion and distraction with rebound hyperextension (Fig. 12.8e).

Treatment and outcome. Types 1 and 2 fractures are treated non-operatively with immobilization in a rigid cervical collar for 6 weeks. Occasionally type 2 fractures can be managed surgically with a direct pars repair according to Judet. Types 2a and 3 fractures should be managed surgically with a ventral C2/C3 discectomy and fusion.

12.4 Subaxial Cervical Spine

The subaxial spine shares many similarities with the thoracolumbar spine. Therefore the AO classification which was initially developed for the thoracolumbar spine has also been adopted for the cervical spine. This classification is primarily based upon radiological and morphological characteristics of the injuries. It is based on a two-column concept as described by Nicoll and Holdsworth. The AO classification differentiates three main categories according to the injury pattern: *type A* – vertebral body compression; *type B* – anterior and posterior element injury with distraction; *type C* – anterior and posterior element injury with rotation. Each type has three groups with a further three subgroups; therefore the AO classification covers a broad range of spine injuries and provides an accurate description.

The classification requires a thin sliced CT scan of the cervical spine, active or passive flexion/extension films or/and an MRI. Occasionally only the intraoperative aspect allows for an assignment of the injury to the correct type, group and subgroup.

12.4.1 Type A Fractures of the Cervical Spine

Group A1: impaction fractures

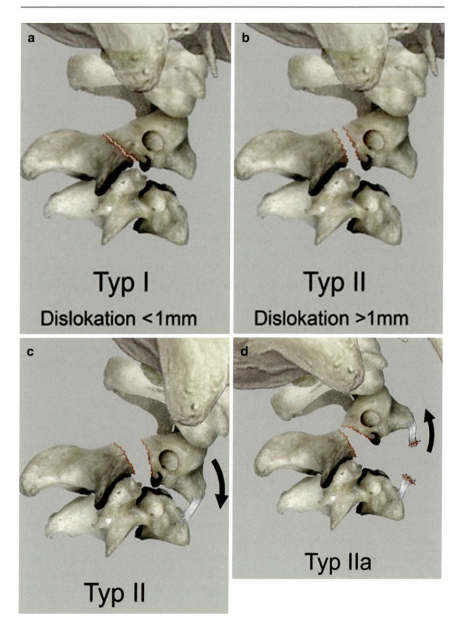

Fig. 12.8 Traumatic spondylolisthesis. The Effendi classification has been modified by Levine and Edwards. (**a**) *Type 1*: fractures through the pars interarticularis with displacement of < than 1 mm and no angulation as a result of a hyperextension and axial load. *Type 1a*: fractures with oblique fracture line often extending into the body on one side (*not shown*). (**b, c**) *Type 2*: fractures with displacement of > than 1 mm and significant ventral angulation (*arrow*), The C2/C3 disc is disrupted, the anterior longitudinal ligament is intact. (**d**) *Type 2a*: fractures with displacement of < than 3 mm and significant dorsal angulation (extension) (*arrow*). The C2/C3 disc and the anterior longitudinal ligament are disrupted. (**e**) *Type 3*: fracture with bilateral locked C2-C3 facet dislocation with ventral angulation (flexion) and displacement. Reprinted with permission from Kandziora et al. 2

Fig. 12.8 (continued)

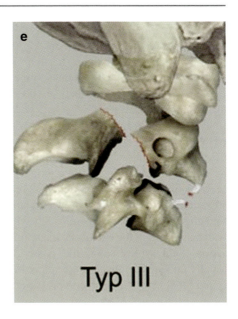

A1.1 end-plate impaction
A1.2 wedge impaction
    A1.2.1 superior wedge impaction
    A1.2.2 lateral wedge impaction
    A1.2.3 inferior wedge impaction
A1.3 vertebral collapse
Group A2: split fractures
    A2.1 sagittal or coronal split fractures
    A2.2 sagittal and coronal split fractures
A2.3 pincer fractures
Group A3: burst fractures
    A3.1 incomplete burst fracture
        A3.1.1 superior incomplete burst fracture
        A3.1.2 lateral incomplete burst fracture
        A3.1.3. inferior incomplete burst fracture
    A3.2 burst-split fractures
        A3.2.1 superior burst-split fracture
        A3.2.2 lateral burst-split fracture
        A3.2.3 inferior burst-split fracture
    A3.3 complete burst fractures
        A3.3.1 pincer burst fracture
        A3.3.2 complete flexion burst fracture
        A3.3.3 complete axial burst fracture

Cervical *type A* injuries show an axial compression with or without flexion. The height of the vertebral body is reduced. An injury of the posterior elements has to be ruled out by MRT or flexion/extension films.

In contrast to the thoracolumbar spine, *type A1* impaction fractures of the cervical spine are rare injuries. There are no signs of subluxation of the facet joints and the vertebral bodies.

Type A2 split fractures can occur in the coronal or sagittal plane. Tear drop injuries correspond to coronal split fractures of the cervical spine and are most often at C5. Tear drop injuries must prompt a thorough evaluation of the posterior elements for an additional injury. Single sagittal or coronal split fracture lines are rare in the cervical spine, although combinations of both are often found. Therefore the classification of this fracture type was modified in comparison to the thoracolumbar fractures. *Type A3* burst fractures always involve the posterior vertebral body wall with narrowing of the spinal canal and possible spinal cord compression. The dislocation of the typical stamp-like posterior wall fragments into the spinal canal is usually not seen in the cervical spine. Most often the whole posterior wall causes spinal canal narrowing and compression of the spinal cord.

12.4.2 Type B Fractures of the Cervical Spine

Group B1: posterior predominantly ligamentous disruptions
    B1.1 with transverse disruption of the disc
        B1.1.1 flexion-subluxation
        B1.1.2 anterior dislocation
        B1.1.3 flexion-subluxation/anterior dislocation with fracture of the articular processes
    B1.2 with type A fracture of the vertebral body
        B1.2.1 flexion-subluxation and type A fracture
        B1.2.2 anterior dislocation and type A fracture
        B1.2.3 flexion-subluxation/anterior dislocation with fracture of the articular processes and type A fracture
Group B2: posterior predominantly osseous disruption
    B2.1 transverse bicolumn fracture
    B2.2 with transverse disruption of the disc
        B2.2.1 disruption through the pedicle and disc
        B2.2.2 disruption through the pars interarticularis and disc (flexion spondylolysis)
    B2.3 with type A fracture of the vertebral body
        B2.3.1 disruption through the pedicle and type A fracture
        B2.3.2 disruption through the pars interarticularis and type A fracture
Group B3: anterior disruption through the disc (hyperextension shear injury)
    B3.1 hyperextension subluxations
        B3.1.1 without injury of the posterior column

B3.1.2 with injury of the posterior column
B3.2 hyperextension spondylolysis
B3.3 posterior dislocation

Cervical type B injuries are characterized by a disruption of the posterior elements as a consequence of a hyperextension or flexion distraction injury mechanism. Group *B1* includes predominantly ligamentous injuries, group *B2* predominantly osseous injuries. Both are caused by a flexion distraction injury mechanism. Group *B3* includes anterior disruptions after hyperextension shear injuries. B1 injuries are frequent and unstable lesions of the lower cervical spine.

12.4.3 Type C Fractures of the Cervical Spine

Group C1: type A (compression) injuries with rotation
    C1.1 rotational wedge fracture
    C1.2 rotational split fracture
        C1.2.1 rotational sagittal split fracture
        C1.2.2 rotational coronal split fracture
        C1.2.3 rotational pincer fracture
        C1.2.4 vertebral body separation
    C1.3 rotational burst fracture
        C1.3.1 incomplete rotational burst fracture
        C1.3.2 rotational burst-split fracture
        C1.3.3 complete rotational burst fracture
Group C2: type B injuries with rotation
    C2.1 B1 injuries with rotation (flexion-distraction injury with rotation)
        C2.1.1 rotational flexion-subluxation
        C2.1.2 rotational flexion-subluxation with unilateral articular process fracture
        C2.1.3 fracture separation of one articular pillar
        C2.1.4 unilateral dislocation
        C2.1.5 rotational anterior dislocation without/with fracture of the articular process
        C2.1.6 rotational flexion-subluxation without/with unilateral articular process fracture and type A fracture
        C2.1.7 unilateral dislocation and type A fracture
        C2.1.8 rotational anterior dislocation without/with fracture of the articular process and type A fracture
    C2.2 B2 injuries with rotation (flexion-distraction injury with rotation)
        C2.2.1 rotational transverse bicolumn fracture
        C2.2.2 unilateral flexion spondylolysis with disruption of the disc
        C2.2.3 unilateral flexion spondylolysis with type A fracture
    C2.3 B3 injury with rotation (hyperextension-shear injury with rotation)

C2.3.1 rotational hyperextension-subluxation without/with fracture of posterior vertebral elements
C2.3.2 unilateral hyperextension spondylolysis
C2.3.3 posterior dislocation with rotation
Group C3: rotational shear injuries
C3.1 slice fracture
C3.2. oblique fracture
C3.3 complete separation

Type C injuries constitute an inhomogeneous injury group. Typical features of type C injuries are rotational displacements, translational displacements in the coronal plane, unilateral fractures of the articular and transverse processes and lateral avulsion fractures of the endplate. Since the uncinate and transverse processes of the cervical vertebrae provide a strong resistance against rotational forces in type A injuries, C1 injuries are very rare. C2 injuries are a result of flexion, distraction and rotation and are quite frequent with up to 40 % of all cervical spine injuries. C3 injuries are very unstable and are also very rare.

12.4.3.1 Therapy

Surgery is indicated if the fracture is considered as unstable, if a compromise of the spinal canal with neurological deficit is present and if a closed reduction cannot be carried out. Types A1 and A2 injuries are usually stable. A2 injuries sometimes develop a non-union with dislocation of posterior wall elements into the spinal canal, which has to be addressed surgically. A3 injuries often compress the spinal cord and/or nerve roots, also an indication for surgery. The majority of types B and C injuries are unstable and need to be treated surgically.

12.5 Sacral Fractures

12.5.1 Aetiology

The sacrum is the most caudal structural segment of the spine. Its five vertebrae start to fuse at the age of 15 years in a caudocranial direction. The fusion is complete at about 25 years of age. From an aetiological standpoint, sacral fractures can be divided into direct injuries caused by direct impact to the sacrum (blow or projectile) and indirect injuries caused by forces acting indirectly on the pelvic ring. Indirect injuries are thought to have more impact on the spinopelvic stability than direct injuries. Injuries to the neural foramina have a high incidence of neurological deficits.

12.5.2 Classification

There have been a number of classifications for sacral fracture described in the literature. The most widely used classification is the one presented by Denis and

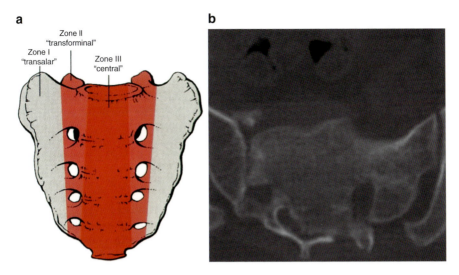

Fig. 12.9 (a) Sacral fractures. The most widely used classification is that presented by Denis and co-workers. Zone 1 is the sacral area lateral to the neuroforamina, zone II encompasses the neural foramina and its contents and zone III is the area in the medium part of the sacrum inclusive the spinal canal. Zone 1 fractures = fractures of the sacral ala are located lateral to the sacral foramina. Zone 2 fractures = fractures of the sacral foramina run through the sacral foramina and may affect the sacral nerve roots. (b) Zone 3 fracture = central sacral fractures run medial from the sacral foramina through the sacral canal. Reprinted with permission from Bühren and Josten [4]

co-workers. He divided the sacrum into three zones. Zone 1 is the sacral area lateral to the neuroforamina, zone II encompasses the neural foramina and its contents and zone III is the area in the medium part of the sacrum including the spinal canal (Fig. 12.9a).

Zone 1 fractures = fractures of the sacral ala are located lateral to the sacral foramina. Lateral compression fractures of the pelvis usually affect the sacral ala. Luxation fractures of the sacro iliac joint often show an avulsion of the sacral ala.

Zone 2 fractures = fractures of the sacral foramina run through the sacral foramina and may affect the sacral nerve roots. About 30 % of patients show neurological deficits.

Zone 3 fractures = central sacral fractures run medial from the sacral foramina through the sacral canal. Therefore neurological complications are seen in up to 60 % of patients.

Zone 1 (transalar) and zone 2 (transforminal) fractures are usually vertical sacrum fractures, while central sacrum fractures show both vertical and horizontal fractures (Fig. 12.9b).

For the evaluation of the stability of sacral fractures the classification of pelvic injuries according to Tile is more suitable.

Type A. Stable injuries of the pelvic ring including isolated horizontal sacral fractures.

Type B. Compression fractures of the pelvis are associated with a rotational instability but are stable in the vertical axis. Occasionally they are combined with ventral sacral fractures in zones 1 and 2 according to Dennis.

Type C. Unstable fractures of the sacrum with a complete separation between spine and pelvis and rotational and vertical instability. The fractures usually run through zones 1 and 2.

12.5.3 Prevalence

Sacral fractures are generally seen in accidents with high impact forces such as falls from great heights, high velocity traffic accidents and running down of pedestrians. Therefore sacrum fractures show a first peak of incidence in younger patients. A second peak is observed in the eighth decade of life. In older patients, osteoporosis is the leading cause of sacral fractures where a simple fall can lead to a sacral fracture.

12.5.4 Symptoms

Sacral fractures are often seen in the setting of polytrauma and an associated pelvic injury. Pelvic injuries might cause symphyseal hematomas, bloody discharge from the rectum and urethra and fixed subluxation position of the legs in a medial or lateral rotation. Complete or incomplete causa equine syndromes might be seen as well as isolated damage to sacral nerve roots and the plexus lumbosacralis.

12.5.5 Diagnosis

Clinical examination should rule out a pelvic instability. If the patient is awake, a neurological examination should rule out damage to the cauda equine, single sacral nerve roots and the plexus lumbosacralis. On plain X-rays, sacral fractures are usually difficult to see. For a general evaluation, inlet and outlet films are helpful. If a sacral or pelvic fracture is seen on plain radiograms, or if there is evidence from the clinical examination, a CT scan is indicated.

12.5.6 Therapy

Stable sacrum fractures are treated conservatively (initial bedrest followed by mobilization under analgesic medication). Unstable sacrum fractures are type c injuries of the pelvis and need a surgical stabilization of the posterior pelvic ring.

12.5.7 Outcome

The general outcome is largely dependent on the concomitant injuries (pelvic, abdominal, traumatic brain injury). The specific outcome is dependent on the presence and extent of neurological injury.

12.6 Traumatic Spinal Cord Injury

12.6.1 Aetiology

Traumatic spinal cord injury (SCI) is a dramatic incident with devastating consequences for the rest of the life of the patients and their relatives. In 40 %, SCI is caused by fractures of the cervical spine and in 15–20 % by fractures of the thoracic and the upper lumbar spine. Traffic accidents (45 %) are the leading cause of SCI followed by falls (housekeeping, work, sport) and criminal violence.

12.6.2 Prevalence

In industrial countries the incidence per year of SCI is estimated to be 10–50 per 1,000,000 citizens. SCI frequently affects younger people, 70 % of all new SCI victims being 15–30 years of age and 70–80 % of the patients male.

12.6.3 Symptoms

Severe SCI frequently leads to spinal shock with flaccid paralysis, areflexia, and vegetative dysfunction, including the loss of bowel and bladder control. Major symptoms of vegetative dysfunction are arterial hypotension, bradycardia and loss of thermoregulation. Spinal shock symptoms usually recede within several days to 6 weeks. After subsiding of the spinal shock, the typical symptoms for a central paralysis with spasticity and hyperreflexia develop. Even after this period, SCI patients are at risk of severe vegetative derailments with excessive hypertension, especially in lesions higher than T5. Paralysis in SCI patients can be complete or incomplete. To understand the neurological deficits in SCI patients, knowledge of the anatomy and spinal cord is essential. During ontogenesis a progressive shifting between the vertebral segment and the associated spinal cord segment occurs, resulting in an "ascent" of the spinal cord. In adults the spinal cord diminishes in thickness below TH12 and ends at the lower endplate of L1. Lesions higher than C4 cause, beside a tetraparesis, a complete paralysis of breathing. Lesions below the cervical spinal cord affect the trunk and the legs with a pure diaphragmatic respiration. Below the affected segment the muscles are paralyzed with hyposensibility and a loss of bowel and bladder control, as well as sexual dysfunction.

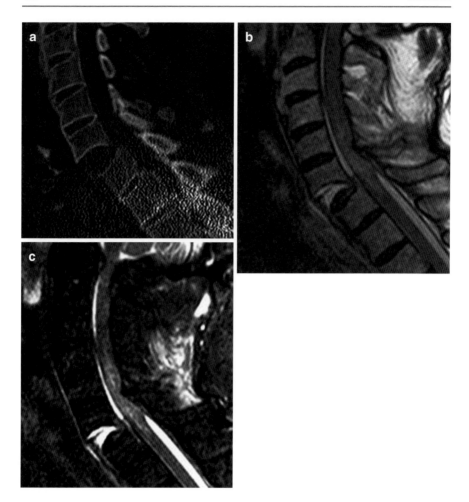

Fig. 12.10 (a) Patient with a clinical complete spinal cord injury with a sensorimotor level of C6. CT shows a "bamboo" spine as a result of ankylosing spondylitis and disruption of the C6/7 disc. (b, c) MRI shows the discoligamentous injury with increased signal intensity of the disc as well as an edema of the spinal cord

Accidents usually cause functional "disruption" rather than anatomical. Complete transection of the spinal cord is very rare (Fig. 12.10a–c).

Traumatic SCI leads to characteristic time dependent biochemical and pathological changes. The initial damage (primary injury) is caused by the direct impact of forces on the spinal cord. Within 24 h a progressive pathophysiological cascade develops and causes further damage to the neural tissue (secondary injury). Unlike the primary injury, the secondary injury is (at least theoretically) amenable to therapeutic intervention.

12.6.4 Diagnosis

In SCI patients an immediate thorough neurological examination is necessary as a baseline for further follow-up examinations. For documentation of the strength of muscles, the six grade scale of the British Medical Research Council should be used. For the classification and documentation of the neurological status the American Spinal Injury Association and the International Medical Society of Paraplegia developed a scheme for a standardized documentation of the neurological status which has gained a wide acceptance. The ASIA Impairment Scale (AIS) which differentiates five grades (A–E) is based on muscle, sensory and anorectal examination and is predictive for the prognosis of SCI. A detailed description of the examination can be found at http://www.asia-spinalinjury.org.

12.6.5 Therapy

To date there is no specific therapy available for the treatment of SCI. Over many years the early (<8 h) administration of methylprednisolone (MPS) has been the standard therapy after the efficacy and benefit of this substance on the outcome of SCI patients has been demonstrated in three large multicenter studies. MPS is an anti-inflammatory and anti-edematic acting substance, inhibits the release of glutamate and acts as a free radicals scavenger. Because of often (for patients) functionally irrelevant improvement and the severe, sometimes life threatening, complications, MPS has come under criticism and in many countries the general administration of MPS in SCI is no longer recommended. From animal studies there is convincing evidence that early decompression in the setting of SCI improves the neurological outcome. However, because of conflicting results from clinical studies, the effect of early decompression in patients with SCI has remained uncertain. A recent multicenter, prospective cohort study (Surgical Timing in Acute Spinal Cord Injury Study: STASCIS) could demonstrate that early decompression prior to 24 h after SCI can be performed safely and is associated with improved neurological outcome.

12.6.6 Outcome

Since the therapeutic options in SCI are still very limited, the prognosis is dependent on the extent of the injury according to the AIS (incomplete vs complete) and whether an initial improvement is observed. Complete SCI without any improvement after 24–48 h has a bad prognosis. If an initial improvement is observed, the improvement usually proceeds fastest in the first 3 months and comes to an end around 12 months after the injury.

References

1. Kandziora F, Schnake K, Hoffmann R (2010a) Verletzungen der oberen Halswirbelsäule Teil 1: Ligamentäre Verletzungen, 2010, Springer, Berlin Heidelberg, Unfallchirurg 113:931–943
2. Kandziora F, Schnake K, Hoffmann R (2010b) Verletzungen der oberen Halswirbelsäule Teil 2: Knöcherne Verletzungen, 2010, Springer Berlin, Heidelberg, Unfallchirurg 113:1023–1041
3. Tscherne H, Blauth M (eds.) Unfallchirurgie Wirbelsäule 1998, Springer, Berlin, Heidelberg
4. Bühren V, Josten C (Hrsg.) (2013) Chirurgie der verletzten Wirbelsäule Frakturen, Instabilitäten, Deformitäten, Springer, Berlin, Heidelberg
5. Harris JH, Carson GC, Wagner LK, Kerr N (1994) Radiologic diagnosis of traumatic occipitovertebral dissociation: 2. Comparison of three methods of detecting occipitovertebral relationships on lateral radiographs of supine subjects. AJR Am J Roentgenol. 162:887–892
6. Traynelis VC, Marano GD, Dunker RO, Kaufman HH (1986) Traumatic atlanto-occipital dislocation. Case report. J Neurosurg. 65:863–870.

Further Reading

1. Aebi M, Arlet V, Webb JK (2007) AO manual, vol 1 and 2. Thieme, Stuttgart/New York
2. Grauer JN, Shafi B, Hilibrand AS, Harrop JS, Kwon BK, Beiner JM, Albert TJ, Fehlings MG, Vaccaro AR (2005) Proposal of a modified, treatment-oriented classification of odontoid fractures. Spine J 5(2):123–129
3. Magerl F, Aebi M, Gertzbein SD, Harms J, Nazarian S (1994) A comprehensive classification of thoracic and lumbar injuries. Eur Spine J 3(4):184–201
4. Schwab JM, Brechtel K, Mueller CA, Failli V, Kaps HP, Tuli SK, Schluesener HJ (2006) Experimental strategies to promote spinal cord regeneration – an integrative perspective. Prog Neurobiol 78(2):91–116
5. Vaccaro AR, Lehman RA Jr, Hurlbert RJ, Anderson PA, Harris M, Hedlund R, Harrop J, Dvorak M, Wood K, Fehlings MG, Fisher C, Zeiller SC, Anderson DG, Bono CM, Stock GH, Brown AK, Kuklo T, Oner FC (2005) A new classification of thoracolumbar injuries: the importance of injury morphology, the integrity of the posterior ligamentous complex, and neurologic status. Spine (Phila Pa 1976) 30(20):2325–2333
6. Vaccaro AR, Oner C, Kepler CK, Dvorak M, Schnake K, Bellabarba C, Reinhold M, Aarabi B, Kandziora F, Chapman J, Shanmuganathan R, Fehlings M, Vialle L, AOSpine Spinal Cord Injury & Trauma Knowledge Forum (2013) AOSpine thoracolumbar spine injury classification system: fracture description, neurological status, and key modifiers. Spine (Phila Pa 1976) 38(23):2028–2037

Meningeal Disorders

13

Marlies Wagner and Johannes C. Klein

Contents

13.1 Introduction 271
13.2 Spinal Meningitis 272
    13.2.1 Bacterial Meningitis 272
    13.2.2 Subdural Abscess/Empyema 275
    13.2.3 Tuberculous Meningitis 276
    13.2.4 Neurosarcoidosis 276
    13.2.5 Guillain-Barré Syndrome 279
13.3 Neoplastic Meningeosis 280
13.4 Other Pachy- and Leptomeningeal Diseases 286
    13.4.1 Spinal CSF Leakage 286
    13.4.2 Spinal Cord Herniation 291
    13.4.3 Subdural Hematoma 293
    13.4.4 Idiopathic Hypertrophic Spinal Pachymeningitis 294
    13.4.5 Arachnopathy 296
Further Reading 299

13.1 Introduction

Meningeal disorders of the spine form a heterogenous group of diseases, affecting the spinal cord and its nerve roots through their intimate contact. Meningeal disease can, at times, present with back pain only. However, neurological symptoms are the more common manifestation leading to diagnosis, be it through compression of the

M. Wagner
Institute of Neuroradiology, Goethe-University,
Schleusenweg 2-16, D-60528 Frankfurt, Germany
e-mail: marlies.wagner@kgu.de

J.C. Klein
Brain Imaging Center (BIC), Department of Neurology, Goethe-University,
Schleusenweg 2-16, D-60528 Frankfurt, Germany
e-mail: klein@med.uni-frankfurt.de

spinal cord or of the spinal nerves. MRI is the imaging modality of choice when meningeal disease of the spine is suspected. Wherever possible, imaging studies should precede diagnostic lumbar puncture, because contrast enhancement of the dural sac can occur subsequent to lumbar puncture. If imaging is performed after lumbar puncture, it may be impossible to distinguish between enhancement through meningeal disease and transient changes subsequent to opening of the dural space.

In this chapter, we will introduce typical imaging findings of meningeal disorders. There is significant overlap between radiological presentations of different disorders. Clinical information on the evolution of symptoms, the pace of disease progression, and CSF findings help interpret imaging findings and establish the correct diagnosis.

13.2 Spinal Meningitis

Infectious spinal meningitis is a significant cause of morbidity and mortality. Pathogens include "typical" bacteria such as *S. aureus* (acute onset), syphilis, mycobacteria (*M. tuberculosis*, "atypical" mycobacteria such as *M. bovis*, *M. fortuitum*, etc., predominantly in immunocompromised patients), viruses (subacute onset), and fungi (fluctuating symptoms, chronic manifestation). In Western countries, parasitic infections are comparatively rare (cysticercosis, amoebae, toxocara, etc.).

Predisposing factors include immunodeficiency, old age, and physical disability. Diagnosis is suspected on the basis of clinical symptoms and CSF analysis. Treatment includes organism-specific antibiotic/virustatic therapy, dexamethasone to inhibit inflammation, and supportive care. Other causes of spinal meningitis include specific granulomatous diseases like Wegener's granulomatosis, sarcoidosis, and inflammation of unknown origin such as idiopathic hypertrophic spinal pachymeningitis. Clinically important complications of spinal meningitis include subdural or epidural abscess formation, development of syrinx, and arachnopathy.

Imaging: The imaging modality of choice is MRI with intravenous application of contrast materials. CT myelography is an alternative in patients with contraindications for MRI. Differential diagnoses with similar imaging findings include neoplastic meningeosis, arachnopathy, intracranial hypotension, idiopathic hypertrophic spinal pachymeningitis, and Guillain-Barré syndrome.

13.2.1 Bacterial Meningitis

Aside from the extension from cranial infection via CSF, other common pathways for the spread of bacterial meningitis include hematogenous or direct extension from extraspinal foci of infection. Routes include sinus, meningocele, or CSF leaks and iatrogenic routes from surgical procedures or lumbar puncture. Since the late 1990s, the rate of bacterial meningitis decreased in the Western world, mainly due to *Haemophilus influenzae* type b conjugate vaccine for infants. Nowadays, the most common infective species causing bacterial meningitis are *Streptococcus pneumoniae* and group B *Streptococcus* (B-S). Other common pathogens of bacterial meningitis are *Neisseria meningitidis* and *Listeria monocytogenes*. A recent study estimates the incidence of bacterial meningitis in the USA with 1.38 per 100,000 population; however, there is an uneven distribution with by far the highest incidence in newborns (B-S). Clinically, spinal bacterial meningitis might manifest by acute headache, back pain, fever, neck stiffness, decreased consciousness, seizures indicating cerebral involvement, and focal neurological symptoms.

Imaging (Figs. 13.1 and 13.2): On T2WI, the arachnoid surrounding the spinal cord and nerve roots might be thickened, and an irregular contour of the dural sac might be seen. The spinal cord might show focal inflammatory myelopathy with increased signal and swelling. On T1WI, an increased signal of the CSF might be seen which is caused by high protein content. On contrast-enhanced T1WI, typical findings include diffuse, less frequently focal enhancement of the leptomeningeal structures that can be smooth or nodular. CSF might enhance homogeneously, indicating leakage of contrast materials from the vasculature.

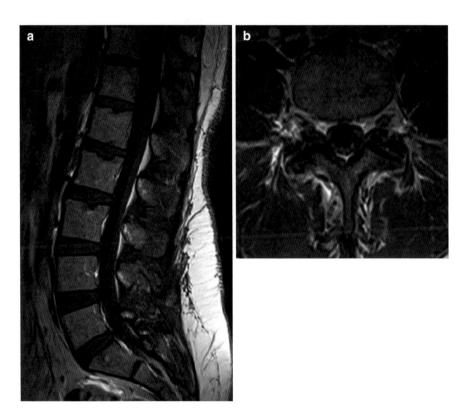

Fig. 13.1 Bacterial spinal meningitis. Patient with bacterial spinal meningitis (*S. pneumoniae*) extended from cranial meningitis. Contrast-enhanced T1WI shows diffuse smooth enhancement of the conus medullaris and equina cauda (sagittal, **a**); the equina cauda is slightly thickened (sagittal and axial, **a** and **b**)

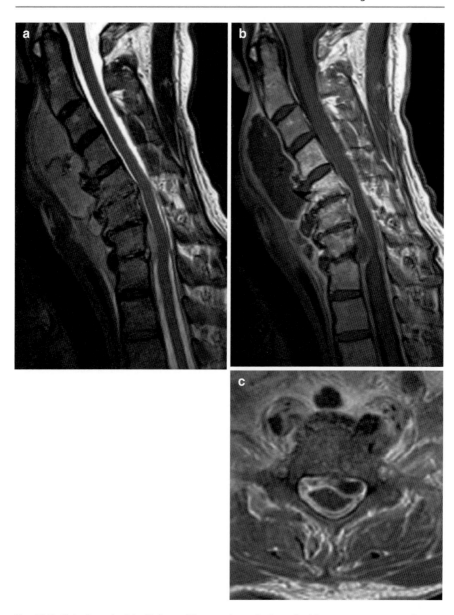

Fig. 13.2 Spinal meningitis. Patient with extensive spinal meningitis as a consequence of spondylodiscitis (C5/6, 6/7, and C7/Th1, **a** and **b**); other complications shown include prevertebral and epidural abscesses. T2WI (sagittal, **a**) shows pachymeningeal thickening; abscesses show intermediate signal. Intervertebral spaces C5/6, 6/7, and C7/Th1 and adjacent vertebra show hyperintense signal caused by inflammatory edema. Contrast-enhanced T1WI (sagittal and axial, **b** and **c**) shows massive enhancement of pachy- and leptomeningeal structures and rim-enhancing abscesses. There is diffuse enhancement of the surrounding soft tissue as well (axial)

13 Meningeal Disorders

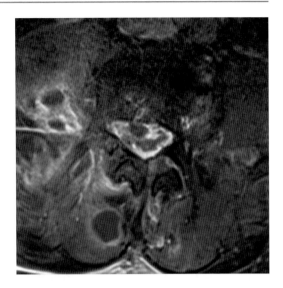

Fig. 13.3 Subdural abscess. Contrast-enhanced T1WI shows neurosurgically confirmed subdural abscess with circumscript intraspinal hypointense fluid collection and massive enhancement of the meninges. The adjacent subarachnoid space is compressed. Note further abscesses and diffuse enhancement of the surrounding soft tissue (right psoas muscle and autochthonous back muscles)

13.2.2 Subdural Abscess/Empyema

Collections of pus in the potential subdural spinal space between the dura and arachnoid are rare, and only less than 100 cases of spinal subdural empyema extending over multiple spinal levels have been reported in the literature. Patients are usually of higher age (60–70 years), and women are more often affected than men (2:1). Etiologically, subdural abscesses/empyemas usually result from invasion of pathogens due to surgical procedures or trauma or from a continuous spread from adjacent inflammatory processes. Less common subdural abscess/empyema is caused by hematogenous spread or idiopathically. The most common pathogens are *Streptococci* and *Staphylococcus aureus*.

Spinal subdural abscesses/empyemas are most commonly located in the lumbar region, followed by the cervical region. Clinically, patients present with signs of meningeal irritation, increased intracranial pressure, fever, and back pain. The symptom onset is usually rapid and sometimes fulminant. Due to its potential rapid compressive effect, spinal subdural abscess/empyema represents an extreme medical and neurosurgical emergency. Treatment of choice is surgical drainage followed by appropriate antibiotic therapy; dexamethasone should be added postsurgically.

Imaging (Fig. 13.3): On MRI or CT, thin intradural extramedullary fluid collection with potential gas accompanied by diffuse subdural thickening should be considered subdural abscess/empyema. Spinal cord displacement, impingement, and edema might be seen also. T2WI shows hyperintense fluid; its presence might be suggested by mass effect on the spinal cord and obliterated subarachnoid space. Contrast-enhanced T1WI shows heterogeneous, diffuse subdural enhancement and hypointense, rim-enhancing fluid collection. Axial imaging confirms subdural localization.

13.2.3 Tuberculous Meningitis

Tuberculous meningitis of the spine can present as primary tuberculous radiculomyelitis. More frequently, it is secondary to cranial meningitis or vertebral involvement. Although tuberculous meningitis is the least frequent presentation of extrapulmonary tuberculosis, it is the most severe form in terms of mortality and morbidity. The so-called atypical mycobacteria may present identically in terms of clinical and radiological manifestation; pathogens include *M. avium* complex (most common atypical form), *M. kansasii, M. peregrinum, M. scrofulaceum, M. gordonae*, and *M. fortuitum*. Clinical symptoms include fever, back pain, radicular symptoms, focal neurological deficits, and fatigue. In contrast to typical bacterial meningitis of acute onset, symptoms of tuberculous meningitis usually manifest chronically and fluctuate in terms of severity and location.

Imaging (Figs. 13.4 and 13.5): The typical imaging findings of tuberculous meningitis are similar to those of typical bacterial meningitis. However, involvement of the pachymeninges is more common. There are frequent nodular enhancement and nerve root thickening, caused by acute edematous swelling or chronic adhesions. On T2WI, the arachnoid surrounding the spinal cord and nerve roots can be thickened, and an irregular contour of the dural sac might be seen. The spinal cord can exhibit focal inflammatory myelopathy with increased signal and swelling. On T1WI, an increased signal of the CSF might be seen which is caused by high protein content. On contrast-enhanced T1WI, mycobacteriosis typically presents with diffuse enhancement of the meninges, including the posterior fossa. Less frequently, focal nodular enhancement of the pachy- and leptomeningeal structures can be observed. The CSF can enhance homogeneously. If nodular thickening is extensive, it can be seen on CT myelography.

13.2.4 Neurosarcoidosis

Neurosarcoidosis is a rare manifestation of sarcoidosis (5–15 %) that can affect the spinal meninges. If present, meningeal involvement is usually secondary to spinal cord involvement. Less commonly, meningeal involvement can occur as the primary spinal presentation (10–20 %). Sarcoidosis typically presents between the third and fourth decades of life; the overall disease prevalence of neurosarcoidosis is estimated at 4 per 100,000. African Americans are affected three to four times more frequently than Caucasians. Pathologically, sarcoidosis is characterized by noncaseating granulomatous inflammation of unknown origin. Elevated angiotensin converting enzyme and other systemic manifestations help with diagnosis. When neurosarcoidosis occurs without other organ manifestations, diagnosis is problematic, and biopsy of neural tissue remains the gold standard of diagnosis. The typical signs of meningitis aside, clinical symptoms depend on the anatomic location and can range from asymptomatic manifestation (10 %) to focal neurological signs and neuropsychiatric symptoms. Acute meningitis due to neurosarcoidosis responds

13 Meningeal Disorders

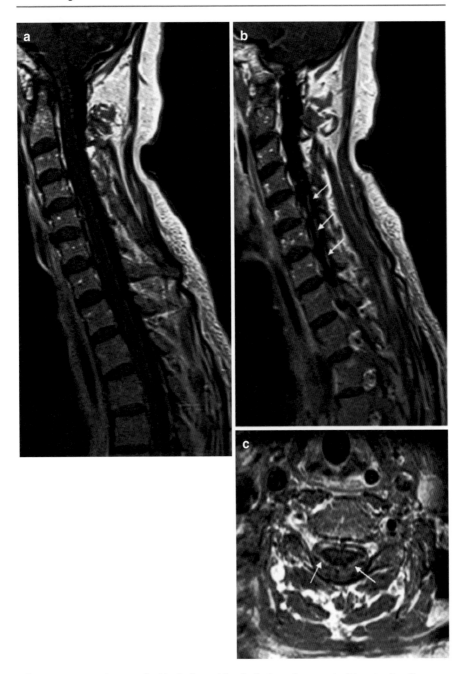

Fig. 13.4 Tuberculous meningitis. Patient with spinal tuberculous meningitis extending from cranial manifestation. Contrast-enhanced T1WI (**a**, **c**) shows extensive nodular enhancement of the leptomeninges (including cerebral basal meningitis) surrounding the spinal cord and massive thickening and enhancement of nerve roots (**b** and **c**)

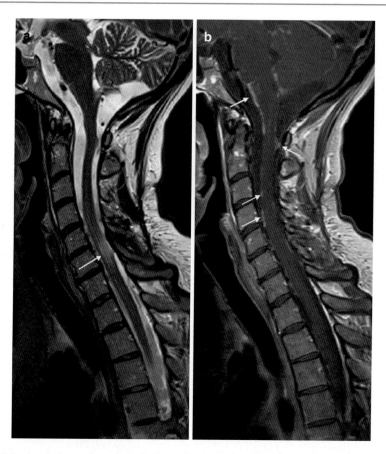

Fig. 13.5 Atypical mycobacteriosis. Patient with atypical mycobacteriosis (*M. fortuitum*). T2WI (sagittal, **a**) shows slight deformation of the upper cervical spinal cord and a short dilation of the central canal; circumscript myelopathy is visible at level C6. Furthermore, small hypointense nodules of the meninges are seen at levels C5 and C6. Contrast-enhanced T1WI (sagittal, **b**) shows diffuse and nodular leptomeningeal enhancement

well to systemic corticosteroids and other immunosuppressants including azathioprine and methotrexate; however, chronic meningitis is usually persistent and requires long-term therapy.

Imaging (Fig. 13.6): MRI shows leptomeningeal and nerve root enhancement, mimicking spinal bacterial or tuberculous meningitis, and swelling of the spinal cord with myelopathic edema. T2WI might reveal nodular hypointense thickening of the arachnoid and fusiform hyperintense swelling of the spinal cord close by. On contrast-enhanced T1WI, nodular leptomeningeal enhancement is typically found. This can include the cranial basilar meninges and the nerve roots. The adjacent spinal cord can show focal fusiform hypointense swelling and focal enhancement.

13 Meningeal Disorders

Fig. 13.6 Neurosarcoidosis. Contrast-enhanced, fat-saturated T1WI shows nodular enhancement of leptomeningeal structures including the cauda equina. Fusiform swelling and irregular enhancement of the conus medullaris reveal spinal cord involvement

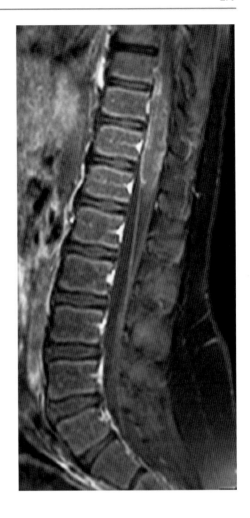

13.2.5 Guillain-Barré Syndrome

The incidence of Guillain-Barré syndrome (GBS) ranges between 1 and 2 per 100,000. Men are more frequently affected than women (2:1). Most patients had suffered from upper respiratory tract infection or diarrhea some weeks before, and GBS is suspected to be caused by an autoimmune response affecting the peripheral nerves and their roots. The most common infectious agent associated with GBS is *Campylobacter jejuni*, a pathogen causing diarrhea. GBS is classified into two subtypes: acute inflammatory demyelinating polyneuropathy and acute motor axonal neuropathy. Initially, typical clinical symptoms include ascending paralysis beginning with progressive symmetric paraparesis with hypo- or areflexia, distal paresthesia, and, possibly, urinary retention. During progression, meningeal, muscular, radicular, and arthralgic pain, respiratory insufficiency, life-threatening cardiac arrhythmia, and psychiatric symptoms may occur. Diagnosis is more likely in the presence of albuminocytologic dissociation. Patients should be kept under hospital observation until there is no more evidence for disease progression. Patients should be monitored regarding cardiac and pulmonary dysfunction. Treatment includes intravenous immune globulin or plasma exchange, if patients are not able to walk unassisted, while corticosteroids are not effective.

Imaging (Fig. 13.7): Contrast-enhanced T1WI may demonstrate diffuse enhancement of conus medullaris and cauda equina including leptomeningeal structures, and nerve root thickening might be present.

13.3 Neoplastic Meningeosis

Neoplastic meningeosis is the result of malignant cells seeding into the leptomeninges. It occurs in 1–5 % of patients with solid tumors (*Meningeosis carcinomatosa*), in 5–15 % of patients with leucemia (*Meningeosis leucemica*) or lymphoma (*Meningeosis lymphomatosa*), and in 1–2 % of patients with primary brain tumors (glioblastoma, medulloblastoma/PNET, ependymoma, etc.).

Meningeosis neoplastica: homogenous or nodular thickening of the leptomeninx and nerve roots
- *Meningeosis carcinomatosa*
- *Meningeosis leucemica*
- *Meningeosis lymphomatosa*
- Spread of primary brain tumors

The solid tumors most commonly spreading to the leptomeninges are melanoma (20 % of leptomeningeal metastases), small-cell lung cancer (11 %), and breast cancer (5 %). Leptomeningeal metastases usually occur as one manifestation of widespread metastatic disease. Sometimes, it may even be the first clinical manifestation of the underlying malignancy. Tumor cells may invade via the bloodstream; via direct extension from an extrameningeal focus, such as tumors of perineural or perivascular location; or via the CSF from an intracranial tumor. Clinical symptoms depend on location and the amount of CSF blockage and include back pain, intracranial hypertension, and neurological deficits such as paralysis, loss of sensation, and cauda equina symptoms.

Diagnosis should be made in patients with a known malignancy through CSF analysis. The median survival for patients without treatment is 4–6 weeks. Treatment options are mainly palliative and include surgery, radiation- and chemotherapy, and supportive care.

13 Meningeal Disorders

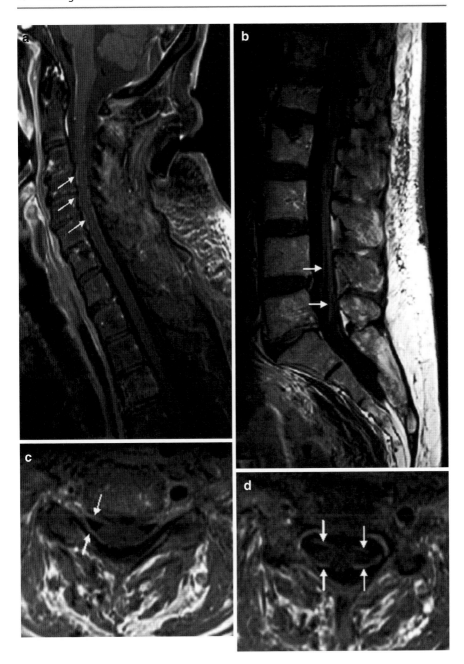

Fig. 13.7 Guillain-Barré syndrome. Patient with GBS showing massive thickening and enhancement of nerve roots (**c, d**) and cauda equina (**b**), extending from the cervical to sacral spinal canal on contrast-enhanced T1WI (sagittal **a, b** and axial **c, d**)

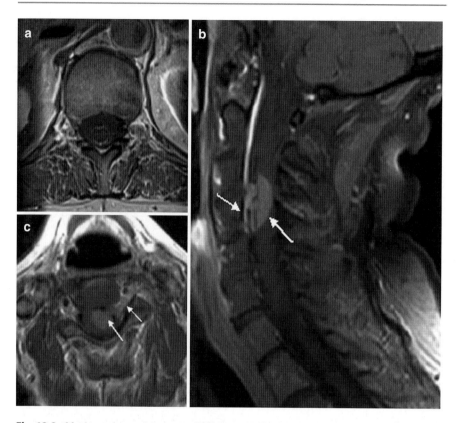

Fig. 13.8 *Meningeosis carcinomatosa*. Different manifestations of *Meningeosis carcinomatosa* in two different patients suffering from lung cancer. Axial contrast-enhanced T1WI (**a**) reveals homogenous enhancement of leptomeningeal structures. Contrast-enhanced axial and sagittal T1WI (**b, c**) shows an enhancing intramedullary mass (medullar metastasis) with lepto- and pachymeningeal involvement and extension along the left nerve root C4 (**c**)

Imaging (Figs. 13.8, 13.9, 13.10, 13.11, 13.12, and 13.13): The entire spinal axis has to be included, such as not to miss manifestations outside the clinically apparent areas. It is of special importance to visualize the complete dural sac including its caudal end, which is a focal point for the so-called drop metastases. In *Meningeosis neoplastica*, the spinal ganglion is commonly involved, as can be demonstrated by nerve conduction studies, which is rare in arachnoiditis due to other pathologies.

> Check the entire dural sac including its caudal end, which is a focal point for the so-called drop metastases

T2WI can show hypointense nodular metastases in the subarachnoid space adjacent to leptomeningeal structures or as "drop metastases" in the caudal dural sac.

Homogenous or focal thickening of dural (especially in leucemia) or leptomeningeal structures may also be seen. However, those changes might be difficult to find in T2WI. The cauda equina might be distributed asymmetrically in the spinal canal in carcinomatous arachnoiditis. However, asymmetry of nerve roots is not specific and seen in all other leptomeningeal disorders as well. Contrast-enhanced T1WI shows enhancement of nodular metastases. Typically, strong enhancement of the thickened leptomeninges ("zuckerguss" appearance, German for sugar icing) can be observed. CT myelography might reveal filling defects accordingly, an option for patients with contraindications to MRI.

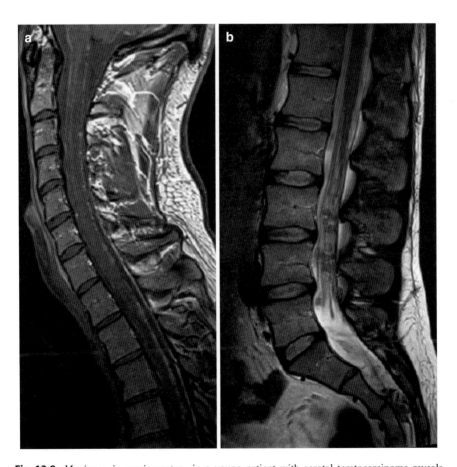

Fig. 13.9 *Meningeosis carcinomatosa* in a young patient with scrotal teratocarcinoma reveals nodular thickening and enhancement of the leptomeninges of the cervical spinal cord (contrast-enhanced T1WI, **a**). T2WI (**b**) of the lumbar spine reveals nodular metastases of the subarachnoid space, affecting the cauda equina. Metastasis at the caudal end of the dural sac might be missed if this region is not included during planning of the MR study. Sagittal contrast-enhanced T1WI (**c**) shows intense enhancement of subarachnoid metastases that extend down to the caudal end of the dural sac. Axial contrast-enhanced T1WI (**d**) shows asymmetrical distribution and thickening of the enhancing cauda equina (carcinomatous arachnoiditis)

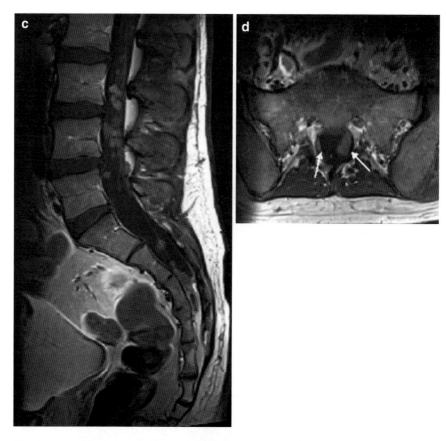

Fig. 13.9 (continued)

Fig. 13.10 *Meningeosis leucemica.* Sagittal contrast-enhanced T1WI reveals circumscript, nodular, contrast-enhancing leptomeningeal metastasis at the back of the cervical spinal cord at level C1. Also note the leptomeningeal involvement of the posterior fossa

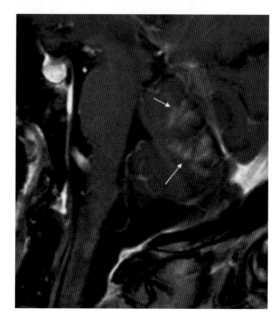

13 Meningeal Disorders

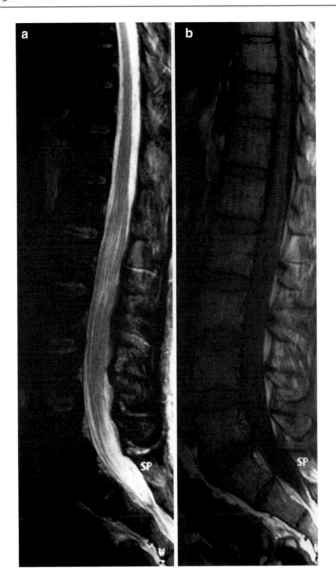

Fig. 13.11 *Meningeosis lymphomatosa.* Sagittal and axial T2WI (**a**, **d**) shows thickening of the cauda equina with unusual distribution of nerve roots. Native (**b**) and contrast-enhanced T1WI (**c**, **e**) reveals enhancement of the conus medullaris and cauda equina

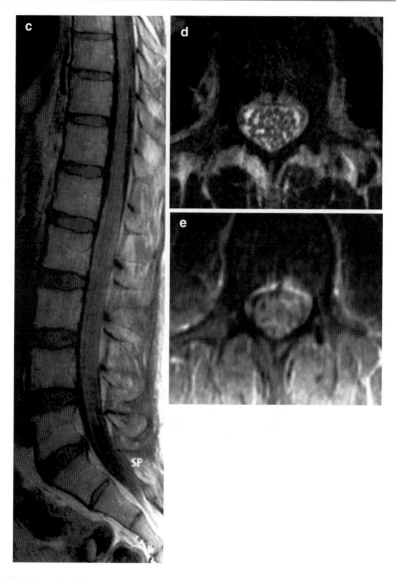

Fig. 13.11 (continued)

13.4 Other Pachy- and Leptomeningeal Diseases

13.4.1 Spinal CSF Leakage

Spinal CSF leaks are caused by even unremarkable trauma in approximately 30 % of cases, such as coughing, sporting activities, falls, or chiropractic manipulation. Also, spinal CSF leaks occur postsurgically. However, in the majority of patients, the cause of CSF leakage remains unclear and is thus called idiopathic. Women are

13 Meningeal Disorders

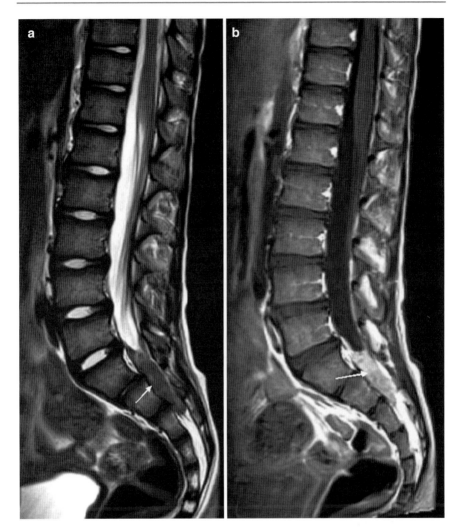

Fig. 13.12 Metastases from medulloblastoma. A 6-year-old boy with cerebellar medulloblastoma. Sagittal T2WI (**a**) shows singular hypointense solid drop metastasis in the caudal dural sac. Sagittal contrast-enhanced T1WI (**b**) reveals strong enhancement of this drop metastasis

more commonly affected than men. Patients usually are around 30–50 years of age. The most common location of spinal CSF leak is the thoracic spine. The leading clinical symptom is orthostatic headache; other symptoms include neck stiffness, tinnitus, nausea and vomiting, or even psychiatric symptoms. Diagnostic procedures should include measurement of CSF opening pressure in the sitting position (<60 mm H_2O) and CSF analysis expecting moderately increased protein but otherwise normal values. Subarachnoid hemorrhage must be excluded. Most cases respond well to conservative therapy including bed rest, oral hydration, and administration of corticosteroids or caffeine. In patients with persisting symptoms, an

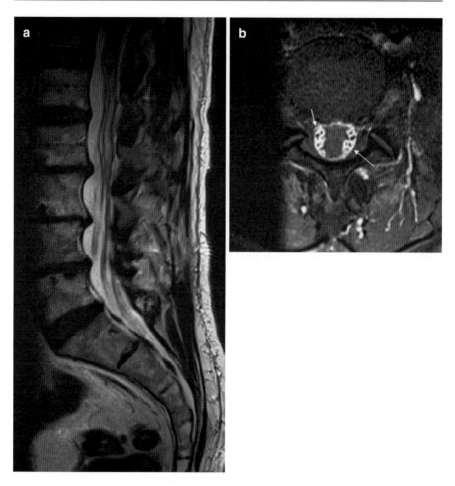

Fig. 13.13 Metastases from glioblastoma. Patient with cerebral glioblastoma. Sagittal T2WI (**a**) shows thickening and atypical distribution of the cauda equina. Axial contrast-enhanced T1WI (**b**) reveals circular enhancement of the cauda equina, which is distributed around the margin of the dural sac (*Meningeosis gliomatosa*)

epidural blood patch is an established treatment option, which is more effective if the exact position of the CSF leak is known.

Imaging (Figs. 13.14 and 13.15)**:** The spinal CSF leak may be difficult to detect with any imaging modality. On MRI, indirect signs of CSF leak include diffuse smooth dural thickening and enhancement due to venous engorgement, cerebellar tonsillar descent, an effaced prepontine space in the posterior fossa, and subdural hematoma. To localize the CSF leak, the first step is conventional MRI of the spinal axis using fat-saturated T2WI. In case of diagnostic failure, CT myelography or MR myelography using intrathecal gadolinium application might be considered. However, the intrathecal use of gadolinium is still off-label use, and inadequate dosing might lead to temporary or persisting toxic damage of the spinal cord. After correct intrathecal application of gadolinium (see current protocols in the literature) via lumbar puncture, sagittal and axial T1WI MRI with spectral fat saturation should be performed.

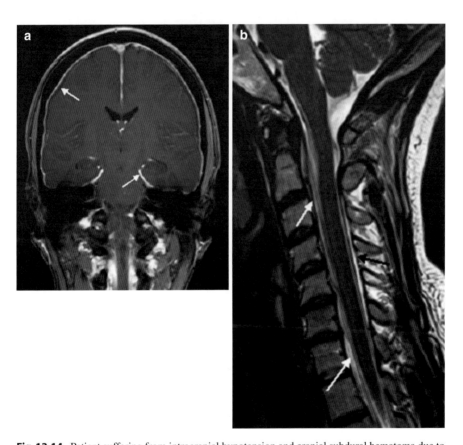

Fig. 13.14 Patient suffering from intracranial hypotension and cranial subdural hematoma due to spinal CSF leakage. Contrast-enhanced coronal T1WI MRI of the brain (**a**) reveals small subdural hygroma bilaterally and enhancing dura. T2WI MRI (sagittal, **b**) revealing spinal subdural hygroma. MR myelography (fat-saturated T1WI sagittal, **c**) revealing the leakage at right nerve root Th 6. T2WI MRI (axial, **d**) revealing spinal subdural hygroma. MR myelography (fat-saturated T1WI sagittal, **e**) revealing the leakage at right nerve root Th 6. Axial CT (**f**) shows therapeutic epidural blood patch (contrast enhanced)

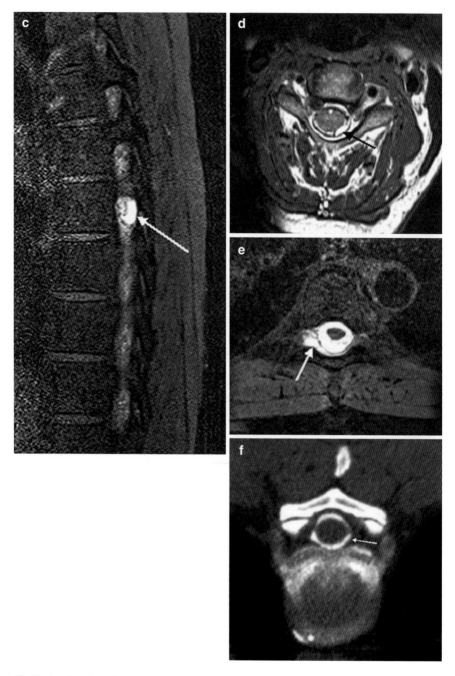

Fig. 13.14 (continued)

Fig. 13.15 Postsurgical CSF leakage extending subcutaneously. T1WI shows hypointense fluid extension with connection to the dural sac

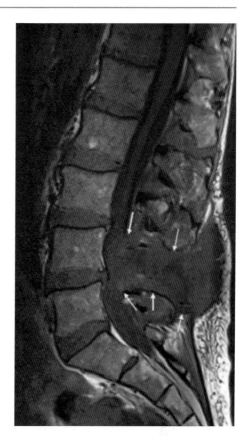

13.4.2 Spinal Cord Herniation

Spinal cord herniation is rare. Herniation of the spinal cord usually occurs through an anterior defect of the dura, typically at thoracic level. Women are slightly more commonly affected than men, and the disease is found in all adult age groups. Clinical manifestations include progressive myelopathy with according neurological deficits, such as Brown-Séquard syndrome. The treatment of choice is surgical repositioning of the herniated myelon; symptoms might improve or at least might not aggravate.

Imaging (Fig. 13.16)**:** Besides the ventral displacement of the spinal cord through the defect, typical imaging findings include signal abnormalities of the spinal cord in T2WI above herniation and scalloping of the adjacent vertebral body.

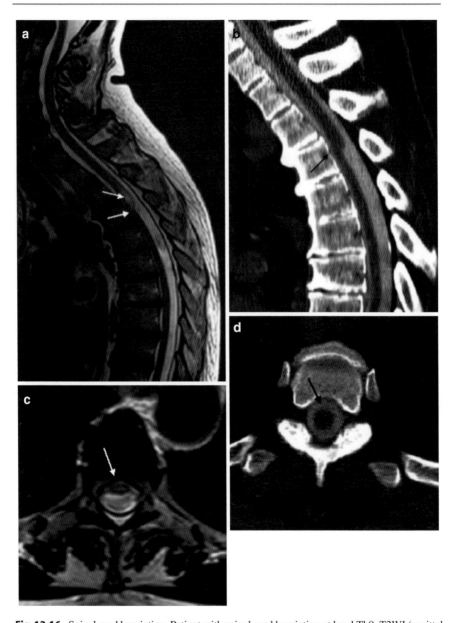

Fig. 13.16 Spinal cord herniation. Patient with spinal cord herniation at level Th9. T2WI (sagittal and axial, **a**, **c**), revealing circumscript anterior myelon herniation at level Th9 and focal myelopathy at level Th8/9. CT myelography (**b**, **d**, **e**) confirms anterior myelon herniation. **d** shows the normal position of the spinal cord surrounded by contrast-enhanced CSF; **e** shows ventral displacement of the spinal cord

Fig. 13.16 (continued)

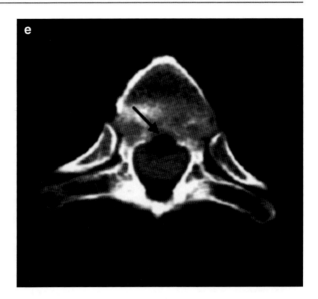

13.4.3 Subdural Hematoma

Spinal subdural hematoma describes the extravasation of blood into the potential compartment of the spine between the dura and arachnoid. Subdural hematoma can be located at any level of the spine, showing fusiform, oval, or tubular morphology. Typically, it will affect multiple segments. Patients of higher age and men are more often affected (m:f ratio 3:2). Spinal subdural hematoma is a rare condition, and only few cases of spontaneous spinal subdural hematomas have been described in the literature. Commonly, spinal subdural hematoma is associated with coagulopathies, administration of anticoagulants, surgery, or trauma. Depending on its size, clinical symptoms of spinal subdural hematoma include signs of cord displacement or compression with sudden back pain and neurological deficits depending on the level of manifestation. Clinical presentations include para- or tetraplegia, bladder dysfunction, sensory deficits, and nerve root symptoms. The treatment of choice is surgical evacuation. The timing of surgery and anatomic location of the spinal subdural hematoma determine functional outcome. Nonsurgical options might be considered only in patients with minor neurological signs.

Imaging (Fig. 13.17): Typical imaging findings include eccentric, multilocular, or inhomogeneous multisegmental collections pinching the CSF space due to its subdural location. On non-contrast CT, subdural hematoma might present with high

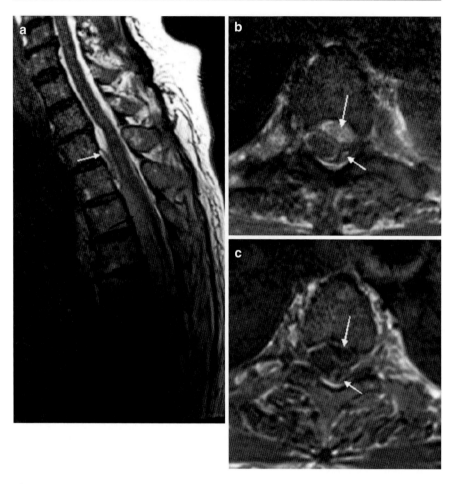

Fig. 13.17 Spontaneous subdural hematoma. Patient presenting with spontaneous subdural hematoma. Sagittal T2WI (**a**) shows thoracic subdural collection with hyperintense to intermediate signal, displacing the spinal cord backward. Axial T2WI (**b**) clearly reveals subdural location ventrally and left sided and shows right and backward displacement of the thoracic spinal cord. Contrast-enhanced axial T1WI (**c**) shows rim enhancement surrounding subdural collection

density. On MRI, spinal subdural hematoma shows hypo-, iso-, or hyperintense signal (depending on age of hematoma) in T1WI; in T2WI, it shows inhomogeneous low (if acute) or high signal (if subacute) intensity. Contrast-enhanced T1WI might show enhancement of the hematoma's margin.

13.4.4 Idiopathic Hypertrophic Spinal Pachymeningitis

Idiopathic hypertrophic spinal pachymeningitis is characterized by fibrous inflammatory thickening of the spinal dura, affecting the spinal cord and nerve roots

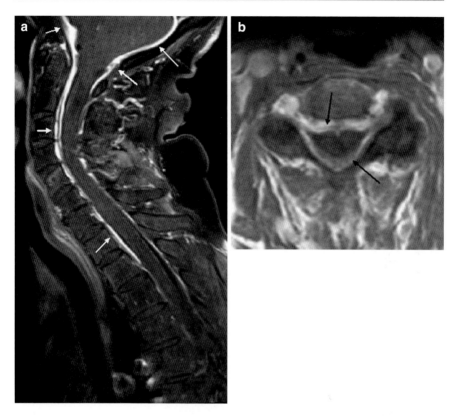

Fig. 13.18 Idiopathic hypertrophic spinal pachymeningitis. Contrast-enhanced T1WI (sagittal **a**, axial **b**) reveals massive thickening and enhancement of the spinal pachymeninges, extending intracranially. At some levels, the spinal cord is no more surrounded by CSF

through compression. The etiology of spinal idiopathic hypertrophic pachymeningitis is unknown. Different etiologies have been discussed including autoimmune inflammatory disease, trauma, infection, and sclerosing disease. It is a rare disease, usually presenting around the sixth or seventh decade of life. Idiopathic hypertrophic spinal pachymeningitis preferably occurs in the cervical and thoracic spine, although manifestation throughout the entire spine has been described. Clinical symptoms include intermittent focal neurological symptoms such as paralysis, paresthesia, progressive numbness, ataxia, increased reflexes, or bladder dysfunction. Treatment relies on surgical decompression and immunosuppressant therapy. Idiopathic hypertrophic spinal pachymeningitis is a diagnosis of exclusion. The diagnosis requires demonstration of spinal dural involvement with or without cranial involvement. The dorsal dura is commonly thickened more strongly than ventrally. Radiographic and pathological confirmation is strongly suggested to exclude differential diagnoses, such as *Meningeosis neoplastica*.

Imaging (Fig. 13.18): Typical imaging findings include thickened dura with iso- to hypointense signal on T1WI and T2WI and a marked post-contrast enhancement.

On CT scanning, idiopathic hypertrophic spinal pachymeningitis might present as slightly hyperdense shadow around the cord.

13.4.5 Arachnopathy

Spinal arachnopathy can result, inter alia, from all of the above-mentioned meningeal diseases, or it might be a complication of their diagnostic procedures or treatments. Furthermore, it may appear subsequent to diseases such as subarachnoid hemorrhage, intervertebral disk herniation, or spinal stenosis. Pathologically, spinal arachnopathy can be classified into three stages including radiculitis, accumulation of collagen, and adhesion and nerve root atrophy. Spinal arachnopathy almost always affects the cauda equina and results in clumped nerve roots, forming a

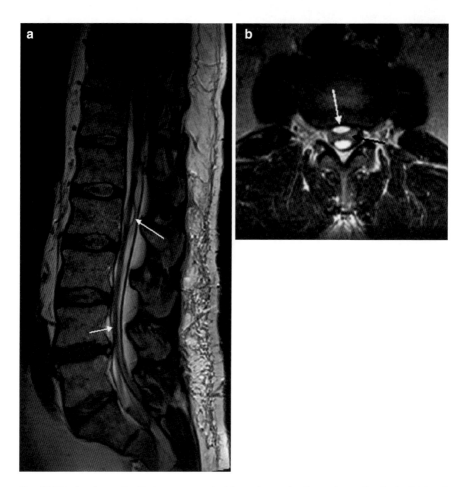

Fig. 13.19 Arachnopathy. Patient presented with posthemorrhagic arachnopathy. Sagittal (**a**) and axial (**b**) T2WI reveals typical signs of central mass caused by loculated CSF. Note hypointense signal of intradural septa due to hemosiderin

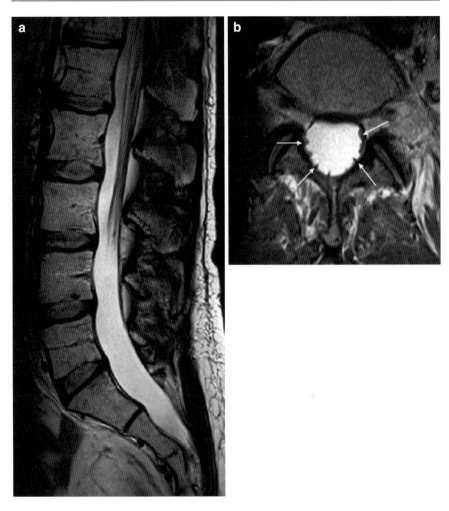

Fig. 13.20 Arachnopathy. Patient with postinflammatory arachnopathy. T2WI (sagittal **a**, axial **b**) shows typical "empty sac," as the cauda equina is attached to the dural sac

central mass or multiple "strands," and loculated (trapped) CSF. Arachnopathy is incurable. It can mimic symptoms of other diseases, causing minor to severe focal neurological symptoms depending on its anatomic location. Syringomyelia might occur as a complication of spinal arachnopathy.

Imaging (Figs. 13.19, 13.20 and 13.21)**:** Imaging features can be divided into three subtypes: The cauda equina forms a central mass in the dural sac, the cauda equina is attached to the dural sac forming the typical "empty thecal sac sign," or the dural sac is filled with a soft tissue mass replacing the subarachnoid space.

Axial and sagittal T2WI can identify the three subtypes. Contrast-enhanced T1WI might reveal diffuse enhancement of the leptomeninges. Finally, CT myelography is a useful imaging method in patients with contraindications against MRI.

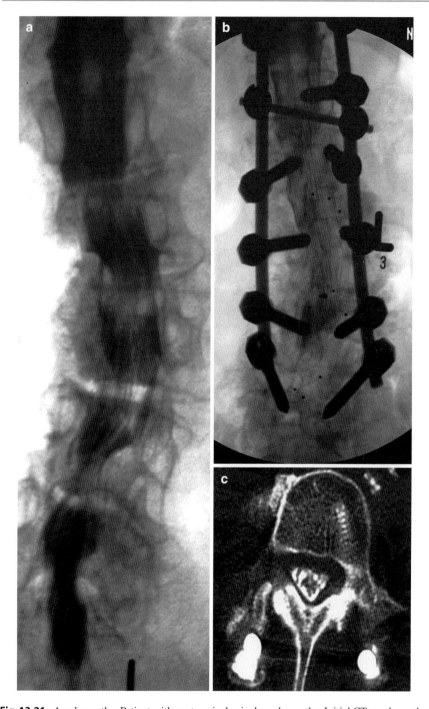

Fig. 13.21 Arachnopathy. Patient with postsurgical spinal arachnopathy. Initial CT myelography (**a**) reveals normal distribution of cauda equina (disk herniation with spinal stenosis at the levels L2/3 and 3/4). One year later, CT myelography (**b–e**) reveals filling defects of the caudal dural sac caused by granulomatous soft tissue

13 Meningeal Disorders

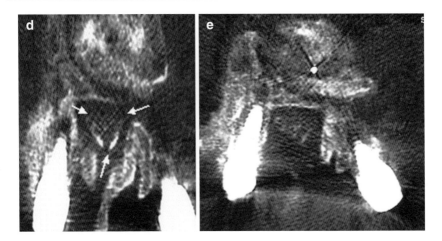

Fig. 13.21 (continued)

Further Reading

1. Chamberlain MC (2008) Neoplastic meningitis. Oncologist 13:967–977
2. Dampeer RA (2010) Spontaneous spinal subdural hematoma: case study. Am J Crit Care 19:191–193
3. Nozaki K, Judson MA (2012) Neurosarcoidosis: clinical manifestation, diagnosis and treatment. Presse Med 41:331–348
4. Prada F, Saladino A, Giombini S et al (2012) Spinal cord herniation: management and outcome in a series of 12 consecutive patients and review of the literature. Acta Neurochir (Wien) 154:723–730
5. Ranasinghe MG, Zalatimo O, Rizk E et al (2011) Idiopathic hypertrophic spinal pachymeningitis. J Neurosurg Spine 15:195–201
6. Ross JS et al (2004) Diagnostic imaging spine, 1st edn. AMIRSYS Inc, Salt Lake City. ISBN 0-7216-2880-X
7. Terushkin V, Stern BJ, Judson MA et al (2010) Neurosarcoidosis: presentations and management. Neurologist 16:2–15
8. Thigpen MC, Whitney CG, Messonnier NE et al (2011) Bacterial meningitis in the United States, 1998–2007. N Engl J Med 364:2016–2025
9. Van Goethem JWM, van den Hauwe L, Parizel PM (2007) Spinal imaging. Springer, Berlin/Heidelberg/New York. ISBN 978-3-540-21344-4
10. Yuki N, Hartung HP (2012) Guillain-Barré syndrome. N Engl J Med 366:2294–2304

Part V
Diseases of the Spinal Cord

Pathophysiological Regards

14

Michael Nichtweiß

Contents

14.1 Introduction 303
14.2 Diagnostically Important White Matter Tracts 303
14.3 Space-Occupying Centromedullary Lesions 306
14.4 Extramedullary Cause of Myelopathy 309
14.5 Relating Radiological and Clinical Findings 311
14.6 Bladder Disturbances 313
References 314

14.1 Introduction

This part of the book deals with intramedullary diseases of neoplastic and inflammatory origin. Here we would like to recall some indispensable anatomical facts in order to facilitate the interpretation of prototypical findings.

14.2 Diagnostically Important White Matter Tracts

The anatomical description in the following is simplified and shortened as far as possible, allowing for the interpretation of some imaging findings. For further details, anatomical textbooks are recommended [1, 2].

The most significant among the descending pathways is the corticospinal tract.

The fibres forming it originate from the motor and premotor cortex of the frontal lobe and bring about the execution of voluntary movements. At the level of the foramen magnum most of the fibres decussate the neuraxis and form the lateral

M. Nichtweiß
Department of Neurology, Hanse Klinikum Wismar; Wellengang 21,
D-23968 Wismar, Germany
e-mail: michael.nichtweiss@gmail.com

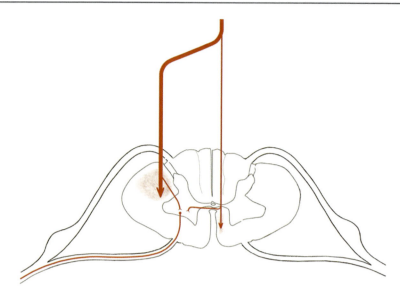

Fig. 14.1 Topography of the corticospinal tract in the spinal cord. Whereas the majority of fibres cross at the level of the decussatio pyramidum, a smaller number of fibres run downward anterior paramedian near the anterior fissure and cross segmental

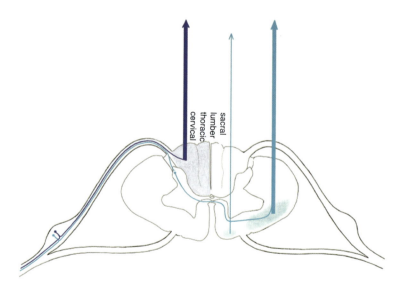

Fig. 14.2 Topography of the gracile and cuneate fascicles and the spinothalamic tracts. Whereas the fibres of the gracile and cuneate fascicles run upward ipsilateral in the dorsal columns, the fibres of the spinothalamic tracts cross segmental and run anterior and anterolateral to the brainstem

corticospinal tract situated within the lateral column (Fig. 14.1). Approximately 15% of the fibres run uncrossed, forming the anterior corticospinal tract which typically ends at cervical levels.

14 Pathophysiological Regards

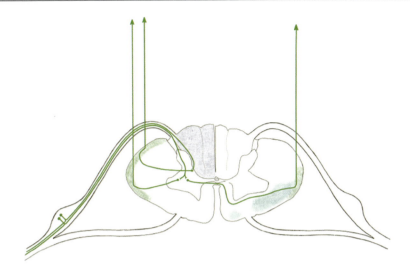

Fig. 14.3 Topography of the spinocerebellar tracts

Two of the ascending fibre tracts whose functions are tested in every neurological examination are depicted in Fig. 14.2. All the fibres ascending in the posterior column represent axons belonging to "pseudounipolar" neurons which are located in the spinal root ganglia. This means processes leading to damage of these cells or of their axons running through the dorsal roots result in degeneration of the corresponding fibre bundles. The afferent fibres of ganglion cells form the peripheral somatic nerves. The medial part of the posterior column is named fasciculus gracilis and contains fibres from the lower body, arranged in a somatotopic fashion (Fig. 14.2). The laterally situated fasciculus cuneatus appears above T6 and is prominent in the cervical cord. The fibres of these fascicles, being thick and myelinated, convey conscious position sense, fine touch and vibratory senses.

Other modalities of somatic perception, the senses of pain and temperature, are carried almost exclusively in the lateral spinothalamic tract (Fig. 14.2). Likewise, the peripheral conducting neurons are located in the spinal ganglia. However, their axons branch and connect with neurons of the posterior grey horn, running several segments up and down the spinal cord in the dorsolateral fascicle adjacent to the posterior horn (tract of Lissauer). They synapse with second-order neurons which send axons across the midline, through the anterior commissure, forming the lateral spinothalamic tract. Sensations of pressure and simple or light touch are conveyed in the ventrolateral spinothalamic tract.

The spinocerebellar tracts represent two further ascending pathways (Fig. 14.3), reaching the cerebellum via the inferior and superior cerebellar peduncles. They provide signals of unconscious position sense. This information arrives via the peripheral nervous system and, again, is transmitted via spinal root ganglia cells. However, the axons of the corresponding cells terminate on neurons of the spinal grey matter and the fibres forming the spinocerebellar tracts originate from these second-order neurons (see Chap. 16).

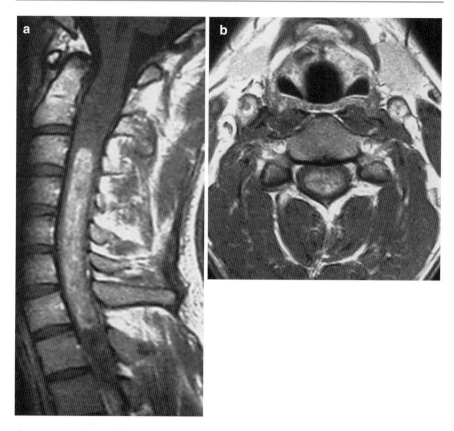

Fig. 14.4 T1 WI post contrast (pc) (**a** sag.; **b** ax.) showing an extended intramedullary space occupying lesion with relatively homogeneous enhancement, i.e. ependymoma, level C2–C7. The 25-year-old man suffered from episodic pain between the shoulders for several months and clinical examination disclosed dissociated anaesthesia in the left arm and slight proximal paresis of the upper extremities

14.3 Space-Occupying Centromedullary Lesions

Sometimes a remarkable discrepancy is to be observed between the extension of an intramedullary spinal mass and neurological deficits being minor only. This may be the case with ependymoma. When located cervically these tumours originate from the central canal, grow slowly and compress rather than infiltrate. The first and possibly only deficits result from the damage of crossing fibres of the spinothalamic tract adjacent to the central canal, leading to segmental anaesthesia of the dissociated type in the upper extremities or just below on the torso (Figs. 14.2, 14.4 and 14.5).

Similarly, cavities within the spinal cord may exert pressure effects.

Hydromyelia was the term originally applied to describe regular moderate extensions of the central canal, possibly extending throughout the entire cord and communicating with the fourth ventricle. It might be viewed as a normal variation and should

14 Pathophysiological Regards

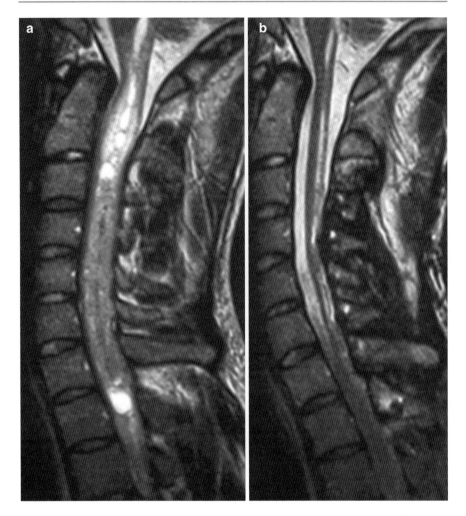

Fig. 14.5 Preoperative sagittal T2 WI (**a**, **b** postoperative) showing a large intramedullary space occupying cervical lesion with inhomogeneous hyperintense signal changes and cystic aspects. Despite obvious atrophic changes and longitudinal hyperintense signal changes with relationship to the central canal on postoperative MRI (**b**), gait was possible without assistance, and bladder as well as bowel function showed no disturbances

not be symptomatic. However, if associated anomalies are verified (for instance hydrocephalus or hindbrain malformation), further distension and deficits may result.

In the case displayed in Figs. 14.6 and 14.7), a communication of the central canal with the fourth ventricle seems unlikely. The channel is striking because it is filled with an abnormally composed fluid containing fat. Distensions not communicating with the fourth ventricle are associated with obstructions of the cerebral spinal fluid-circulation at or below the foramen magnum, spinal arachnoiditis or tethered cord (see Fig. 14.7) [3].

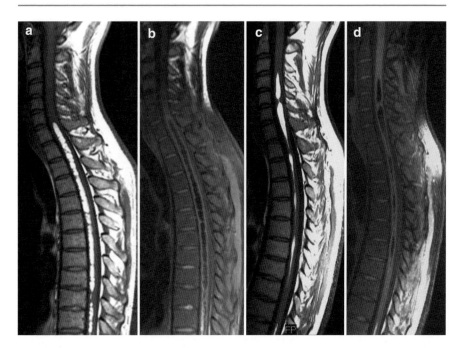

Fig. 14.6 First (**a**, **b**) and follow-up MRI 17 months later (**c**, **d**); sagittal T1 WI without (**a**, **c**) and with fat saturation (**b**, **d**) showing a channel filled with a fluid containing fat in a 33-year-old man

When the central canal expands, strange symptoms such as painless burning of the hand might be the single noticed abnormality for a long time. Signs and symptoms may arise in a way similar to ependymoma.

First symptoms in the case displayed were episodes of tachycardia and chest pain radiating into the left arm. There were no motor findings, but subtle sensory disturbances. The distension of the lumen decreased spontaneously and the complaints no longer occurred. The origin of the vegetative symptoms mentioned is open to speculation, the intermediate horn of the thoracic grey matter with corresponding nuclei [1, 2] being a good candidate.

Originally the term *syringomyelia* was used when an intramedullary hole had originated behind the central canal, with or without communication [4]; now all intramedullary cystic spaces are summarized under this heading [3].

They may result as an epiphenomenon of certain intramedullary tumours. In the case displayed in Figs. 14.8 and 14.9 the cavity resembles a cleft following the course of the left posterior tract, barely discernible from surrounding oedema which is confined to the posterior column. Causative is a richly vascularized nodular mass at T8, several segments away from the cervical spinal cord, possibly representing hemangioblastoma. Symptoms in the left arm and torso have existed for several years.

There is an overwhelming amount of literature concerning the different aspects and diverse associated conditions of hydro- and syringomyelia, but until now no unifying and well-accepted pathophysiological concept has existed. The interested

14 Pathophysiological Regards

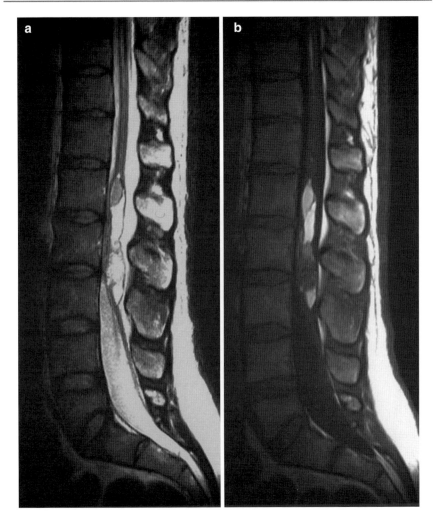

Fig. 14.7 Sagittal T2 WI (**a**) and T1 WI (**b**) demonstrating a tumour with inhomogeneous signal, e.g. dermoid at the level L1–L3 and in addition a tethered cord. Beside absence of the Achilles tendon reflex on the right the patient (same as in Fig. 14.6) showed no neurological symptoms

reader is referred to Milhorat [3] for classification, Bonafé and Aubin [3, 4] for historical aspects and Greitz for pathophysiology [5].

14.4 Extramedullary Cause of Myelopathy

Exceptionally, clinical and imaging findings suggest myelopathy, but cause (and remedy) may be located outside the dura mater. This is the case with compressive myelopathy (see Sect. 10.3) [5, 6]. Long, fusiform, T2 hyperintense lesions

displayed cervically had led to confusion with transverse myelitis. Two out of five cases in that paper showed some swelling of the cord. The authors emphasize that the diagnoses can be distinguished by:
1. The time course of progressive dysfunction, taking several months in compressive myelopathy and about 2 weeks in myelitis to reach a nadir.
2. In all five cases, gadolinium enhancement was limited to the region of maximal spinal cord compression in contrast to inflammatory myelopathy where enhancement occurs characteristically over a longer segment.

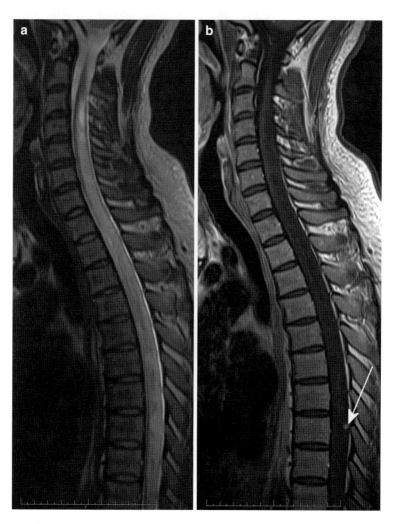

Fig. 14.8 T2 WI (**a** sag.; **c** ax.) and T1 WI pc (**b** sag.; **d** ax.): circumscribed contrast enhancing intramedullary lesion with relationship to the dorsal columns paramedian left at the level T8, e.g. hemangioblastoma in a 38-year-old male (*arrow*; **b**, **d**); impressive swelling of nearly the whole spinal cord up to level C3 with inhomogeneous hyperintense signal changes on T2 WI (**a**, **c**)

14 Pathophysiological Regards

Fig. 14.8 (continued)

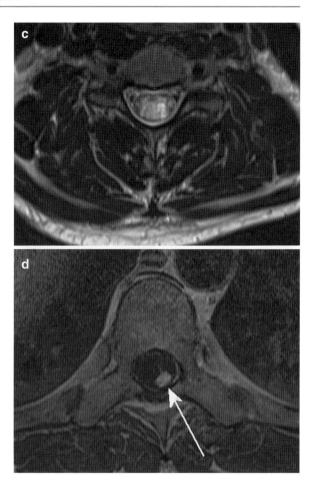

They demonstrated that the deficits are at least partially reversible – despite a prolonged presurgical course as in the case displayed (Fig. 14.10). With regard to spinal arteriovenous fistula, see Sect. 19.4.

14.5 Relating Radiological and Clinical Findings

Similar to cases of enlarged space-occupying centromedullary mass, there may be an obvious discrepancy between minor deficits and extension of the "lesion" as exemplified in Figs. 14.8 and 14.9, suggesting vasogenic oedema. T2 hyperintensity represents increased water content and/or cellular reaction. Therefore, if spread seems nearly unrestricted along the course of fibre tracts, subtle mass effects are of particular importance to differentiate between swelling and demyelination.

Fig. 14.9 Sag. (**a**) and ax. T2 WI (**b**) in the same patient as shown in Fig. 14.8: cranial extension of the intramedullary signal changes up to level C2; note relationship to dorsal columns (**b**, *arrow*)

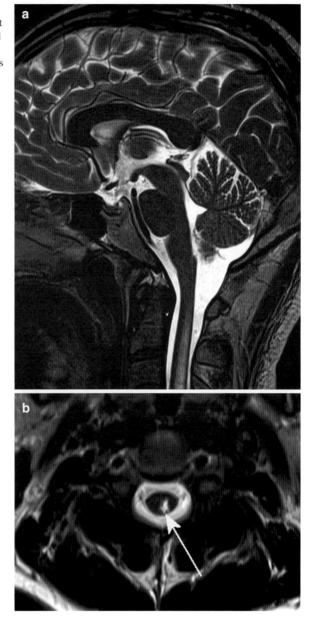

More often, the biological significance of T2 hyperintensity cannot be derived from the image and suggestions for the underlying pathology are given by history with clinical and paraclinical tests. Accordingly, lengthwise extended hyperintensity of the spinal cord should not be considered as "longitudinally extensive transverse myelitis" ("LETM"). Such findings may be indicative for, but are not synonymous with, myelitis.

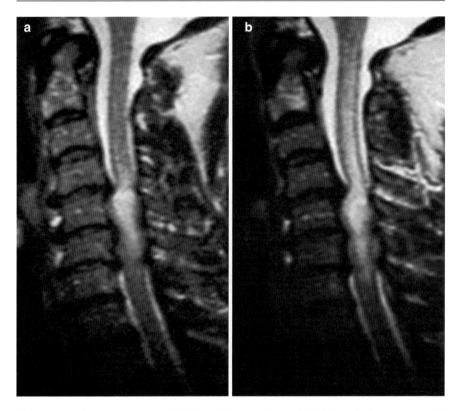

Fig. 14.10 Follow-up MRI (sag. T2 WI; **a, b**) over a time period of 6 weeks in a woman with minor gait disturbance exhibiting progressive intramedullary hyperintense signal conversion (**b**) in compressive myelopathy

If, the other way round, clinical examination demonstrates unequivocal evidence of a spinal cord process and the spinal cord MRI appears normal, various reasons come to mind, including limits of spatial resolution and the non-use of contrast media [7, 8], (see Sect. 15.1.1, Chap. 16).

14.6 Bladder Disturbances

Complaints of urgency and urge incontinence are symptoms frequently associated with known chronic spinal cord disease, and seem to have minor diagnostic significance. But surprisingly, in selected cases neurogenic bladder may be the presenting symptom at the beginning, heralding myelopathy years before any other deficit emerges (see Sect. 16.6, covering polyglucosan body disease).

Likewise, in bilhaziosis (schistosomiasis) (see Sect. 15.2.3), which is abundant only in some developing countries, myeloradiculitis is observed with a striking lumbar predilection, and the association with urological symptoms is well recognized.

Not surprisingly, the authors of a small neurosurgical study [9] investigating suspected cauda equina syndrome recommend urgent MRI with new onset. If urinary symptoms appear in the context of lumbar back pain or sciatica, it seems impossible to exclude lesions of the cauda equina on clinical grounds.

Of course, for the purposes of the following chapters, the administration of gadolinium should be considered [8].

Acute injuries of the spinal cord are accompanied by atonic paralysis of bladder and bowel. This is followed by passive distension of the bladder and ultimately overflow incontinence, vasomotor tone, sweating and piloerection are lost.

The two functions of the lower urinary tract, continence and micturition, are mediated and controlled by neural circuits whose complete anatomy is not understood. However, the presence of a pontine micturition region has been confirmed in man, and in the intermediate grey of the lumbar and sacral cord are groups of neurons which are known to take part in these functions [2]. If this part of the spinal cord is damaged in isolation, an atonic bladder coupled with a preserved sense of needing to void may ensue. In rare cases, this knowledge could gain special importance (see Sect. 15.3.5 covering systemic lupus erythematodeus, SLE).

References

1. Kahle W, Frotscher M (2009) Colour atlas of human anatomy 3: nervous system and sensory organs, 6th edn. Thieme, Stuttgart
2. Nieuwenhuys R, Voogd J, van Huijzen C (2008) The human central nervous system, 4th edn. Springer, Berlin/Heidelberg/New York
3. Milhorat TH (2000) Classification of syringomyelia. Neurosurg Focus 8:1–6
4. Bonafé A, Aubin ML (1992) Syringomyelia. In: Manelfe C (ed) Imaging of the spinal cord. Raven Press, New York, pp 751–770
5. Greitz D (2006) Unraveling the riddle of syringomyelia. Neurosurg Rev 29:251–264
6. Kelley BJ, Erickson BJ, Weinshenker BG (2010) Compressive myelopathy mimicking transverse myelitis. Neurologist 16:120–122
7. Schmalstieg WF, Weinshenker BG (2010) Approach to acute or subacute myelopathy. Neurology 75(Suppl 1):S2
8. Herrlinger U, Weller M, Küker W (2002) Primary CNS lymphoma in the spinal cord: clinical manifestations may precede MRI detectability. Neuroradiology 44:239–244
9. Bell DA, Collie D, Statham PF (2007) Cauda equina syndrome – what is the correlation between clinical assessment and MRI scanning? Br J Neurosurg 21:201–203

Inflammation of the Spinal Cord

15

Michael Nichtweiß, Elke Hattingen, and Stefan Weidauer

Contents

15.1	Introduction	316
	15.1.1 Preliminary Remarks	317
15.2	Myelopathies Associated with Infection	319
	15.2.1 Known Infectious Agents Associated with Acute Myelopathy, Viruses	320
	15.2.2 Known Infectious Agents Associated with Subacute Myelopathy, Bacteria	326
	15.2.3 Known Infectious Agents Associated with Subacute Myelopathy, Fungi, Parasites	328
	15.2.4 Idiopathic Acute Transverse Myelitis (Possible, but not Proven Virus Infection)	330
	15.2.5 Parainfectious Myelitis, Post-infectious Myelitis	330
	15.2.6 Myelopathy Associated with Subacute and Chronic Infections	332
15.3	Immune-Mediated Myelopathies	334
	15.3.1 Multiple Sclerosis	334
	15.3.2 Adverse Effects of Tumor Necrosis Factor Alpha-Blockers	345
	15.3.3 Neuromyelitis Optica	346
	15.3.4 Acute Disseminated Encephalomyelitis, Postvaccination Myelopathies	351
	15.3.5 Myelopathy Associated with Systemic Autoimmune Disease (SAD) and Sarcoidosis	358
15.4	Concluding Remarks	362
References		365

M. Nichtweiß (✉)
Department of Neurology, Hanse Klinikum Wismar; Wellengang 21, D-23968 Wismar, Germany
e-mail: michael.nichtweiss@gmail.com

E. Hattingen
Institute for Neuroradiology, Goethe-University,
Schleusenweg 2-16, D-60528 Frankfurt, Germany
e-mail: elke.hattingen@kgu.de

S. Weidauer
Department of Neurology, Sankt Katharinen Hospital,
Seckbacher Landstr. 65, D-60389 Frankfurt, Germany
e-mail: stefan.weidauer@sankt-katharinen-ffm.de

Abbreviations

ADEM	Acute disseminated encephalomyelitis
ATM	Acute transverse myelitis
Gd	Gadolinium
LETM	Longitudinally extensive transverse myelitis
NMO	Neuromyelitis optica
NMOSD	NMO spectrum disorders
SAD	Systemic autoimmune disease
TMCWG	Transverse Myelitis Consortium Working Group
VM	Vacuolar myelopathy
WI	Weighted images

15.1 Introduction

With respect to therapeutic measures in acute and subacute myelopathy, further differentiation is urgently needed, to be carried out almost exclusively by MRI, while the exclusion of cord compression and space-occupying lesion may be done with (myelo-) CT.

However, because of a notorious lack of specificity, proper interpretation of MRI findings is based on pathological and clinical knowledge. Therefore, not only imaging features of myelopathy are described, but further aspects of infectious and important immune-mediated diseases are detailed. As part of the radiological work-up, cerebral imaging is mandatory in the majority of cases, since some of the inflammatory processes may affect the cerebrum as well. This approach helps to characterize the diseases better, including the potential to relapse.

Inflammatory diseases of the spinal cord can occur at any age; they typically present with an acute or subacute myelopathy. In an attempt to give uniform diagnostic criteria for the prototypical acute transverse myelitis (ATM), the Transverse Myelitis Consortium Working Group (TMCWG) described the nosology in 2002 [1] (Table 15.1). For the onset a progression of deficits to a nadir between 4 h and 3 weeks was regarded as typical and now seems to be generally accepted for broader use in the description of inflammatory spinal cord disease [1–3]. The term "idiopathic" ATM was coined by the TMCWG, as opposed to ATM, secondary to a proven underlying disease, suggesting an established medical treatment. The clinical and laboratory investigations to diagnose causes other than "idiopathic" are detailed in [3], including the aquaporin 4 antibody, described in 2004, which is a major contribution (see Sect. 15.3.3).

The tasks of the radiological department at this point are first to rule out cord compression or tumor. Second, infarction and vascular malformation are to be differentiated. Third, the advantage of MRI as a tool to detect and differentiate inflammatory lesions in the spinal cord and elsewhere has become apparent and appreciated. This chapter aims to describe those findings and the underlying diseases. Because the diseases represent great variety, the literature cited may seem extensive – nevertheless a simplified classification of spinal cord inflammation has been used.

15 Inflammation of the Spinal Cord

Table 15.1 Diagnostic criteria for transverse myelitis

	TMCWG	Complete acute transverse myelitis	Acute partial transverse myelitis
Deficits attributable to the spinal cord	Sensory, motor, or autonomic dysfunction	Moderate or severe symmetrical weakness and autonomic (bladder) dysfunction	Mild sensory and motor dysfunction, bilateral or unilateral; when severe, marked asymmetry is observed
	Bilateral signs and/or symptoms (not necessarily symmetric), clearly defined sensory level	Symmetric sensory level	Sensory signs or symptoms attributable to a sensory level or hemi-level or MR lesion typical of myelitis
Signs of inflammation	Demonstrated by CSF findings or Gd.-enhanced MRI	CSF or MRI evidence of inflammation within the spinal cord may or may not be present	
Development		Progression to nadir between 4 h and 21 days following the onset of symptoms	
Exclusion criteria		Radiation within 10 years, vascular disease, brain abnormalities suggestive of MS or other demyelinating disease, presence of NMO, ADEM, connective tissue diseases, sarcoidosis and proven infection with known agents	

Modified from [1, 3] Transverse Myelitis Consortium Working Group (TMCWG)
NMO neuromyelitis optica, *ADEM* acute disseminated encephalomyelitis

15.1.1 Preliminary Remarks

Scott [1] proposes further differentiation of the spinal cord syndrome (Table 15.1). The mere description gives some clues as to the further course:

The rate of transition to clinically definite multiple sclerosis (CDMS) in patients presenting with a complete transverse myelitis as defined in Table 15.1 seems to be less than 2 %. In cases following the definition of an acute partial transverse myelitis, the rate of conversion to CDMS is estimated to be anywhere between 20 and 30 % at approximately 5 years follow-up – despite negative cerebral MRI [1]. Likewise, severe initial symptoms suggesting spinal shock seem to be highly predictive of a poor outcome [4].

From a radiological point of view, it is worth noting that clinical diagnosis of myelopathy is not always straightforward:

1. There are symptoms which are ambiguous by nature. Weakness of the lower extremities may be caused by disease of the muscle, the nerves or the neuromuscular junction. Muscle stiffness resulting from an autoimmune or paraneoplastic syndrome could be mistaken for spasticity, and gait disturbances of bilateral frontal lobe lesions may mimic myelopathy.
2. One should take into account that there may be some overlap between syndromes. For example, two prototypical acute inflammatory diseases, transverse myelitis, and polyradiculitis (Guillain–Barré–Strohl syndrome) have heralding

infection, ascending symptoms, pain and an elevated protein content of cerebrospinal fluid in common. Moreover, simultaneous inflammation of spinal cord and roots seems to occur in several cases [5].
3. Chronic but hitherto undetected disease can show sudden worsening, often precipitated by viral illness or minor trauma. Examples of this include primary progressive multiple sclerosis, motor neuron disease including primary lateral sclerosis, vitamin B12 or copper deficiency myelopathy ([3]; see Schmalstieg in Chap. 14). Therefore it is not infrequent that imaging leads to surprising findings which stimulate the clinician to targeted history taking.
4. The above-mentioned definition of the TMCWG rules out cases which reach the maximum deficit within less than 4 h. As a result, only a few cases of peracute idiopathic myelitis may be excluded, but it is likely that some vascular myelopathies fulfill the given time criterion for myelitis. Spinal infarction may even show some contrast enhancement if scanned repeatedly as proposed to demonstrate inflammation. Nevertheless, signs which strongly indicate myelopathy form the criteria embraced in Table 15.1.

ATM has an incidence rate of one to four new cases per million people per year (TMCWG), roughly a fifth occurring in the young, below the age of 18 years [6]. One small, more recent study from North Canterbury, New Zealand – a region with a known high incidence of multiple sclerosis (MS) – differentiates between acute complete and partial myelitis, giving an annual incidence of 6.2 cases per million for the first and of 24.6 cases per million for both complete and partial myelitis [7].

Whenever acute and subacute myelopathies are taken as a whole, non-inflammatory etiologies (i.e. vascular, postradiation and toxic) are to be taken into consideration as well. As shown by a large French series of 170 consecutive cases, a definite diagnosis is determined in part by observation of the further course of the disease: 55 of 101 (54.4 %) myelopathies initially classified as uncertain of cause were ultimately diagnosed as multiple sclerosis ($n=45$), systemic disease ($n=5$), neuromyelitis optica ($n=5$) [2].

Spinal cord lesions as depicted by MRI are highly unusual in healthy individuals including older age groups (Thorpe 1993, in [20]) and thus the demonstration of intramedullary abnormality is of high value in a newly evolving disease.

On the other hand, one has to take into account that the detection rate for spinal lesions is far from ideal, because of motion artifacts and resolution with an insufficient discrimination of detail on axial slices [8]. A comparison of lesion numbers and volumes on images from 1.5 and 3 T scans of MS has concluded that there seems to be no real gain from higher field strength [9].

High sensitivity of spinal MRI to detect ATM

In the case of ATM, however, sensitivity seems to be high: only 2 out of 38 cases in a series of children and adolescents recruited between 2000 and 2004 showed a normal MRI scan of the spinal cord [6]. A large multicenter study of ATM in adults, where patients were recruited between 1994 and 2004, gives a detection rate of 43/45 (95.2 %) for ATM lesions [4].

The possibility remains that there are more complex acute cases ([5], see Sect. 15.3.4), and in subacute or chronic myelopathy there is additional ambiguity in attempting to recognize a clear-cut abnormality (see [20]). Moreover, the abundance of vertebral changes and the ease with which osteophytic compression of the spinal cord is depicted by MRI altogether encompass the risk of mistaking those findings as the most relevant, disregarding more subtle or questionable intramedullary alterations.

15.2 Myelopathies Associated with Infection

Myelopathies associated with infection are rare when considering the rough incidence numbers (given above) for both complete and partial myelitis. Debette et al. [2], investigating the course of acute and subacute myelopathies, consolidated all infection-associated cases into the one heading of "parainfectious myelopathy" and estimated that 12.4 % (21/170) belong in this group. It is pertinent to note that in all of these rare instances a timely and accurate diagnosis is crucial to improve outcome.

Infections affecting the spinal cord lead to signs and symptoms in different ways: their consequences may be caused by cytolysis of neural cells induced by viral invasion, by destructive bacterial inflammation, by space-occupying effects as in the case of granuloma or by vascular complications. However, even in the case of proof for an infectious agent in CSF, the interpretation of the phenomena should extend beyond that of mere local tissue destruction, and instead take into account molecular mimicry, superantigen-mediated inflammation or humoral derangements as well [10]. For instance, the development of paraplegia within hours and the diffuse extension of signal abnormality over large parts or the entire length of the spinal cord could advocate in favor of an immunopathogenesis. The term 'myelopathy' is chosen as an umbrella term, encompassing direct tissue damage on the one hand, and more complex, mostly concealed steps in immunopathogenesis on the other. Table 15.2 provides a short and inevitably incomplete overview of infectious agents which are named with respect to frequency, predilection, or therapeutic significance. Myelitis is viewed as an emergency case in the clinic and for the calculation of antimicrobial therapy some very unusual agents must also be considered, depending on immuno competence and epidemiological factors. For instance, *Listeria monocytogenes* is a widely unknown cause of myelitis in most parts of the world, but, if present, some standard antibiotics fail as it is an intracellularly replicating bacterium.

Table 15.2 Infectious myelopathies –agents

Viruses:	DNA:	Herpesviruses (HSV-2, HSV-1, VZV, CMV, Epstein-Barr, HHV-6, -7)
	RNA:	Flaviviruses (Japanese e., St. Louis e., Tick-borne e., Dengue v., West-Nile v.)
		Orthomyxoviruses (Influenza A)
		Paramyxoviruses (Measles, Mumps)
		Picornaviruses (Coxsackievv., Echovv., Enterovv. Hepatitis A,C, Poliovv., vaccine- associated: Sabin)
Retroviruses:	HIV, HTLV-1 (chronic myelopathies)	
Bacterial:	Mykoplasma pneumonia	
	Borrelia b., Treponema p., Mycobact. tuberc., Tropheryma whipple	
	Listeria, Brucella (contaminated dairy products)	
	Staphylococcus, Streptococcus., Escherichia c., (also:)	
	Nocardia, Actinomyces	
Fungal:	Blastomyces, Coccidioides, Aspergillus, Candida	
Parasites:	Bilharziosis (Schistosomiasis) (Far East, South America, Africa),	
	Neurocysticercosis (China, Southeast Asia, India, Mexico, Central, South America)	
	Gnathostomiasis (Southeast Asia)	
	Strongyloides (tropical, subtropical areas, southern United States)	
	Toxocara (worldwide, housing of dog)	
	Toxoplasmosis (AIDS)	

See [3, 11–13]
Japanese e Japanese encephalitis, *Coxsackievv* Coxsackievirus A and B

15.2.1 Known Infectious Agents Associated with Acute Myelopathy, Viruses

Viruses are the most common agent causing acute infectious myelopathy [2], but definite proof by serological tests and polymerase chain reactions more often fails to give a definite diagnosis [3, 11]. Given the definition above, all such cases could be viewed as "idiopathic" ATM [3]; see Sect. 15.2.4. On the other hand, because of the implementation of novel diagnostic techniques in the last two decades, the spectrum of diseases caused by infection from known viral agents have been able to be better characterized [12].

The most common neurologic disease caused by any of the herpes viruses is zoster. Infection with the *varicella zoster virus* (VZV) usually takes place during the first two to three decades of life, leading to varicella (chicken pox). The viral genome persists in the dorsal root ganglia (the trigeminal or geniculate ganglia as well) and may be reactivated later in life, then causing shingles. Typically, individuals above 60 years of age and immunocompromised patients become ill. Both chicken pox and shingles may be complicated by neurological diseases including myelitis [13]. In the latter case, a partial transversal syndrome may result days to weeks after a painful rash in one or several dermatomas, caused by spreading of the virus from the spinal ganglion. If sensation is impaired bilaterally, the upper level should be compatible with the segment of VZV reactivation. Dermatomal pain syndromes caused by VZV from reactivation in thoracal dorsal root ganglia, but without rash (zoster sine herpete) might be under-recognized.

15 Inflammation of the Spinal Cord

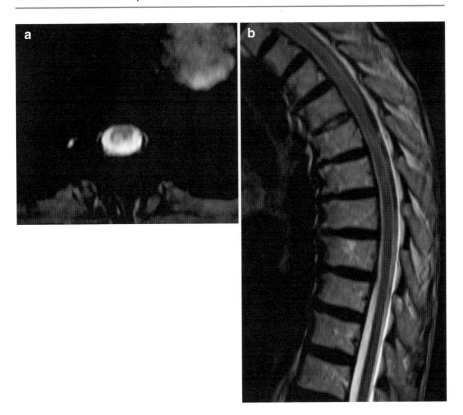

Fig. 15.1 A 77-year-old female with chronic state after zoster in the dermatomes D 6 and D 7 and with gait disturbance. Sagittal T2WI (**a**) and axial T2*WI (**b**) showing signal increase of the dorsal spinal cord. At the time of exanthema there was no gait disturbance

Imaging. In the acute stage, more extensive alterations may dominate longitudinally [3] and intramedullary, as well as the occurrence of radicular enhancement [13]. If remote spinal lesions ensue, they are interpreted as a consequence of multifocal small vessel vasculitis, thought to be caused by the hematogenous spread.

At times, especially in the further course of the disease, lesions can be recognized as being more circumscribed, referring to implicated roots (Fig. 15.1, Table 15.3). Recurrent protean manifestations of VZV infection (meningoencephalitis, vasculopathy, myelitis) may occur with or without a rash.

Herpes simplex virus (HSV)-2, the etiological agent of genital herpes, is known to be a common cause of aseptic meningitis in adult women, often occurring without a rash. It also accounts for 6 % of necrotizing frontotemporal encephalitis and has been reported to lead to sacral radiculitis [11] as well as to acute and subacute myelitis (Nakajima 1998, cited in [12, 13]). Typically, a corresponding localized dermatomal rash occurs [13]. First symptoms of this necrotizing myelitis may be sensorimotor disturbances of the lower extremities and bladder dysfunction, followed by ascension over the course of several weeks. Prognosis varies, in some cases leading to tetraplegia and death despite timely therapy. Moreover, recurrences have been reported.

Table 15.3 ATM – five imaging findings that lessen differential diagnoses

Segmental distribution (Fig. 15.1):
Intramedullar lesions affecting white and gray matter, corresponding to dermatomal rash or pain
Varicella- Zoster virus (VZV)
DD: HSV- 2, without rash: diverse!

"Poliolike": (Fig. 15.3)
Lesions affecting the gray matter of the anterior horn and surroundings
Polio-, St. Louis-, West-Nile-, FSME- viruses
DD: spinal infarction, "Kira Hopkins Syndrome"

Granulomatous: (Figs. 15.5, 15.29 and 15.31)
Enhancing nodular lesions, located in the leptomeninx and/or intramedullary, possibly T2 iso- or hypointensity
DD: sarcoidosis, tuberculosis, lues cerebrospinalis, parasitic infections, metastasis

Longitudinally extensive transverse myelitis (LETM): (Figs. 15.2, 15.6, 15.7, 15.24–15.28)
Lesions with extensive homogenous T2-hyperintensity lengthwise, affecting the central gray matter structures, often with some swelling. In case of NMO enhancement is more frequently intense and homogeneous
DD: viral myelitides, NMO, SAD, ADEM, Gnathostomiasis, spinal vascular disease (see Chap. 17)
If the circumstances of lesion formation are unknown instead of "myelitis", "hyperintensity" is preferred (Figs. 15.27 and 15.28)

Short segment ovoid or peripherally located (Figs. 15.13–15.17): Lesions affecting predominantly white matter, with or without enhancement and possibly slight space-occupying effects: "CIS" (see Sect. 15.3.1) DD: diverse, but alltogether less probable, brain imaging is mandatory

HSV-1 causes the classic necrotizing encephalitis (which spreads from the temporal lobe) and, less frequently, brainstem encephalitis. Besides this, HSV-1 may lead to an acute or subacute myelitis in immunocompetent adults, but, as reported, less frequently than HSV-2. Nakajima et al. cited in [12, 13]) demonstrated a parenchymal high signal both on T1WI and T2WI, suggesting hemorrhagic necrosis as known from temporal HSV-1 encephalitis.

Imaging. MR imaging may demonstrate longitudinally extensive T2-hyperintense lesions (longitudinally extensive transverse myelitis, (LETM), Table 15.3) with variable intra-medullary and, possibly, meningeal and radicular enhancement on contrast-enhanced T1WI [14].

In *HIV* patients as well as in healthy adults, the cytomegalovirus (*CMV*) is certainly highly prevalent, but remains asymptomatic. In the case of infection or reactivation, it causes retinitis or encephalitis selectively in the immunocompromised, evidenced by enhancement along the ventricular border, polyradiculitis, multifocal neuropathy and myeloradiculitis, often concomitantly [12, 13]. Among spinal diseases which are known to complicate AIDS, CMV-radiculitis was the most common intradural disease (Thurnher, cited in [14]).

Imaging. Typically thickening, clumping and enhancement of nerve roots ensue, quite similar to what is shown in Guillain–Barre syndrome (see Fig. 13.7), often with involvement of the conus as well [13, 14].

CMV myelitis may occur in isolation: a case of Moulignier et al. (cited by [13]) showed some swelling in the conus medullaris and ring enhancement intramedullary, mimicking a tumor. CSF analysis exhibited pleocytosis. Moreover, Moulignier et al. mention a 7-year-old, perinatally HIV infected girl with a similar lesion in the cervical spinal cord. Histology provided evidence of necrotizing myelitis and positive CMV immunostaining, but the spinal roots did not show any signs of inflammation.

In contrast, immunocompetent adults manifesting neurological disease associated with CMV are rare, occurring as transverse myelitis or myeloradiculitis. Concerning the pathogenesis, some scattered case reports give the impression of considerable heterogeneity, with negative PCR when tested in the CSF, and several normal MR reports. Therefore Fux et al. [15] argued in favor of an immune-mediated rather than a directly virus-induced pathogenesis and pointed to the absence of intrathecal production of specific CMV antibodies in their particular case. Karacostas et al. [16] reported on a 16-year-old student who developed paraplegia days after a temporary improvement of an illness starting with a sore throat, malaise and fever. T2WI demonstrated an increased signal from the lower cervical to the thoracic cord (LETM). Contrast-enhanced MRI was unrevealing and the further course was very favorable, showing complete recovery within 2 months. In the CSF, the cell count was normal and no viral DNA was detected. Again, this case could serve as an example for a probable immune-mediated pathogenesis (see Sect. 15.2.5).

The Epstein–Barr virus (*EBV*) causes infectious mononucleosis, which is complicated by neurological manifestations in 1–5 % of all cases, whereby this rate may possibly be an underestimation [13]. Severe complications are rare, but protean: among others, they include meningoencephalitis, acute disseminated encephalomyelitis (ADEM), radiculitis, encephalo-myeloradiculitis and myelitis [12, 13].

Imaging. Potential patterns of radiculitis on contrast-enhanced T1WI include leptomeningeal and root enhancement along the intrathecal course of spinal nerves, with or without thickening.

These findings are preferentially depicted with fat suppressed T1WI after intravenous application of gadolinium (see Chap. 13).

The pathogenesis of inflammatory CNS-disease associated with EBV infection is controversial, either favoring a direct virus invasion, or an immune-mediated lesion caused by cytotoxic CD 8+ cells [13]. An example possibly supporting the first interpretation is given by Gruhn [17]: a 16-year-old boy had received unrelated bone marrow transplantation. Nineteen months later he presented with a partial transversal syndrome and pleocytosis; PCR for EBV was positive in the CSF. On T2WI an intramedullary edema throughout the cervical and thoracic cord was demonstrated with some spotty hyperintensities which showed strong enhancement on contrast-enhanced T1WI. They were interpreted as inflammatory foci by the authors. The boy was treated with gancyclovir and hyperimmune globulin and recovered completely. An example of postinfectious EBV myelitis has been presented by de Seze et al. [4], corresponding to a long-segment diffuse T2 hyperintensity cervicodorsal (LETM, Table 15.3). The case imaged with Fig. 15.2 was interpreted as infection with HHV-6, proven by PCR, again showing LETM.

If in the context of viral infection rapidly flaccid paresis arise in the absence of sensory disturbances, either radiculitis or a "poliomyelitis-like" syndrome might be the cause. In such cases proof of a spinal lesion is of interest.

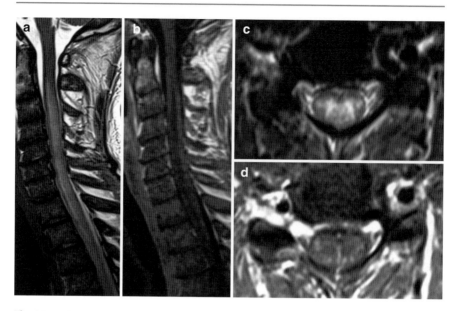

Fig. 15.2 HHV 6 infection. A 47-year-old man with acute lymphocytic leukemia, bone marrow transplantation 5 months ago and ataxia. Sagittal T2 WI (**a**) reveal extended hyperintense signal changes especially in the cervical spinal cord pronounced in the dorsal columns (**c**; axial T2 WI) with mild swelling (**a, c**) and slight enhancement (**b, d**: sagittal and axial T1 WI post contrast (pc) medium administration)

Poliomyelitis is nearly eradicated and today only occasional cases are reported in association with oral vaccination.

Imaging. MRI shows obvious similarities to ischemic or degenerative loss of anterior horn cells (see Figs. 20.7 and 20.8). Lesions are radiologically and neuropathologically confined to the anterior two-thirds of the spinal gray matter [18]. Similarities to these patterns are seen in infections by some flaviviruses and enteroviruses [3].

In such cases the clinical syndrome and imaging studies suggest a preferential rather than an isolated destruction of anterior horn cells (Fig. 15.3, Table 15.3).

Equally, some similarities are given to Hopkins syndrome and atopic myelitis. The former was described as a "poliomyelitis-like" condition following asthma attacks, associated with elevated serum IgG levels. Affected children (and in a few cases adults) showed an acute onset of flaccid pareses of one or two limbs, days to weeks after an asthma attack [19].

In recent years the flavivirus *West Nile virus*, predominantly transmitted by mosquitoes, has attracted attention, causing outbreaks with higher incidence of severe neuroinvasive disease in North America, totaling 8,606 cases between 1999 and 2005. As further detailed in a review of Kramer [20], the virus was first isolated in 1937 in the West Nile province of Uganda and has spread rapidly throughout the Western world. While the majority of infected individuals stay asymptomatic, less

15 Inflammation of the Spinal Cord

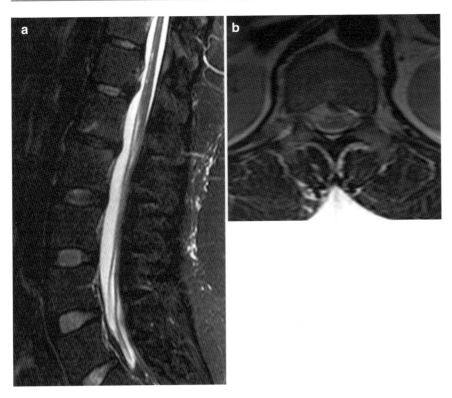

Fig. 15.3 Chronic state after tick-borne myelitis at the age of 13. Sensory level at dermatome 9, initially flaccid paralysis and absent tendon reflexes of the legs. Later on, walking with minimal restrictions, but plantar response being extensor. Sagittal (**a**) and axial T2 WI (**b**) showing ventral accentuated slight hyperintense lesions

than 1 % develops meningitis, encephalitis or flaccid paralysis, sometimes overlapping in the same patient. However, flaccid paralysis may occur in the absence of meningitis or an encephalitis syndrome as well. Pareses are often asymmetric, reaching a nadir within hours. Bladder and bowel function are disturbed in some patients, but on neurological examination substantial sensory deficits might be absent.

Imaging: Focal changes have been described on cerebral MRI scans: these are patchy and located in the white matter, but can affect pons, substantia nigra and the thalami as well, and may result from cytolytic effects of the virus. Spinal MRI may show gray matter lesions of the anterior horn, documented by prolonged T2-relaxation time, uni- or bilaterally, possibly longitudinally extended. Occasionally, spinal root or patchy parenchymal enhancement is reported [14].

Of course, referring to the above-mentioned question, only the gray matter findings are decisive. Interestingly, as shown with another flavivirus infection, the appearance of brain abnormalities later in the course of spinal disease may indicate ADEM as well [21].

15.2.2 Known Infectious Agents Associated with Subacute Myelopathy, Bacteria

Bacterial inflammation of the spinal cord parenchyma may spread from bacterial meningitis as described in Chap. 13, hematogenous or from adjacent infection, forming an abscess, granulomas, or causing vascular damage (see Chap. 13). However, such cases represent rarities, as stated by Kurita et al. [22], who collected 25 well-documented cases of intramedullary spinal cord abscesses worldwide within 10 years. The most common presentation was deficit occurring in all patients, followed by fever, pain, and bladder disturbances. The radiological findings were similar to those known from brain abscesses.

Moreover, as discussed in Sect. 15.2.5, bacteria may act abruptly and "parainfectiously" on the spinal cord, a process which is poorly understood.

More often observed are spinal cord syndromes caused by bacterial inflammation, taking a more protracted course, as in borreliosis or tuberculosis.

Lyme disease, or borreliosis, are the most frequently recognized arthropod-borne infections of the nervous system in the USA and in Europe. Upwards of 25 % of the healthy European population is seropositive for anti-borreliosis antibodies, yet has never been sick with the disease. Proof of an infection affecting the central nervous system therefore rests on examination of the cerebrospinal fluid. In Europe, meningopolyradiculitis represents the manifestation most often seen.

Imaging. On T1WI a prominent enhancement in the leptomeninges is to be expected, and radicular enhancement is even more typical for borreliosis.

Several case reports of "myelitis" highlight aspects of pathogenesis and are of interest for differential diagnosis: described and displayed are (1) a prominent long segment swelling of the spinal cord in a 12year-old child, even without neurological deficit, possibly with some patchy intramedullary enhancement [23], (2) a circumscribed, prominent intramedullary enhancement surrounded by swelling [24], and (3) a painless "polyomyelitis-like syndrome" of the upper extremities [25], together with the well-known meningeal and radicular enhancements. In this particular case a T2-hyperintense, enhancing lesion was identified, exactly confined to the cervical anterior horn bilaterally, extending in longitudinal direction only.

More typically, patients complain of persistent, radiating pain as in the case displayed (Fig. 15.4). Therapy leads to cure and subtle spinal symptoms are easily missed – therefore the incidence of myelitis remains unclear.

The other well-known spirochaetal disease with prominent neurological sequelae is *syphilis*.

In an attempt to cover a rare illness with diverse manifestations, some simplification seems inevitable. Therefore, following Conde-Sendin [26], meningeal, meningovascular and ocular forms are considered early and general paresis (progressive paralysis) and tabes dorsalis late forms of syphilis. Accordingly, myelitis is classified as early and dealt with in this section, but tabes dorsalis is viewed as chronic and covered under Sect. 15.2.6. These authors report an incidence number for new cases of syphilis of 1.77/100,000 over the year 2000 in Spain.

15 Inflammation of the Spinal Cord

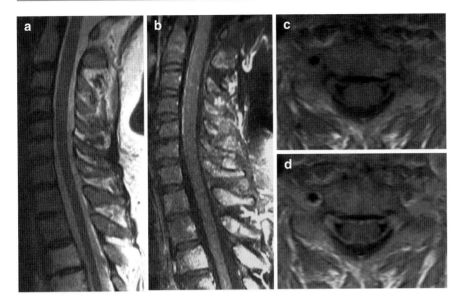

Fig. 15.4 Borreliosis in a 67-year-old female. Numbness, pain, and flaccid paraparesis in both arms and unsteady gait for 2 weeks. Sagittal T2 WI (**a**) showing no clear-cut intramedullary abnormalities, but T1 WI pc (**b**, sagittal; **d**, axial) disclosed thickened and enhancing roots (**c**: T1 WI axial)

Meningeal inflammation, the formation of granuloma (gumma), infarction as a consequence of arteritis and myelitis may occur concurrently. Concerning meningomyelitis, latencies varying from 1 to 30 years from the onset of infection are given [11]. The radiological spectrum of meningomyelitis may well be illustrated by scattered case reports, again with respect to differential diagnosis: in a 25-year-old patient, a small space-occupying lesion in the dorsal cervical spinal cord caused a partial transversal (Brown Sequard) syndrome and was interpreted as an isolated demyelination, where brain MRI was unremarkable. Based on a biopsy 2 years later, the lesion was diagnosed as gumma [27]. On T2WI the center of the nodule was isointense. In the case of Tsui et al. [28], brain MRI was normal as well: a 57-year-old woman developed an acute complete transversal syndrome within 5 days. An extensive high signal involving the whole spinal cord was present on T2WI. A nodular hypointensity in the thoracic cord was depicted (possibly gumma) but not commented on. This small mass was surrounded by focal enhancement, and CSF pleocytosis was shown. Kikuchi et al. [29] described a case of syphilitic meningomyelitis. A 36-year-old man first evolved a cervical pain and, within months, weakness and sensory loss in the upper extremities, followed by difficulty in walking and pyramidal signs on both sides at the time of neurological evaluation. Spinal cord MRI revealed swelling of the entire spinal cord and the leptomeninges showed enhancement. The superficial parts of C3 to 5 and Th3 to 4 showed intense enhancement, giving a "candle guttering appearance" on sagittal images. The abnormal enhancing parenchyma showed hypointensity in T2WI, named by the authors as "flip-flop sign". The latter finding may be interpreted as caused by lipids and the release of free radicals by macrophages, corresponding to the composition of granulomata. Unfortunately, axial slices were neither described nor displayed. Brain MRI showed two small intensely enhancing lesions. All three individuals described were immunocompetent. In the case of pathological examination, luetic meningomyelitis shows thickened, inflamed meninges with predominance at the cervical region (hypertrophic pachymeningitis, [11]), a description fitting the findings mentioned above quite well. To sum up, syphilis may lead to an inflammation resembling other granulomatous diseases (see sarcoidosis, Sect. 15.3.5, Table 15.3).

Authors from Pakistan [30] who reported a prevalence of 405/100,000 for *tuberculosis* in their country, compared clinical and neuroimaging features of ten of their own patients with tuberculous myelitis. Most patients presented as radiculomeningitis (Figs. 13.4 and 13.5), but isolated myelitis or polyradiculitis are not uncommon.

Imaging. The involvement of spinal cord may resemble glioma or lymphoma, more than 80 % affecting the thoracic spine. Besides intramedullary localization, tuberculoma intradural-extramedullary and isolated involvement of the cauda equina were observed. The MRI signal characteristics of tubercular lesions are related to the histological stage, T1-hyperintensity and T2 shortening being representative of caseous necrosis with a large amount of lipids and macrophages. A majority of the lesions variably enhance contrast on T1WI, showing diffuse, nodular, ring-like or tumor-like patterns, but the absence of enhancement does not exclude the disease.

Spinal cord tuberculoma usually responds to medical treatment; syrinx formation, spinal infarction and atrophy do occur in the course of the disease.

15.2.3 Known Infectious Agents Associated with Subacute Myelopathy, Fungi, Parasites

Fungi as a cause of myelitis may occur during the course of known diseases. Cryptococcus neoformans, for instance, is known to be a prominent source of opportunistic infections in patients suffering from AIDS, but they play no role in presenting spinal symptoms in developed countries and thus are not addressed here (see [11, 31]).

Likewise, exposure to parasitic diseases is limited in developed regions, but other than fungi, parasites may cause serious infection in immunocompetent individuals. In times of mass tourism and globalization, they are worth mentioning with some degree of importance not only in the countries where they are endemic. Some index of suspicion is given by contexts outlined in Table 15.2. Another hint may result from eosinophilia in the blood or CSF.

In *cysticercosis*, spinal involvement rarely occurs, below 5 % [14] of all cases. Surprisingly in a series of 16 cases with spinal cysticercosis from four centers [32], all had evidence of simultaneous cranial manifestations.

Imaging. The patients with intramedullary involvement showed either solitary focal cystic lesions within the spinal cord (6/16), or syrinx formation related to chronic arachnoiditis (2/16). Evidence of intradural-extramedullary disease included cystic structures within the subarachnoid space or meningeal enhancement.

Saleem et al. [33] from Egypt were able to present eight cases of spinal *schistosomiasis* with pathological correlation. All patients were male and the site of involvement was the lumbar intumescence of the spinal cord in all cases.

Imaging. Involvement of the lumbar intumescence with swelling and intramedullary nodular enhancement, correlating to multiple schistosomiasis microtubercles. Meningeal enhancement was present in all and some radicular enhancement in four cases.

A similar striking male preponderance in another series [34] was believed to result from greater exposure of men to schistosomal infestation in agriculture. The invariable involvement of the lumbar cord is explained by the existence of valve free venous plexus anastomoses between intraabdominal and spinal veins and raised intraabdominal pressure, which permits the eggs of the worm to migrate through these vessels. The highly antigenic structure of the ova provides an extensive immune reaction.

A common cause of paraparesis with eosinophilic CSF in Northeast Thailand is the infection with *Gnathostomiasis*, caused by the consumption of raw fish or other intermediate hosts. Depicted in a case report of [35] is diffuse cord enlargement with high signal on T2WI of the cervical and thoracic spinal cord, encompassing the gray matter. Small intracerebral or subarachnoid hemorrhages seem to be common.

In a case of *toxocara* infection (Fig. 15.5) [36] there were several, areas of raised T2 signal intramedullary and leptomeningeal as well as some punctuate intramedullary enhancement. Diagnostic confirmation in such cases depends on positive CSF or serum antibody titers.

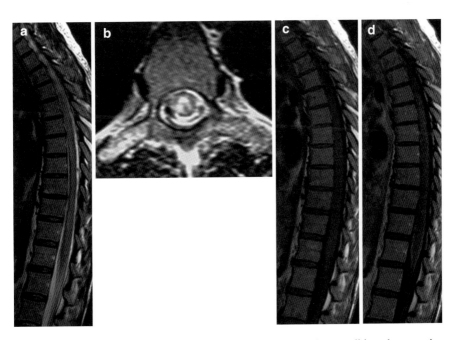

Fig. 15.5 A 44-year-old woman (dog owner) with eosinophilic meningomyelitis and progressive paraparesis caused by parasitic infection (neurotoxocariosis). Spinal MRI showing hyperintense lesions of the thoracic cord (**a, b**; sagittal and axial T2WI) with diffuse leptomeningeal and faint punctuate intraparenchymal contrast enhancement (**c, d**; sagittal T1WI)

15.2.4 Idiopathic Acute Transverse Myelitis (Possible, but not Proven Virus Infection)

Applying the definition of idiopathic ATM, some cases are to be characterized that differ neither in clinical nor in radiological detail from infections with proven viral etiology [3, 4, 14], begging the question whether the causative agent is merely missed or unknown.

In 2002 the TMCWG addressed the problem whereby neuromyelitis optica (Devic's disease; see Sect. 15.3.3) could not be differentiated sufficiently. In the meantime, a potent serological marker was found and recent series of ATM [6] rule out neuromyelitis optica not only by follow-up of the patients but by defining aquaporin-4 antibody.

Lastly, the question as to whether there is a pure spinal form of acute disseminated encephalo-myelitis fulfilling the definition of idiopathic ATM remains unanswered and are discussed in Sect. 15.3.4. Bearing this in mind, neither heterogeneity of outcome nor a diversity of radiological features [14] in this group is surprising. The moderate detection rate of earlier series might be explicable by technical limitations of older MR scanners, so the notion of Goh et al. [14]: "MR imaging demonstrates T2-hyperintense lesions in almost all reported cases" could be the adequate description of currently available imaging results.

Imaging. T2-hyperintense lesions are seen in almost all cases with extension lengthwise over more than three segments, centrally located and involving most of the cross section (LETM). The cervical or thoracic spinal cord, and less often lumbar or several parts, are involved.

This pattern is known from several infectious and non-infectious causes [14], as well as some swelling [4]. In children, lesions are possibly more extended and swelling may be more pronounced.

15.2.5 Parainfectious Myelitis, Post-infectious Myelitis (see Sect. 15.3.4)

The terms 'parainfectious,' and likewise 'post-infectious' myelitis, are used to stress the point that the causative agents for these spinal cord syndromes are factors other than the direct destructive outcomes of an infectious agent [10, 11]. In fact, trigger and effector mechanisms in respective cases are not well-known and cytolitic viral action vs neural injury resulting from immune-mediated mechanism may be impossible to differentiate on clinical grounds [10, 14]. Some examples given above show there may be blurring margins even in established etiologies. The terms are descriptive and used when a close temporal relationship exists between a systemic infection and the acute or subacute occurrence of myelitis [10].

An example of parainfectious myelitis – as well as the technical problems of imaging – is given in Fig. 15.6: during an acute septicemia with Staphylococcus, a transversal syndrome evolved within hours. The first MRI study was performed

15 Inflammation of the Spinal Cord

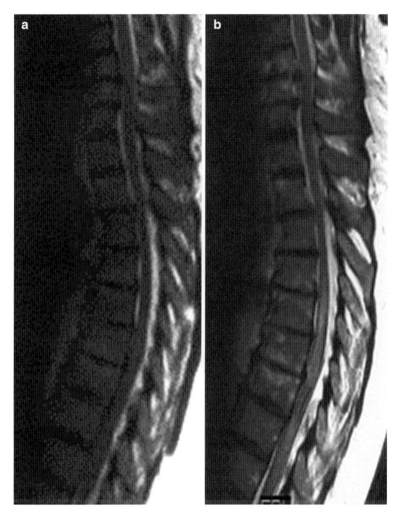

Fig. 15.6 Parainfectious myelitis in a 62-year-old woman with complete paraplegia within less than 4 h. Cerebrospinal fluid (CSF) showed pleocytosis, cultures from blood and spinal fluid positive for Staphylococcus. First MRI (**a**, T2 WI sag.) was performed 2 h after paraplegia and second MRI (**b**, T2 WI sag.) 4 days later, revealing swelling and long sectional hyperintense signal of the thoracolumbar spinal cord

about 2 h after complete paraplegia, which did not show any substantial improvement during the disease progression. This rapid catastrophic course was possibly elicited by microbial superantigens [10]. Another case (Fig. 15.7) made a favorable recovery in spite of early and extended radiological findings corresponding to LETM.

The term acute disseminated encephalomyelitis (ADEM) is often in use interchangeably. We tried to specify ADEM as a postinfectious CNS complication, with the onset of symptoms between 2 and 21 days after initial infection ([37]; see Sect. 15.3.4).

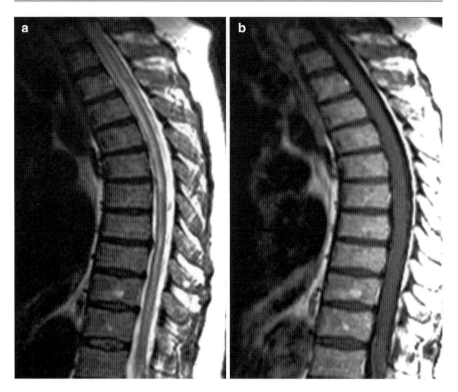

Fig. 15.7 Longitudinally extended transverse myelitis (LETM) 1 day after incomplete paraparesis during urosepsis (Table 15.3), e.g. parainfectious myelitis. Sagittal T2WI (**a**) showing a central accentuated hyperintense lesion over the whole thoracolumbar spinal cord without intramedullary enhancement (**b**, T1 WI sag. pc)

15.2.6 Myelopathy Associated with Subacute and Chronic Infections

The most commonly observed spinal cord lesion of AIDS patients on necropsy is vacuolar myelopathy (VM). This is in contrast to clinical series where apparent myelopathy is an infrequent experience in the order of 1 % of neurological complications [11]. Although VM is notoriously linked with the AIDS pandemic, it has been observed in patients with cancer and other immuno-suppressive conditions [11]. Accordingly, VM occurs independently from HIV infection of the spinal cord parenchyma and highly active antiretroviral therapy does not seem to alter the course. VM shows striking similarities to the subacute degeneration of the spinal cord following vitamin B12 deficiency, and, because both conditions probably have parts of their pathogenesis in common, they are discussed together in Sect. 16.3.

HIV myelitis must be taken into consideration, when under circumstances of known or suspected HIV infection a myelopathy appears, probably with a more protracted course than with an infection caused by the various above-mentioned agents.

Imaging. In contrast to VM, HIV myelitis shows parenchymal and leptomeningeal enhancement without swelling [38, 14].

Notably, in the case report of Michou et al. [38], highly active antiretroviral therapy showed efficacy.

Another retrovirus, Human T-cell Lymphotrophic Virus (*HTLV*), poses a health problem affecting high-risk individuals and those in endemic areas such as southern Japan, equatorial Africa, the Caribbean, and parts of South America. It is transmitted by transfusion, through breastfeeding, or sexually, but less effectively than HIV. The virus is associated with adult T-cell leukemia and a chronic progressive disease of the central nervous system. It was termed HTLV-1 – associated myelopathy or tropical spastic paraparesis, depending on the location where it was observed [39]. The causal relationship of HTLV-II and myelitis [11, 40] is not yet clear.

The classic course of this myelopathy is chronic, taking several years to develop, and bladder dysfunction may precede the onset of paraparesis [40]. The disease affects mainly the thoracic part of the spinal cord, but may also involve the cervical segment or both regions concurrently [39].

Imaging. The chronic course is manifested by atrophy of the lateral columns, following degeneration and demyelination of pyramidal, spinocerebellar, and spinothalamic tracts.

These lesions are associated with perivascular and parenchymal lymphocytic infiltration, proliferation of astrocytes, and fibrillary gliosis. Unlike VM and HIV, there seems to be an association between the presence of myelopathy and viral load in the spinal cord and CSF [11].

Less commonly, the disease develops within several months.

Imaging. In these more subacute cases, or alternatively during an initial inflammatory phase of chronic cases, extended lesions can be observed consisting of high signal intensity on T2WI with or without swelling [40]. The lesions can be found in the center of the spinal cord, bilaterally, or in the posterior columns.

When these lesions were surveyed [39], swelling and T2-lesions decreased and were followed by atrophy. Two out of eleven patients in the series of Umehara et al. [39] showed enhancement in the lateral columns, which was believed to reflect severity of inflammation. Periventricular and subcortical white matter lesions are present in 80 % of cases on brain MRI [40].

Prior to the development of antibiotics, syphilis was the most frequent cause of spinal disease, but occurred rarely in the absence of involvement at other sites of the nervous system.

Historically, *tabes dorsalis* has been viewed as the prototypical spinal disorder associated with syphilis [11], occurring on average 10–15 years after infection. It is characterized by "lancinating" or "lightning" pain, ataxia, loss of proprioception, trophic abnormalities, and autonomical dysfunction, most often attributed to selective degeneration of the dorsal spinal roots, the spinal root ganglia, and Wallerian degeneration of the posterior columns (Fig. 15.8). The pathogenesis of the lesions in the spinal roots is not well known, but chronic meningeal inflammation around the spinal roots is indicated. Unlike the cerebral cortex in "general paralysis of the insane," there is no demonstrable inflammation in the spinal cord and *Treponema*

Fig. 15.8 Tabes dorsalis, myelin stain: Wallerian degeneration in the posterior columns, note atrophic dorsal roots; *arrow*: perivascular infiltration (From: Mennel and Solcher [74] with kind permission)

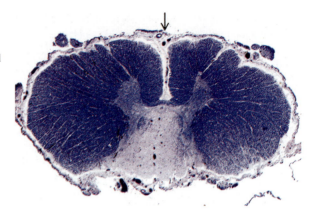

pallidum is absent. Radiologists should be cautious: the differential diagnosis of a lesional pattern including the dorsal columns should embrace tabes dorsalis and be followed by a contrast enhanced study of the brain.

Imaging. Affection of the dorsal columns.

Even if there is some similarity to the MRI finding of subacute combined spinal cord degeneration (see Chap. 16), the mode of formation is quite different. The most recent study on neurosyphilis from Nagappa et al. [41] encompasses ten remarkable myelopathic cases and depicts this lesion of the dorsal columns nicely.

15.3 Immune-Mediated Myelopathies

15.3.1 Multiple Sclerosis

Multiple sclerosis (MS) is a chronic disease with strikingly different prevalence numbers around the world, ranging from near zero at the equator to above 130/100,000 in Northern parts of the USA or Europe. This has led to causative hypotheses stressing environmental factors. However, so far, the disease is better characterized with findings substantiating an autoimmune pathology. Typically, first symptoms appear between the third and sixth decade of life, but the disease has to be considered in childhood and in old age. Throughout all age groups roughly two-thirds of newly diagnosed patients are female.

A clinical definite diagnosis of MS (using the criteria of the Poser committee, 1983) requires two episodes of symptoms separated by at least 1 month and signs on examination of at least two lesions involving anatomically separate regions. In the midst of new and promising therapeutic options there has been a growing effort to reach an early diagnosis. To this end, MRI has been able to provide a key advancement: when a first episode arises, clinically non-apparent lesions besides the symptomatic one can be detected and, moreover, repeating the examination allows for the detection of new lesions early in the course. This has led to the establishment of the "McDonald criteria" which implemented such MRI findings. The last revisions in 2010 are depicted in Tables 15.4 and 15.5 [42, 43]. Notably, it is mandatory for all criteria to consider and exclude alternative explanations for the clinical presentation [44]. In line with the

Table 15.4 MRI criteria for dissemination in space and time for multiple sclerosis (MAGNIMS[a] proposal after [42])

Dissemination in space (on either baseline or follow-up MRI)	
≥1 lesion in at least two of the following areas[b]:	
Periventricular	
Juxtacortical	
Brainstem and cerebellum	
Spinal cord	
Dissemination in time	
Simultaneous presence of asymptomatic Gd-enhancing and nonenhancing lesions at any time	
A new T2 and/or Gd-enhancing lesion on follow up MRI irrespective of timing of baseline scan	

[a]MAGNIMS: Magnetic resonance in MS, (European multicenter collaborative network)
[b]In case of a brainstem or spinal cord syndrome the symptomatic lesions do not contribute to the lesion count

Table 15.5 2010 McDonald criteria for diagnosis of primary progressive multiple sclerosis after [43]

One year of disease progression
Plus 2 of the 3 following criteria:
1. Evidence for dissemination in space: ≥1 T2 lesion in at least one of the following brain areas[a]: periventricular, juxtacortical, infratentorial
2. In the spinal cord: evidence for dissemination based on: ≥2 T2 lesions in the cord
3. Positive CSF (isoelectric focusing evidence of oligoclonal bands and/or elevated IgG index

[a]In case of a brainstem or spinal cord syndrome the symptomatic lesions do not contribute to the lesion count

nature of acute inflammatory demyelization, the first symptoms of the disease in the case of relapsing remitting subtype are termed anatomically related "clinically isolated syndromes" (CIS). These are:
1. Unilateral optic neuritis
2. Brainstem or cerebellar signs such as facial numbness, internuclear ophthalmoplegia, ataxia and multidirectional nystagmus or sixth nerve palsy
3. Spinal cord signs such as partial myelopathy, Lhermitte's symptom, deafferented hand, numbness, urinary urgency, progressive (asymmetric) spastic paraplegia
4. Symptoms from the cerebral hemispheres

Such CIS can be monofocal or multifocal, with or without asymptomatic MRI lesions. In two situations some diagnostic uncertainty remains: a multifocal clinical presentation without MRI detected lesions ("CIS Type 4"). Further follow-up is required to determine whether there is a condition other than MS. Apparently, imaging studies performed for reasons other than "CIS" may be suggestive for MS as well – again, there is the need for follow-up. However, the description of an incidental finding "CIS type 5," as proposed in the paper, defined as "no clinical presentation," appears somewhat contradictory.

To diagnose multiple sclerosis in the case of a spinal cord syndrome according to CIS "c" applying the *revised McDonald criteria 2010* (Table 15.4) needs the minimum proof of two further brain lesions, appropriately located to fulfill the criterion dissemination in space (DIS).

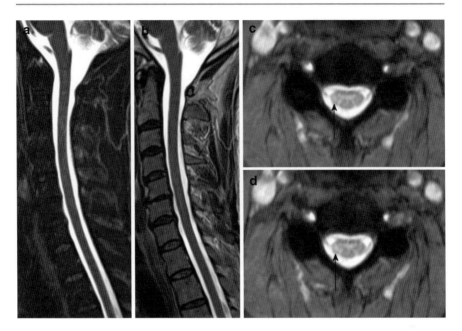

Fig. 15.9 A 57-year-old man with primary progressive MS (PPMS) with right side accentuated spastic paraparesis and a 1 year insidious progression; CSF disclosed positive oligoclonal bands, and cranial MRI showed one juxtacortical and one periventricular lesion (not shown). Sagittal short tau inversion recovery (STIR) (**a**) and axial slices T2* GRE (**c, d**)) at the level C5 showing subtle focal signal increases in the cervical spinal cord (*arrow*), while sagittal T2WI (**b**) is normal

To support the criterion dissemination in time (DIT), the simultaneous presence of asymptomatic gadolinium enhancing and non-enhancing lesions at any time, or a new lesion upon follow-up MRI in reference to the baseline scan, is thought to be sufficient [42]. These criteria are valid only for "CIS" [44].

In contrast to the presentation of a first episode, possibly followed by a relapsing-remitting course, a steady progression of the disease from onset can occur. This phenotype, named primary progressive MS, represents not more than 15 % of MS cases and is found predominantly in elderly patients. The most typical presentation is progressive myelopathy, often in the form of pure spastic paraparesis.

Still today, positive CSF findings are of major interest (Table 15.5) [43]. This is because history lacks specificity and, moreover, radiological findings are more subtle and ambiguous (Fig. 15.9). Unfortunately, CSF findings may be negative in approximately 20 % of cases, especially at the beginning of the disease. Since the presenting symptoms differ, it is even more important to know the radiological details of conventional spinal cord imaging supporting the clinical diagnosis of MS.

Bot et al. [45] described the distribution of focal abnormalities in the spinal cord early in the course of MS. They saw lesions throughout the cord but with clear cervical preponderance, more than 55 % of lesions being located there. Oppenheimer [46], who described the localization of plaques neuropathologically in 1977 based on 18 autopsy cases, categorized three main lesion patterns in the cervical enlargement:

15 Inflammation of the Spinal Cord

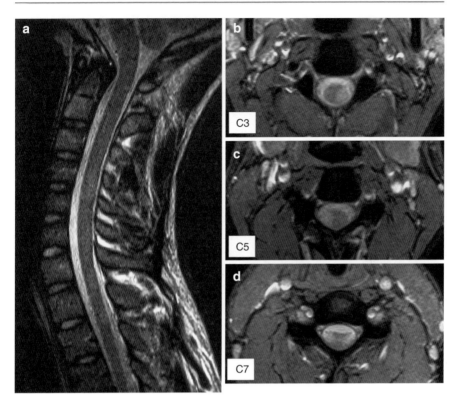

Fig. 15.10 Relapsing-remitting MS (RRMS) in a 35-year-old male suffering from slight gait disturbance. Sagittal (**a**) and axial (**b–d**) T2 WI revealing multiple hyperintense lesions in the cervical spinal cord preferentially in the dorso-lateral circumference without mass effect

1. In the lateral columns, fan-shaped, abutting the lateral surface roughly symmetric on some levels (Figs. 15.10 and 15.11),
2. In the posterior columns, tending to lie in the midline (Figs. 15.12 and 15.13),
3. A narrow band running between the lateral tip of the anterior horn and the lateral surface.

He stated that the form and position of the plaques in the lateral columns strongly suggest that the denticulate ligaments play a part in their formation (which seems arguable for lesions in the posterior columns of the craniocervical junction as well). He reiterated that some lesions are related to veins, and hypothesized that mechanical forces could lead to vascular leakage. The paper of BJ Kelley (reference of Chap. 14) mentions the problem and cites a contribution from CM Poser to the problem of trauma triggering plaque formation.

Two own cases are given to illustrate how mechanical stress could initiate spinal cord symptoms under certain circumstances. Both patients have had physical trauma/local pain at the beginning, followed by a partial spinal cord syndrome, and in both patients CSF analysis showed oligoclonal bands (Figs. 15.14 and 15.15).

As often emphasized [47, 48], focal lesions in MS as seen with MRI should be confined to two vertebral segments in length, as opposed to other inflammatory

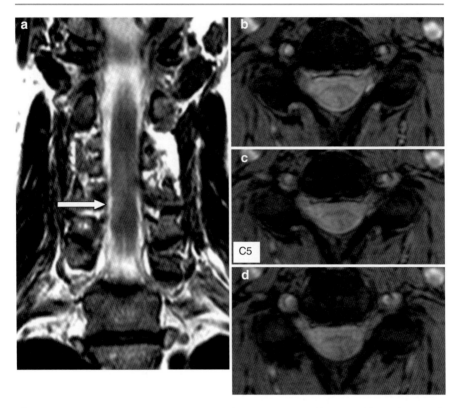

Fig. 15.11 Secondary progressive MS (SPMS) in a 49-year-old man with moderate gait disturbance. Coronal T2W TSE (**a**) and contiguous axial slices in T2*W GRE at level C5 (**b–d**), showing involvement of the gray matter, and possibly minimal shrinkage (**a**, *arrow*)

diseases named in Sects. 15.2 and 15.3. Possible exceptions to the rule are acute lesions in pediatric patients [49]. The authors found longitudinally extended lesions (similar to LETM) in 6/36 patients at first presentation and 4 in the further course of the illness. With regards to more chronic cases, confluence of lesions being of different ages should be considered.

On axial images there are two types of lesions typical for relapsing remitting MS:
1. More often, there is a broad basis abutting the surface of the spinal cord, giving a wedge-shaped aspect as described above. As known from correlative studies, such lesions may involve the gray matter too, disregarding anatomical borders [48, 50]. This interpretation may also be suggested from conventional imaging (Figs. 15.10 and 15.11).
2. In the minority are those where contact with the surface is absent or unclear. They are rounded [47] or ovoid, possibly showing some swelling (Figs. 15.13, 15.15, and 15.16).

Enhancement of spinal lesions often seems less prominent and accentuated along the surface of the spinal cord (Figs. 15.16 and 15.17). In the brain, new enhancing lesions are up to ten times more common than in the spinal cord [48]. Nevertheless,

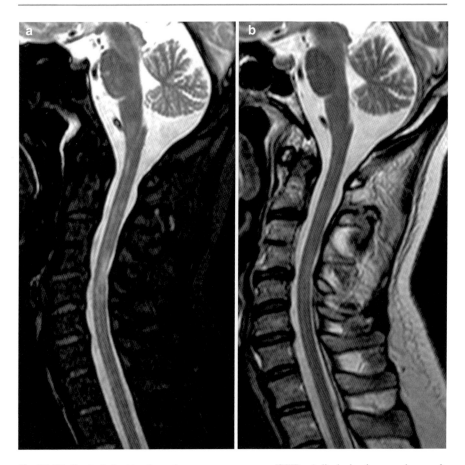

Fig. 15.12 Sagittal short tau inversion recovery sequence (STIR; **a**) disclosing improved recognition of hyperintense demyelination lesions in comparison to sagittal T2W TSE (**b**) in the cervical spinal cord as well in the brain stem (same patient as showed in Fig. 15.11)

13/25 patients in the study of Trop I and her colleagues (cited in [51]) who examined MS patients with signs and symptoms of myelopathy who had enhancing lesions in the cord on their first scans. In the further course, 70 % of these patients showed enhancing lesions with new clinical manifestations. They were best seen 15–22 min after contrast administration and mostly had a nodular appearance with homogeneous enhancement. Some lesions showed patchy enhancement, and sometimes an increase in size and change from ring-like to homogenous enhancement were observed within some minutes. Within 1 year, in 35 % of examinations, MRI findings showed lesion progression in spite of clinical improvement or stability.

In the case of primary progressive MS (PPMS), the clinical presentation with slowly progressing spastic paraparesis is more ambiguous and the radiological findings more subtle. In 1997 Lycklama à Nijeholt et al. described the investigations of 16 patients with primary progressive MS (citation in [48]). Besides patients with a few demyelinating non-enhancing lesions, 7/16 patients only showed diffuse

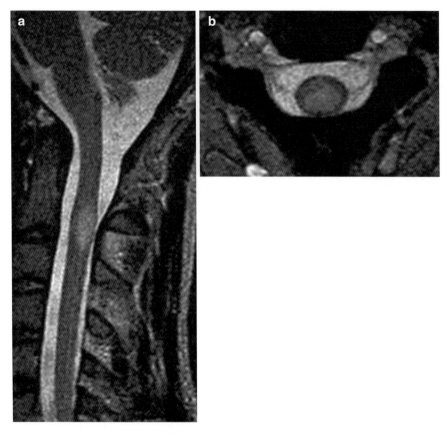

Fig. 15.13 Clinical isolated syndrome (CIS) in a 30-year-old woman. Sag. T2 WI TSE (**a**) and axial T2* GRE (**b**) showing a slightly swollen lesion of the cervical spinal cord at the level C2/3

abnormalities. They were depicted on proton-weighted sagittal images and are not seen on T2WI. Even with post mortem MRI at 1.5 T devoid of the usual motion artifacts, such lesions might be missed [8]: one out of seven patients (three having a primary progressive course) had no spinal cord lesions on conventional in situ sagittal dual echo images. However, high resolution imaging of thoracic cord samples at 4.7 T disclosed two small lesions. Confirmed by histology, they were showing partial and total demyelization. One subject showing diffuse abnormalities only was found to have lesions with intermediate and high signals on axial high resolution images. Nowadays fast short tau inversion recovery sequences (Fig. 15.12) are in use as an alternative to proton-density imaging [47].

In clinically definite MS, brain imaging shows negative results in up to 5 % of cases [48]. More often, it is the primary progressive variety of the disease where brain imaging shows minimal or no abnormalities (Thorpe 1996, cited in [48]). As summarized by Hu and Lucchinetti [52], some studies suggest that neurodegeneration occurs independently from focal inflammation in progressive MS and axonal injury may be prominent in the normal appearing white matter. On the other hand,

15 Inflammation of the Spinal Cord

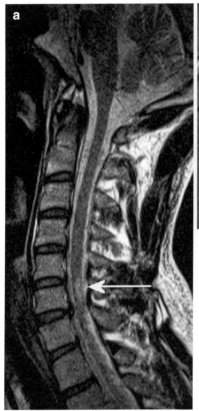
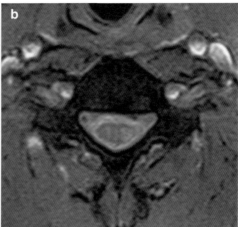

Fig. 15.14 CIS, 47-year-old man suffering 2 days after cervical trauma during judo exercise from numbness evolved in the left hand. Sag. (**a**) and axial (**b**) T2 WI disclosing a intramedullary hyperintense lesion just above a protruded disc. Cranial MRI (not shown) revealed in addition two cerebral lesions in the deep white matter and periventricular (see text). *Arrow* points to the same lesion as displayed in **b** on the left

it is worth noting that spinal cord lesions may occur asymptomatically, found in 30–40 % of patients with clinically isolated syndromes [48, 49]. Similarly, in 43 % of recently diagnosed MS cases there are no clinical signs pointing to spinal lesions as proven by MRI [45].

MRI has proven to be a sensitive instrument not only in detecting focal MS lesions in the brain, but, by doing so, in recognizing subclinical progression of the disease. However, the correlation of focal cerebral abnormalities as shown by conventional MRI with clinical impairment is low. Several technical and clinical theories have been brought forward to explain this so-called "clinico-radiological paradox" [53], but the most obvious idea to look for an association of impairment with spinal T2-lesion load showed no correlation [51].

Probably a major factor in explaining this inconsistency is the weakness of conventional MRI in making subtle, non-focal tissue loss visible. There is, for instance, a correlation between impairment and "black holes" depicted in the brain,

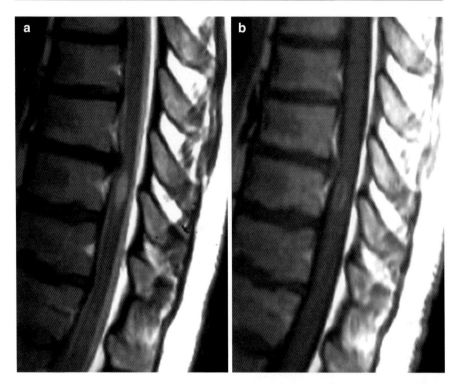

Fig. 15.15 CIS, 37-year-old female. After thoracic pain for several days a mild sensory bilateral deficit evolved. Sag. T2 WI (**a**) and T1 WI pc (**b**) showing a moderate broad-based medial disc herniation at the level D 8/9 and a intramedullary hyperintense (**a**) enhancing (**b**) lesion just below (see text). Additional cranial MRI (not shown) disclosed one periventricular lesion

but in spinal imaging comparable focal lesions are lacking. As known from more recent neuropathological studies [50, 52], demyelinating lesions appear not only in white but also in gray matter. In the spinal cord they dissect and diminish axons in the course of tracts and lead to reduced numbers of motorneurons and interneurons. There are now several, equally promising and demanding techniques available, based on changes in magnetization transfer, diffusibility or N-acetyl-aspartate levels [47, 48], possibly suitable for measuring tissue destruction leading to impairment. However, even with conventional technology, Loseff and colleagues [54] showed clear correlations between impairment and spinal cord atrophy, as determined with measurements of cross-sectional areas at the C2 level. Although subtle, their findings have since been confirmed repeatedly by different groups and measurements [51]. A key problem of these measurements is the poor resolution of axial images and artifacts from surrounding tissues. The Queen Square Working Group [54] introduced a semi-automated technique to define the spinal cord border, improving the scan–rescan reproducibility. Compared to simple procedures (Fig. 16.10), the variation is much lower, reaching a standard deviation of 0.79 % for scan – rescan measurements. Volume measures of the cervical spinal cord show even greater differences between controls and the disease subtypes of MS [51].

15 Inflammation of the Spinal Cord

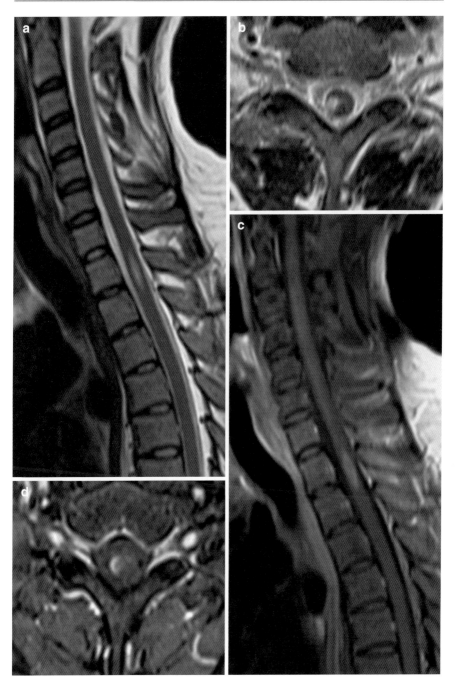

Fig. 15.16 CIS, 40-year-old man. Sagittal (**a**) and axial (**b**) T2WI with an right-sided hyperintense lesion of the cervical spine and marginal strong enhancement on sagittal (**c**) and axial (**d**) T1WI pc with fat suppression. Note the enhancement along the cerebral spinal fluid interface on the right. Cerebral MRI (not shown) disclosed two juxtacortical lesions and oligoclonal bands were positive in the CSF

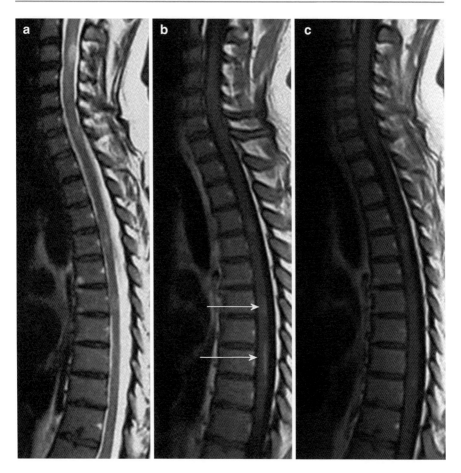

Fig. 15.17 Relapsing-remitting MS (RRMS), 44-year-old woman. The disease started with three bouts of acute partial transverse myelitis. T2 WI sag. (**a**) disclosing multiple hyperintense lesions with inhomogeneous enhancement especially at the CSF interface (**b, c**; T1 WI sag. pc, *arrows*)

> Measuring spinal cord atrophy seems well suited to monitor disease progression in individual cases and to compare disease subtypes on a group level.

Because of the abundance of degenerative vertebral diseases, some coincidence of multiple sclerosis and compressive myelopathy is to be expected.

> Concerning the management of myelopathy, there are in principle three mistakes that should be avoided:

1. The assumption that progressive myelopathy in the course of known MS is caused by the underlying disease, discarding further diagnostic measures. This seems possible especially when compression of the spinal cord occurs without radicular or local pain.
2. Alternatively, ascribing a progressive myelopathy to questionable spondylotic compression, and not to search for other abnormalities by imaging and other measures, CSF studies included.
3. Not to consider surgery if a patient exhibits radiological findings of both MS and compression of the spinal cord. A caveat is given by bladder disturbances. They occur late in the course of compressive myelopathy and are a daily occurrence in the care of MS patients.

There are several small sets of MS patients who were operated on for compression of the spinal cord (cited in [55]) showing stable improvement and minor or no complications. This contribution corresponds to inflammatory diseases of the spinal cord and therefore the description of MS is limited to the context of clinically isolated syndromes and progressive myelopathy. In both situations complementing brain MRI may be afforded either to describe further manifestations of another inflammatory disease or, if there is no other explanation than spinal manifestation of MS, to look for lesions that are suitable as diagnostic criteria. Moreover, concerning prognosis, especially in young patients, brain imaging may prove to be helpful because lesion load at the time of diagnosis seems to reflect the future course [56], supporting clinical decisions.

15.3.2 Adverse Effects of Tumor Necrosis Factor Alpha-Blockers

Tumor necrosis factor (TNF, formerly known as TNF alpha) is a proinflammatory cytokine involved in the regulation of immune cells and in systemic inflammatory reactions. It is thought to play an important role in the pathophysiology of several inflammatory diseases such as rheumatoid arthritis, ankylosing spondylitis, Crohn's disease, inflammatory bowel disease, psoriatic arthritis, and MS. A variety of cell types produce TNFs, among them macrophages, as well as microglia, astrocytes, and some neurons [57]. TNFs may mediate demyelination, but also seem to have protective effects. With the advent of two monoclonal antibodies (adalimumab, infliximab) and a soluble TNF receptor-Fc fusion protein (etanercept) all acting as TNF antagonists, there were several observations of associated neurological disease. These include demyelinating neuropathies, optic neuritis, MS, aggravating or new onset and only few cases of myelopathy, possibly representing a first episode of demyelization with favorable prognosis. Notably, anti-TNF agents have been associated with the development of systemic lupus erythematosus, including antinuclear and anti-DNA antibodies (Vadikolias et al., cited in [57]). In the particular case cited, an enhancing lesion

was observed, reaching from D9 to the conus. The diagnosis of neuromyelitis optica was discussed, but rejected on the basis of a lack of visual symptoms (see below). In a meta-analysis, including postmarketing studies of the anti-TNF drugs (Ramos-Casals et al., cited in [57]), demyelinating events were rare, ranging between 0.05 and 0.2 %. Following the definition of drug-induced illness, some criteria are fulfilled:
1. Temporal association
2. Stabilization/improvement of the disease by discontinuing exposure to the drug
3. Reappearance after re-exposure
4. Similar disorders reported after similar exposure

Nevertheless, the overall number of cases reported appears not to be superior to the incidence seen in patients untreated with these drugs [57]. Little is known about the incidence and prevalence of MS in certain autoimmune diseases; the other way around, there seems to be an increased risk for MS patients and their first-degree relatives to acquire systemic autoimmune diseases [57]. Therefore it may be wise to perform a baseline brain MRI before initiating anti-TNF drugs as has already been recommended. Two own cases are given to demonstrate the problem of differential diagnosis (Figs. 15.18, 15.19, and 15.20).

15.3.3 Neuromyelitis Optica

Neuromyelitis optica (NMO), known as *Devic's disease*, has long been thought of as a variant of multiple sclerosis. is most prevalent in Asia, and is characterized by severe attacks of optic neuritis and myelitis, commonly sparing the brain. However, in 2004 an antibody against the abundant aquaporin-4 protein (NMO-IgG) leading to demyelination in NMO was identified. In the following years this antibody was never detected in MS. Several groups confirmed that assays for NMO-IgG are highly specific [58]. While previously the description of NMO was based on clinical definition alone, diagnosis could be supported by the new serological marker (Table 15.6). Moreover, from now on NMO-IgG was recognizable as a common pathophysiological link in conditions named NMO spectrum disorders (Table 15.6), e.g. in formes frustes or in systemic autoimmune diseases (SAD). Both the deficits from optic neuritis and the MRI imaging of spinal lesions differ compared to those acquired in multiple sclerosis. NMO patients show a higher incidence of non-central scotoma, especially altitudinal hemianopia, which is highly characteristic of ischemic neuropathy ([59]; Figs. 15.21, 15.22, 15.23, 15.24, and 15.25) and the typical spinal lesion, LETM is an exceptional finding in MS, sometimes seen in childhood MS. However, concerning the spinal findings in (most) SAD, differences are neither clinically nor radiologically clear cut. Quite the opposite – the appearance of optic neuritis or LETM with SAD allows for the diagnosis of NMOSD (see Sect. 15.3.5).

15 Inflammation of the Spinal Cord

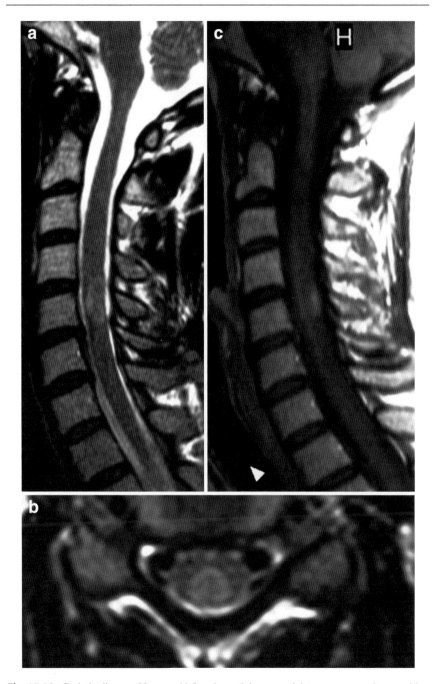

Fig. 15.18 Crohn's disease, 32-year-old female evolving a partial transverse syndrome with a sensory level D 8 following anti tumor necrosis factor (TNF; Infliximab) therapy. Spinal MRI exhibiting a hyperintense lesion on T2 WI (**a**, **b**: sag., ax.) with partial enhancement (**c**, T1 WI pc) (see also Fig. 14.6)

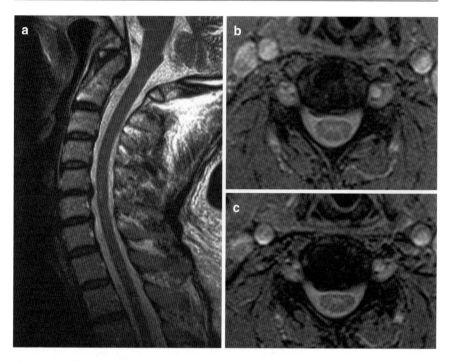

Fig. 15.19 Psoriasis arthritis, 52-year-old man with etarnacept therapy for 2 years, evolving burning paraesthesia in the right arm and dysaesthesia of swelling in both hands. MRI (T2 WI sag. (**a**) and axial (**b**, **c**)) disclosing a subtle intramedullary lesion at C 5/6 located in the gray matter around the central canal

A French multicenter study determined that the delay before a bifocal lesion (the diagnostic prerequisite of NMO) was reached was approximately 1 year [60]. It is entirely possible that NMO-IgG can identify patients at risk, although the sensitivity was found to be lower, as reported before, with 54 % [60].

In the United States the prevalence of NMO was estimated to be 1–2 % of that of MS, and in Denmark a yearly incidence rate of 0.4/100,000 was determined [61]. Among 187 patients with NMO and NMOSD, the classic presentation of simultaneous optic neuritis and transverse myelitis (occurring within 3 month) was found in 10 %, whereas transverse myelitis in isolation occurred as the first event in 50 % of all cases examined [61].

Imaging. Spinal cord lesions affect the cervical and/or thoracic spinal cord, most typically with longitudinally extensive lesions over three or more segments (LETM) (Figs. 15.23, 15.24, and 15.25) [58, 14, 61]. On axial sections, NMO occupy more than half of the cord area and involvement of the central gray matter is prominent (Fig. 15.24) [62]. LETM typically shows enhancement during an acute event ([62], Fig. 15.26).

15 Inflammation of the Spinal Cord

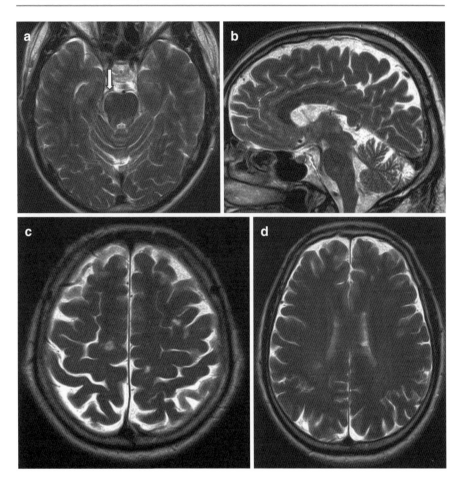

Fig. 15.20 Cranial MRI of same patient as in Fig. 15.19 with spastic paresis on the left, accentuated in the leg showing the possibly causative lesion on the right ventral surface of the pons (**a**, *arrow*; T2 WI ax.); (**b**) (T2 WI sag.): hyperintense lesions in the corpus callosum and beneath the floor of the fourth ventricle; (**c, d**) (T2 WI ax): additional lesions juxtacortical and periventricular (see criteria for dissemination in space, Table 15.4; CSF analysis showed negative oligoclonal banding)

LETM comprise more than 85 % of lesions. In contrast to the distribution of abnormalities in MS (see Sect. 15.3.1), in chronic lesions NMO cases may show T1 hypointensities.

Most relapses of NMO worsen over several days [58] and the persisting disability after a first spinal attack is poorer compared to MS (as severe residual visual loss is more common in NMO [60]). In the above-mentioned American study, the female to male ratio was 6.5:1 (in MS: 2:1) and, other than in MS, patients of African descent constituted roughly 1/3 of the patient population, making up a considerable portion of the study population. Moreover, 24/30 patients who developed brain stem lesions were of African American demographic.

Table 15.6 Neuromyelitis optica (NMO) and neuromyelitis optica spectrum after [58]

Mandatory: *Transverse myelitis* and optic neuritis, simultaneously or sequentially and *at least two* of the following supportive criteria: 1. Spinal cord lesion extending over ≥ three vertebral segments (longitudinally extensive myelitis, LETM)   2. Brain MRI non-diagnostic for multiple sclerosis   3. Seropositive for NMO-IgG
Neuromyelitis optica spectrum after [58]:
1. Neuromyelitis optica
2. Limited forms: Idiopathic single or recurrent events of LETM seen on MRI   Recurrent or bilateral optic neuritis
3. Asian optic-spinal multiple sclerosis
4. Optic neuritis or LETM associated with systemic autoimmune disease
5. Optic neuritis or myelitis associated with brain lesions typical of neuromyelitis optica (see text)

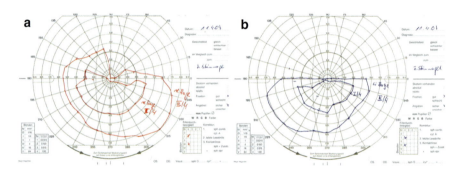

Fig. 15.21 Perimetric investigation in a 37-year-old woman with rapid progression of visual disturbances beginning on the left eye (see Fig. 15.22 and Fig. 15.23). (**a**) Right eye, (**b**) left eye

Acute spinal cord lesions in NMO demonstrate diffuse swelling and softening extending over multiple segments. Necrosis occurs in both white and gray matter [52, 58]. Systematic immunopathological analyses of active NMO lesions revealed a unique vasculocentric pattern of complement activation and eosinophil/neutrophil infiltrates, coupled with prominent vascular hyalinization [52]. All NMO lesions demonstrate a striking loss of aquaporin-4. This protein forms the most prevalent water channel in the central nervous system, located in the astrocytic foot processes surrounding endothelial cells and lining the interface between brain and cerebrospinal fluid. Aquaporin-4 is highly concentrated in the central gray matter of the spinal cord [62]. Moreover, high concentrations are found in periependymal regions around the lateral, third and fourth ventricles, including the tegmentum pontis and the area postrema.

It is in these areas where additional brain abnormalities are known to occur in about 10 % of NMO patients [58, 62]. Possibly, in patients of Asian descent, brain involvement can be found more often [63, 64].

Fig. 15.22 Neuromyelitis optica (same patient as Fig. 15.21) Coronal (**a**) and axial T1 WI pc (**b**) showing intense contrast enhancement of the optic chiasma

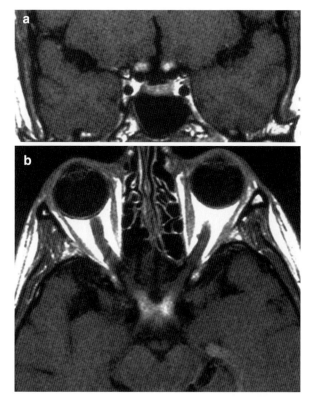

Besides NMO-IgG, two other autoantibody markers might be of interest in cases of ATM: if myelopathy is part of a paraneoplastic disorder, the presentation could resemble that of NMO, showing LETM. The corresponding autoantibodies are CRMP-5-IgG and amphiphysin IgG (Pittock, cited in [3]).

15.3.4 Acute Disseminated Encephalomyelitis, Postvaccination Myelopathies

Acute disseminated encephalomyelitis (ADEM) is thought of as an immune-mediated disease which predominantly affects the white matter of the brain and spinal cord, with an involvement of the latter in up to 28 % [37]. The lesions consist of perivenous foci of demyelination, associated with macrophage-dominated infiltration and, unlike in plaques from MS, the margins are rather indistinct.

Scott [1] stated in 2007 that it is yet to be determined whether or not some cases of acute partial or complete transverse myelitis represent limited forms of ADEM.

In accordance with [5] and several reports thereafter, it is assumed that site-restricted spinal forms of ADEM do exist in this fraction. One should bear in mind that it is essentially the same events which precipitate certain inflammatory diseases

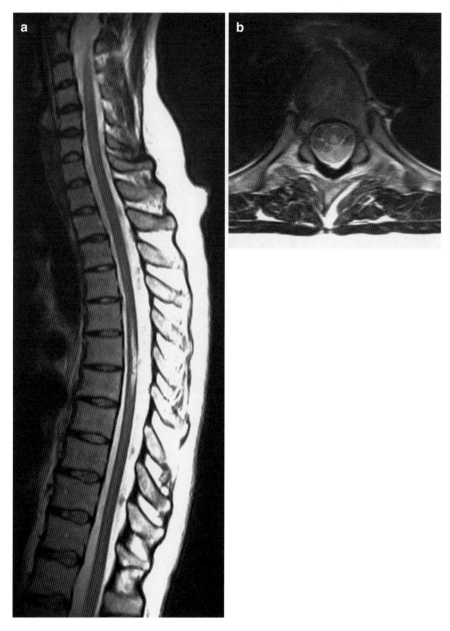

Fig. 15.23 Neuromyelitis optica (same patient as in Figs. 15.21 and 15.22): Sag. (**a**) and axial T2 WI (**b**) revealing a hyperintense lesion located in central and dorsal parts of the spinal cord, extending over three segments and correlating well to bilateral sensory disturbances that had developed 2 months before; aquaporin-4 antibodies were positive

15 Inflammation of the Spinal Cord

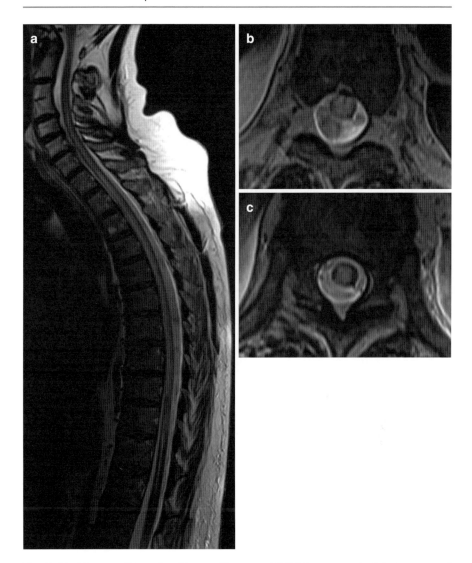

Fig. 15.24 Neuromyelitis optica, 55-year-old woman. T2 WI images acquired during a second spinal attack showing an extension lengthwise between C 4 and D 10 (**a**) The central parts of the cross section are involved predominantly, including gray matter structures (**b, c**)

of the spinal cord and the brain: in the former case, the disorder is usually called transverse myelitis, parainfectious myelitis, or myelopathy (see Sect. 15.2.5; [2, 10]); in the latter it is, self evidently, ADEM and the antecedent infection is viewed as an "antigenic challenge." While vaccination is widely accepted as a precipitating event for ADEM, in the case of an inflammatory disease restricted to the spinal cord, a relationship in fact sometimes is called in question [3].

ADEM may occur at any age, but has a clear peak in incidence during childhood. Among persons less than 20 years old, an incidence rate of 0.4/100,000 is estimated [37]. Classically described as a monophasic disorder, albeit a matter of current debate, symptoms arise typically 2–21 days after an antecedent infection or vaccination and progress within days ([37], Fig. 15.26).

In children the cerebral disease is clearly different from MS, often febrile, with encephalopathy, headaches, and sometimes fits. In the series cited by [37], full recovery was reached in 57–92 % of cases. Infections commonly associated with ADEM include, among others, influenza, enterovirus, measles, mumps, rubella, and the herpesvirus family. Bacterial triggers include Borrelia, Leptospira, beta-hemolytic Streptococcus and *Mycoplasma pneumoniae*.

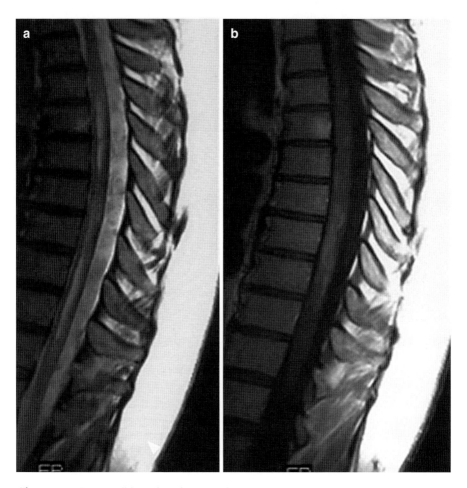

Fig. 15.25 Neuromyelitis optica, 64-year-old woman. Extension and enhancement of spinal lesions during the first (**a**, **b**; T2 WI sag., T1 WI pc sag.) and the second attack (**c**, **d**; T2 WI sag., T1 WI pc sag.)

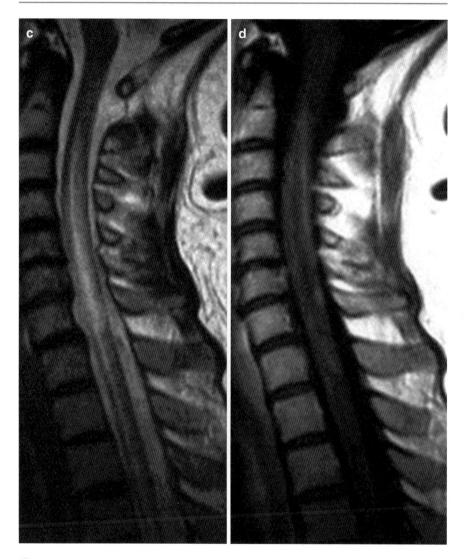

Fig. 15.25 (continued)

The notion of a site-restricted spinal variant of ADEM could be supported with some cases of acute myelitis associated with viral infection (Sect. 15.2.1). For instance, the cases of CMV [16] and EBV [4] infection could well represent ADEM restricted to the spinal cord, showing LETM and a favorable prognosis. In their review of *Mycoplasma pneumonia*-associated myelitis, Tsiodras et al. [65] distinguish ADEM (with cerebral findings) as opposed to acute transverse myelitis (without such findings) but emphasize that a direct CNS invasion with the agent does not play an important role in myelitis. The antecedent respiratory tract infection occurs with an interval of approximately 10 days before the spinal symptoms develop. Notably, the outcome of patients embraced under the term "acute transverse myelitis" was the better one

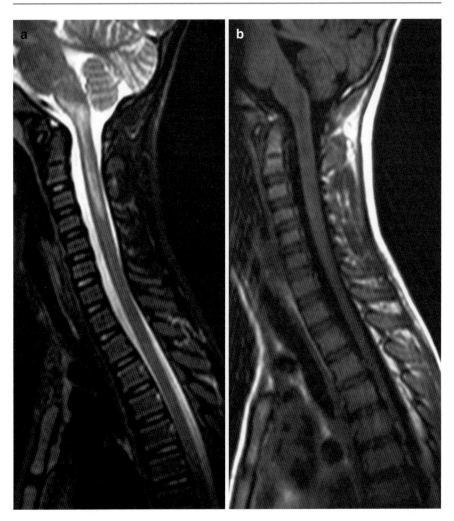

Fig. 15.26 Sag. T2 (**a**) and T1 W1 pc. (**b**) in a child with prototypical ADEM (acute disseminated encephalomyelitis) showing an extended lesion from lower brainstem to the level C4 (Courtesy Prof. M. Thurnher, Vienna)

compared with ADEM (plus cerebral findings). Two adult patients of Goebels et al. (cited in this review) may underline the hypothesis of a site-restricted ADEM variant: after an infection, in the same way as with typical ADEM, spinal symptoms arose, LETM was proven, and in their further course only minor residual deficits were left. Recently, antibodies against myelin oligidendrocyte glycoprotein were found to be elevated in ADEM, and in two LETM cases negative for NMO IgG as well [66].

The large series of 60 postinfectious patients [5] included patients with cerebral, spinal, and radiculoneuritic symptomatology. Thirty three patients showed multifocal lesions on cerebral MRI and 42/60 patients had focal or multifocal lesions depicted on spinal MRI, mostly multisegmental, interestingly, in 11 patients the lesions were asymptomatic. On the other hand, in 6 patients MRI scans were within

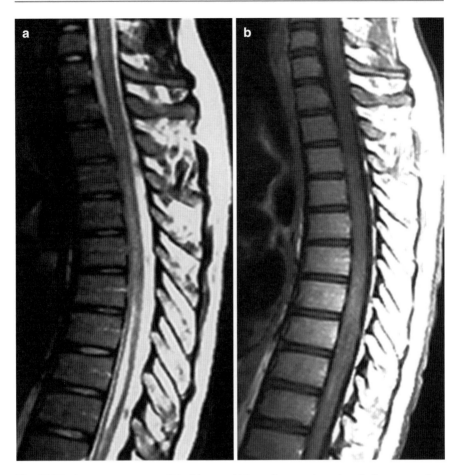

Fig. 15.27 Acute transverse myelitis, 14-year-old boy who experienced again fever some days after an upper airway infection. MRI (**a**, T2 WI sag.; **b**, T1 WI sag. pc) disclosing LETM (longitudinally extensive transverse myelitis) with slight swelling (**a**) and faint enhancement (**b**). Clinical examination exhibit transversal syndrome and meningeal signs; pleocytosis on CSF examination. No infectious agent was proven (cranial imaging not done)

normal limits, despite severe clinically and neurophysiologically proven transverse myelitis.

In conclusion, some cases of "acute transverse myelitis" as described in Sect. 15.2.1 might be interpreted as "acute disseminated encephalomyelitis" rather than caused by direct destructive effects of infectious agents. The possible interpretation of a case as portrayed with Fig. 15.27 remains somewhat arbitrary:

1. Idiopathic
2. Postinfectious
3. Site-restricted spinal variant of ADEM (a normal brain scan assumed) without further assistance from images

The radiological contribution essentially consists of the exclusion of tumor, vascular disease, and ADEM with typical cerebral findings. Other diagnoses (infection,

NMO, SAD) depend on clinical findings, additional laboratory tests and the evaluation of the further course. But if the lesion is small, "CIS" (Sect. 15.1.3, Table 15.1) comes into consideration.

15.3.5 Myelopathy Associated with Systemic Autoimmune Disease (SAD) and Sarcoidosis

The diseases collected here are of autoimmune or unknown etiology, with systemic lupus erythematosus (SLE) and Sjögren's syndrome (SS) being most often quoted. Other diseases associated with myelopathy include mixed connective tissue disease, sclerodermia, Morbus Behçet, and sarcoidosis [3]. Information on the antiphospholipid syndrome (APL) which is also indicated for, is provided by Mayer et al. [67]. Only SLE, SS, Behcet's disease, and sarcoidosis are discussed. Other, even less common, or more questionable diseases (e.g. primary angitis of the central nervous system (PACNS) and inflammatory bowel disease) are not dealt with in this chapter.

Of course, for the purposes of this contribution, an inflammatory pathogenesis of detectable lesions is assumed. To qualify this, however, it should be mentioned that pathogenetic differentiation is limited on clinical and radiological grounds. Inflammation – often badly understood – aside, arterial and venous occlusive disease, swelling, and non-inflammatory demyelination may ensue.

If a lesion emerges in the course of a known illness fulfilling established diagnostic criteria, the corresponding spinal cord syndrome is attributable to SAD. However, unfortunately, as emphasized repeatedly, it is not uncommon for neurological deficits to be the first or only manifestation of SAD, posing diagnostic challenges.

In the series of Birnbaum et al. [68], in 6/22 patients with SLE, spinal cord syndrome was the presenting illness. Similarly, in the large study of Delalande et al. (cited in [69]) conducted on patients with primary SS from an internal medicine and a neurological department, in 17/29 patients the spinal cord syndrome preceded the diagnosis of primary SS. Debette et al. [2], describing the further course of myelopathies, diagnosed 5/14 SAD during follow-up only (SS 8; SLE 4; Sarcoidosis 1; Wegener's disease 1).

Looking at the mode of presentation in partial ATM (Table 15.1), probably the most frequent diagnosis is MS finally. Other causes may be quoted less often but, obviously, accuracy is afforded because therapies differ (e.g. interferon-ß could worsen SLE). In the study of Delalande et al. (cited in [69]) the course in 4/29 patients resembled MS, while others mimicked primary progressive MS. At least in the majority (65 %), imaging disclosed a single spinal lesion as opposed to 35 % LETM being more typical for the presentation with complete ATM. Since the description of NMOSD [58], the list of causes other than MS might be complemented by formes frustes of NMO. However, to satisfy the criteria set (Table 15.6) the length of the lesion has to cover at least three segments.

Complete ATM (Table 15.1) is estimated to affect SLE patients in 1–2 % of cases [68] and in the case of first manifestation, NMO is an important differential diagnosis. Surprisingly, in recent years it has become evident that the antibody NMO-IgG initially believed to be disease specific seems to occur "syndrome specifically" [70]. Therefore, NMO-IgG can be found in rheumatologic diseases when they are complicated by ATM or relapsing optic neuritis, but not when other neurological manifestations emerge.

In a large series of 22 SLE patients, Birnbaum et al. [68] could separate two groups, characterized by history and clinical and paraclinical findings:
1. The first one, designated "gray matter myelitis" was characterized with high inflammatory activity of SLE, mirrored in CSF findings, rapid (<24 h) evolution of ATM, and rare relapses. Ten out of eleven patients remained paraplegic (vs 0/11 in the second group). An unexpected observation was that fever and urinary retention heralded paraplegia in 10/11 cases. Swelling of the spinal cord and LETM was typical (11/12 studies), accompanied by contrast enhancement in not more than 25 %. This was interpreted as a consequence of impaired venous efflux during maximum spinal engorgement.
2. In the second group named "white matter myelitis," NMOSD criteria are often satisfied with optic neuritis, relapses, and positive NMO-Ig-G. Because of several relapses, 23 imaging studies could be reviewed. Swelling was noticed less often, in 21.7 %, and enhancement in nearly 50 % of the studies. In addition, it was this second group where the findings of secondary APL were more prevalent.

A case presenting with complete ATM and fulfilling the definition of both primary SS and NMOSD is described by Kahlenberg [71]. She reviewed the current literature and stated that the high prevalence of NMO-IgG when tested and the occurrence of optic neuritis argue for an overlap of SS and NMOSD. Nevertheless, in primary SS LETM is also rare but well documented, notwithstanding NMO-IgG titers failing to appear [69].

The already mentioned analysis of Mealy et al. [61] comprising NMO and NMOSD cases shows that, similar to SLE and SS, most cases are female and have the potential for recurrence in common. Twenty five of ninety five patients tested were positive for anti SS-A, and 10/92 positive for anti SS-B antibody titers. Interestingly, in the study of SLE patients described [68], anti-Ro (anti SS-A) antibodies were found eight times, despite none of these patients having Sjögren's syndrome, more often being associated with features of NMOSD.

In summary, there seem to be two clearly different groups of ATM in SLE patients, indicating pathogenetic heterogeneity. Although they have LETM in common, they are either with or without NMO-IgG associated (Fig. 15.28). Known from older neuropathological studies are spinal infarction, and lesions compatible with NMO as well as vacuolar myelopathy (see Chap. 16).

Similarly, LETM has been detected in primary SS as well, with or without NMO-IgG association. Moreover, primary SS lesions may be observed to be resembling MS as evidenced by Delalande et al. (cited in [69]) and several other reports thereafter.

Behcet's disease is well known in Mediterranean, Middle East and East Asian countries, highly associated with the presence of HLA B 51, and rarely seen in Northern parts of Europe. It is a multisystem, vascular-inflammatory disorder of

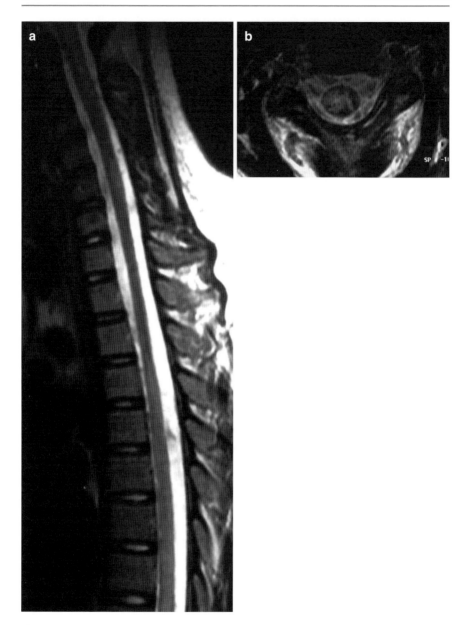

Fig. 15.28 Systemic lupus erythematodes (SLE), 17-year-old woman with partial transverse syndrome, walking ability only marginal restricted. T2 WI (**a**: sag., **b**: ax.) revealing LETM. The examination was performed in the early 2000s when neither NMO spectum diseases were described, nor any tests available. Today, proof of LETM, should prompt laboratory testing – irrespective of further clinical aspects

unknown cause, which affects arteries, small vessels, and veins. Other than in SLE and SS, besides clinical diagnostic criteria, there are some sound neuropathological reports that help to interpret morphological aspects of a given lesion. Most typical, they involve the mesodiencephalic junction asymmetrically and are characterized by edematous swelling extending along fiber tracts. Causative are venous thromboses of small intra-axial veins with insufficient collateral supply.

Imaging. In the acute phase some nodular enhancement is observed and possibly leptomeningeal enhancement originating from venous occlusion as well (Kocer et al., cited in [72]).

In a large series of "Neuro-Behcet" (Akman et al., cited in [72]), 10/200 cases showed an isolated and 13/200 cases a predominantly spinal cord involvement. Some cases collected from the English literature in [72] give the impression of a variable lesion length, often spanning more than three segments, one segment and the entire cord being the extremes. More often, the upper spinal cord seems to be affected. Thus, the extension is "LETM" but, in contrast to the examples of NMO depicted (Figs. 15.25 and 15.26) T2-hyperintensities and some swelling are noncontiguous. Similarly, on T1WI the lesions were mildly or patchily enhanced after application of gadolinium. Fukae et al. [72] emphasize the discrepancy between lesion extension and mild clinical deficits without sensory or sphincter disturbance and a good response to steroids – in line with an interpretation of (less destructive) swelling caused by venous obstruction. The prognosis is variable as known from the more prevalent cerebral lesions and tissue loss resulting in T1-hypointensity, atrophy and Wallerian degeneration may develop, consistent with concomitant inflammation of different parts of the vasculature during the acute phase.

Similar to the aforementioned diseases, sarcoidosis is an inflammatory multisystem disorder of unknown cause. However, in contrast to SAD and Behçet's disease, sarcoidosis and also "neurosarcoidosis", i.e. the affection of the nervous system, can remain unnoticed.

An example is given with bihilar adenopathy detected by chance in a chest radiogram –without any complaints. Vitaly Terushkin (cited in Chap. 13 which describes meningeal disorders) estimates asymptomatic central nervous system involvement being present in at least 10 % of sarcoidosis patients.

Similar to other systemic inflammatory diseases described, a spinal cord syndrome may be the presenting illness. In a recent study involving 31 patients, spinal cord symptoms were the initial manifestation of the disease in not less than 90 %. In the remaining three patients spinal involvement occurred between 2 and 11 years after respiratory symptoms, uveitis and arthritis respectively [73].

The mode of onset in these cases was subacute, symptoms evolving twice within one day. Symptoms did not differ compared to those of a control group consisting of other myelopathies (NMO, SS, MS, infectious, compressive) with the exception of pain (14/31). All MRI studies displayed T2-hyperintense lesions within the spinal cord, being multiple (≥ 2 lesions) in more than 50 % and mostly centrally located as revealed by axial slices. Seventeen of twenty three patients showed contrast medium enhancement.

Enhancing intramedullary lesions are more often nodular or irregular shaped and surrounded by some edema ([4, 40, 73]; Figs. 15.29 and 15.31).

Another form of intramedullary lesion enhances intensely and abuts broad based on the spinal cord surface without space-occupying effects (Kumar and Spencer, cited in [14, 73]; Fig. 15.31), showing similarities to meningovascular syphilis (see Sect. 15.2.2). Associated leptomenigeal and spinal root enhancement is regarded as a common finding, depicted and discussed in Chap. 13.

Depiction of nodules as shown in Fig. 15.29, representing granuloma lessens the number of differential-diagnoses to few other inflammatory diseases and to malignancy (see Table 15.3).

In the investigation of Cohen-Aubart et al. [73], brain imaging was carried out in all cases and found to be abnormal more often when compared to the control group: these were T2-hyperintesities 15 patients, enhancing meninges 3 patients, and pituitary involvement 1 patient. If there is widespread nodular meningeal enhancement detected in a chronic case, only sarcoidosis or tuberculosis should be causative. An example is given by Spencer (cited in [73]). If such spinal findings are associated with intraparenchymatous cerebral perivascular enhancements (Fig. 15.30), this "pattern" seems to be characteristic.

15.4 Concluding Remarks

To complement a spinal MRI with a study of the brain may be prudent in the case of an inflammatory spinal cord syndrome. However, the timing of this examination should depend on the actual condition of the patient and the suspected diagnosis.

For instance, it is simple to exclude a space-occupying cerebral lesion but, on the other hand, delineating cerebral manifestations from sarcoidosis could turn out to be a demanding task and often a second well-planned examination would be more appropriate.

As presented, there are some rare inflammatory conditions where cerebral findings are to be expected and contributing, as in the case of cysticercosis or sarcoidosis.

It would be advisable that, if the suspected diagnosis is MS, ADEM, or NMO, cerebral examination is not dispensible for the radiological description. However, concerning the latter, the most recent consensus seems to be that NMO can no longer be regarded as a disease without any brain involvement. One has to count with confusing findings in the white matter whose prevalence in different populations seems unsettled [63, 64]. How to discriminate them is an issue that remains under discussion.

Concerning the imaging criteria for MS, it should be remembered that clinical differential diagnosis is viewed as a prerequisite to minimize false positive diagnosis ([42, 44], with a comment on "red flags" clinically and radiologically).

The fact should be reemphasized that knowledge of the evolution of symptoms is helpful for both clinical diagnosing and the interpretation of images.

If a myelopathy develops insidiously or continues to progress after 3 weeks, transverse myelitis becomes unlikely and the differential diagnosis of a lesion includes tumor, dural arteriovenous fistula, sarcoidoses, and rare infectious agents. Of course, in all these cases the examination of the cerebrospinal fluid is mandatory.

15 Inflammation of the Spinal Cord

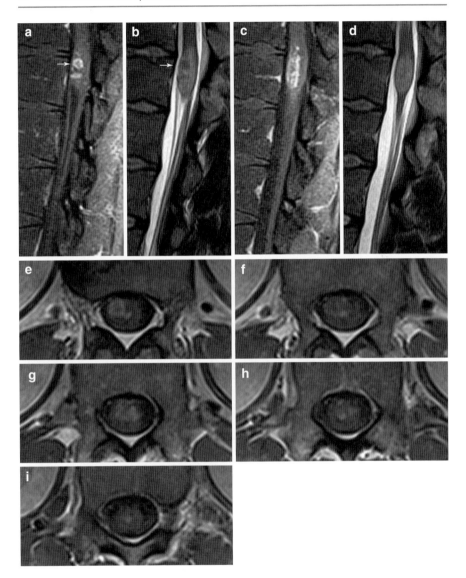

Fig. 15.29 Sarcoidosis in an 11-year-old boy with paraparesis accentuated on right and incontinence, steroid medication. T1 WI sag. pc (**a**, **c**) and T2 WI sag. (**b**, **d**) showing intramedullary inhomogeneous mass lesion of the lumbar spinal cord at D 12 with nodular hypointense signal changes on T2 WI and corresponding nodular enhancement on T1 WI pc (**a**, **b**: *arrow*); linear intramedullary enhancement, probably following the course of the central canal. Moreover, on axial T1 WI pc (**e–i**) slight enhancement in the leptomeninges and along spinal roots are visible

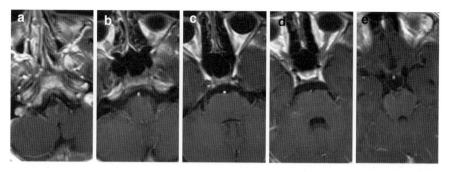

Fig. 15.30 Cranial MRI (**a–e**; T1 WI ax. pc; same patient as in Fig. 15.29) showing "angiocentric" involvement in the right brachium pontis besides meningeal enhancement. Neurological examination disclose visual complaints and impaired adduction of the left eyeball

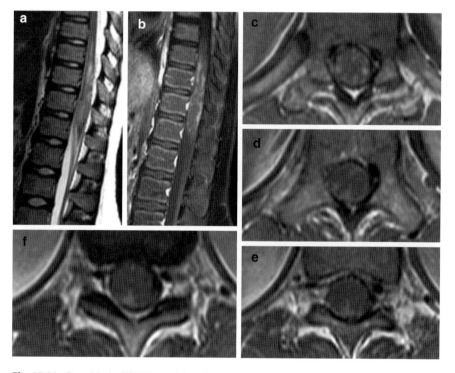

Fig. 15.31 Sarcoidosis. T2 WI sag. (**a**) and T1 WI pc FS (**b**: sag.; **c–f**: ax.) in a 25-year-old man with a history of a half year of sciatic pain without neurological deficits showing nodular and linear enhancement along the pial surface, with some vertical and wedge-shaped extension into the parenchyma (same case as shown in Chap. 13)

References

1. Scott TF (2007) Nosology of idopathic transverse myelitis syndromes. Acta Neurol Scand 115:371–376
2. Debette S, de Seze J, Pruvo J-P et al (2009) Long-term outcome of acute and subacute myelopathies. J Neurol 256:980–988
3. Jacob A, Weinshenker BG (2008) An approach to the diagnosis of acute transverse myelitis. Semin Neurol 28:105–120
4. de Seze J, Lanctin C, Lebrun C et al (2005) Idiopathic transverse myelitis: application of the recent diagnostic criteria. Neurology 65:1950–1953
5. Marchioni E, Ravaglia S, Piccolo G et al (2005) Postinfectious inflammatory disorders subgroups based on prospective follow-up. Neurology 65:1057–1065
6. Pidcock FS, Krishnan C, Crawford TO et al (2007) Acute transverse myelitis in childhood center-based analysis of 47 cases. Neurology 68:1474–1480
7. Young J, Quinn S, Hurrell M et al (2009) Clinically isolated acute transverse myelitis: prognostic features and incidence. Mult Scler 15:1295–1302
8. Bergers E, Bot JCJ, van der Valk P et al (2002) Diffuse signal abnormalities in the spinal cord in multiple sclerosis: direct postmortem in situ magnetic resonance imaging correlated with in vitro high-resolution magnetic resonance imaging and histopathology. Ann Neurol 51:652–656
9. Stankiewicz JM, Neema M, Alsop DC et al (2009) Spinal cord lesions and clinical status in multiple sclerosis: a 1.5 T and 3 T MRI study. J Neurol Sci 279:99–105
10. Kerr DA, Ayetey H (2002) Immunpathogenesis of acute transverse myelitis. Curr Opin Neurol 15:339–347
11. Berger JR, Sabet A (2002) Infectious myelopathies. Semin Neurol 22:133–141
12. Kleinschmidt-DeMasters BK, Gilden DH (2001) The expanding spectrum of herpesvirus infections of the nervous system. Brain Pathol 11:440–451
13. Bulakbasi N, Kocaoglu M (2008) Central nervous system infections of herpesvirus family. Neuroimaging Clin N Am 18:53–84
14. Goh C, Phal PM, Desmond PM (2011) Neuroimaging in acute transverse myelitis. Neuroimaging Clin N Am 21:951–973
15. Fux CA, Pfister S, Nohl F, Zimmerli S (2003) Cytomegalovirus-associated acute transverse myelitis in immunocompetent adults. Clin Microbiol Infect 9:1187–1190
16. Karacostas D, Christodoulou C, Drevelengas A et al (2002) Cytomegalovirus-associated transverse myelitis in a non-immunocompromised patient. Spinal Cord 40:145–149
17. Gruhn B, Meerbach A, Egerer R et al (1999) Successful treatment of Epstein-Barr virus-induced transverse myelitis with gancyclovir and cytomegalovirus hyperimmune globulin following unrelated bone marrow transplantation. Bone Marrow Transplant 24:1355–1358
18. Haq A, Wasay M (2006) Magnetic resonance imaging in poliomyelitis. Arch Neurol 63:778–779
19. Kira J, Isobe N, Kawano Y et al (2008) Atopic myelitis with focal amyotrophy: a possible link to Hopkins syndrome. J Neurol Sci 269:143–151
20. Kramer LD, Li J, Shi PY (2007) West Nile virus. Lancet Neurol 6:171–181
21. Sejvar JJ, Bode AV, Curiel M et al (2004) Post-infectious encephalomyelitis associated with St. Louis encephalitis virus infection. Neurology 63:1719–1721
22. Kurita N, Sakurai Y, Taniguchi M et al (2009) Intramedullary spinal cord abscess treated with antibiotic therapy. Case report and review. Neurol Med Chir 49:262–268
23. Bigi S, Aebi C, Nauer C et al (2010) Acute transverse myelitis in Lyme neuroborreliosis. Infection 38:413–416
24. Koc F, Bozdemir H, Pekoz T et al (2009) Lyme disease presenting as subacute transverse myelitis. Acta Neurol Belg 109:326–329
25. Charles V, Duprez TP, Kabamba B et al (2007) Poliomyelitis-like syndrome with matching magnetic resonance features in a case of Lyme neuroborreliosis. J Neurol Neurosurg Psychiatry 78:1160–1161

26. Conde-Sendín M, Amela-Peris R, Aladro-Benito Y (2004) Current clinical spectrum of neurosyphilis in immunocompetent patients. Eur Neurol 52:29–35
27. El Quessar A, El Hassani R, Chakir N et al (2000) La gomme syphylitique médullaire. J Neuroradiol 27:207–210
28. Tsui EYK, Ng SH, Chow L et al (2002) Syphilitic myelitis with diffuse spinal abnormality on MR imaging. Eur Radiol 12:2973–2976
29. Kikuchi S, Shinpo K, Niino M et al (2003) Subacute syphilitic meningomyelitis with characteristic spinal MRI findings. J Neurol 250:106–107
30. Wasay M, Arif H, Khealani B et al (2006) Neuroimaging of tuberculous myelitis: analysis of ten cases and review of literature. J Neuroimaging 16:197–205
31. Gumbo T, Hakim JG, Mielke J et al (2001) Cryptococcus myelitis: atypical presentation of a common infection. Clin Infect Dis 21:54–56
32. Leite CL, Jinkins JR, Escobar BE et al (1997) MR imaging of intramedullary and intradural-extramedullary spinal cysticercosis. Am J Roentgenol 169:1713–1717
33. Saleem S, Belal AI, el-Ghandour NM (2005) Spinal cord schistosomiasis: MR imaging appearance with surgical and pathologic correlation. AJNR Am J Neuroradiol 26:1646–1654
34. Badr HI, Shaker AA, Mansour MA et al (2011) Schistosomal myeloradiculopathy due to schistosoma mansoni: report of 17 cases from an endemic area. Ann Indian Acad Neurol 14:107–110
35. Sawanyawisuth K, Tiamkao S, Kanpittaya J et al (2004) MR imaging findings in cerebrospinal gnathostomiasis. AJNR Am J Neuroradiol 25:446–449
36. Singer OC, Conrad F, Jahnke K et al (2011) Severe meningoencephalitis due to CNS-toxocariosis. J Neurol 258:696–698
37. Tenembaum S, Chitnis T, Ness J (2007) Acute disseminated encephalomyelitis. Neurology 68(Suppl 2):S23–S36
38. Michou L, Sauve C, Sereni C et al (2002) Rapid efficacy of highly active antiretroviral therapy in a case of HIV myelitis. Eur J Intern Med 13:65–66
39. Umehara F, Nose H, Saito M et al (2007) Abnormalities of spinal magnetic resonance images implicate clinical variability in human T-cell lymphotrophic virus type I-associated myelopathy. J Neurovirol 13:260–267
40. Eckstein C, Syc S, Saidha S (2011) Differential diagnosis of longitudinally extensive transverse myelitis in adults. Eur Neurol J 3:27–39
41. Nagappa M, Sinha S, Taly AB et al (2013) Neurosyphilis: MRI features and their phenotypic correlation in a cohort of 35 patients from a tertiary care university hospital. Neuroradiology 55:379–388
42. Montalban X, Tintoré M, Swanton J et al (2010) MRI criteria for MS in patients with clinically isolated syndromes. Neurology 74:427–434
43. Polman CH, Reingold SC, Banwell B et al (2011) Diagnostic criteria for multiple sclerosis: 2010 revisions to the McDonald criteria. Ann Neurol 69:292–302
44. Miller DH, Weinshenker BG, Filippi M et al (2008) Differential diagnosis of suspected multiple sclerosis: a consensus approach. Mult Scler 14:1157–1174
45. Bot JCJ, Barkhof F, Polman CH et al (2004) Spinal cord abnormalities in recently diagnosed MS patients. Neurology 62:226–233
46. Oppenheimer DR (1978) The cervical cord in multiple sclerosis. Neuropathol Appl Neurobiol 4:151–162
47. Rocca MA, Hickman SJ, Bö L et al (2005) Imaging spinal cord damage in multiple sclerosis. J Neuroimaging 15:297–304
48. Lycklama G, Thomson A, Filippi M et al (2003) Spinal cord MRI in multiple sclerosis. Lancet Neurol 2:555–562
49. Verhey LH, Branson HM, Makhija M et al (2010) Magnetic resonance imaging features of the spinal cord in pediatric multiple sclerosis: a preliminary study. Neuroradiology 52:1153–1162
50. Gilmore CP, Geurts JJG, Evangelou N et al (2009) Spinal cord grey matter lesions in multiple sclerosis detected by post-mortem high field MR imaging. Mult Scler 15:180–188
51. Zivadinov R, Banas AC, Yella V et al (2008) Comparison of three different methods for measurement of cervical cord atrophy in multiple sclerosis. AJNR Am J Neuroradiol 29:319–325

52. Hu W, Lucchinetti CF (2009) The pathological spectrum of CNS inflammatory demyelinating diseases. Semin Immunopathol 31:439–453
53. Barkhof F (1999) MRI in multiple sclerosis: correlation with expanded disability status scale (EDSS). Mult Scler 5:283–286
54. Losseff NA, Webb SL, O'Riordan JI et al (1996) Spinal cord atrophy and disability in multiple sclerosis. A new reproducible and sensitive MRI method with potential to monitor disease progression. Brain 119:701–708
55. Arnold PM, Warren RK, Anderson KK et al (2011) Surgical treatment of patients with cervical myeloradiculopathy and coexistent multiple sclerosis. Report of 15 patients with long-term follow-up. J Spinal Disord Tech 24:177–182
56. O'Riordan JI, Thomson AJ, Kingsley DPE et al (1998) The prognostic value of brain MRI in clinically isolated syndromes of the CNS. A ten –year follow-up. Brain 121:495–503
57. Tristano AG (2010) Neurological adverse events associated with ant-tumor necrosis factor alpha treatment. J Neurol 257:1421–1431
58. Wingerchuk DM, Lennon VA, Lucchinetti CF et al (2007) The spectrum of neuromyelitis optica. Lancet Neurol 6:805–815
59. Nakajima H, Hosokawa T, Sugino M et al (2010) Visual field defects of optic neuritis in neuromyelitis optica compared with multiple sclerosis. BMC Neurol 10:45
60. Collongues N, Marignier R, Zéphir H et al (2010) Neuromyelitis optica in France. A multicenter study of 125 patients. Neurology 74:736–742
61. Mealy MA, Wingerchuk DM, Greenberg BM et al (2012) Epidemiology of neuromyelitis optica in the United States. A multicenter analysis. Arch Neurol 69:1176–1180
62. Nakamura M, Miyazawa I, Fujihara K et al (2008) Preferential spinal central gray matter involvement in neuromyelitis optica. An MRI study. J Neurol 255:163–170
63. Chan KH, Tse CT, Chung CP et al (2011) Brain involvement in neuromyelitis optica spectrum disorders. Arch Neurol 68:1432–1439
64. Kim W, Park MS, Lee SH et al (2010) Characteristic brain magnetic resonance imaging abnormalities in central nervous system aquaporin-4 autoimmunity. Mult Scler 16:1229–1236
65. Tsiodras S, Kelesidis TH, Kelesidis I et al (2006) Mycoplasma pneumoniae-associated myelitis: a comprehensive review. Eur J Neurol 13:112–124
66. Mader S, Gredler V, Schanda K et al (2011) Complement activating antibodies to myelin oligodendrocyte glycoprotein in neuromyelitis optica and related disorders. J Neuroinflammation 8:184
67. Mayer M, Cerovec M, Rados M et al (2010) Antiphospholipid syndrome and central nervous system. Clin Neurol Neurosurg 112:602–608
68. Birnbaum J, Petri M, Thompson I et al (2009) Distinct subtypes of myelitis in systemic lupus erythematosus. Arthritis Rheum 60:3378–3387
69. Trebst C, Raab P, Voss EV et al (2011) Longitudinal extensive transverse myelitis- it's not all neuromyelitis optica. Nat Rev Neurol 7:688–698
70. Wingerchuk DM, Weinshenker BG (2012) The emerging relationship between neuromyelitis optica and systemic rheumatologic autoimmune disease. Mult Scler 18:5–10
71. Kahlenberg JM (2011) Neuromyelitis optica spectrum disorder as an initial presentation of primary Sjögren's syndrome. Semin Arthritis Rheum 40:343–348
72. Ukae J, Noda K, Fujishima K et al (2010) Subacute longitudinal myelitis associated with Behçet's disease. Intern Med 49:343–347
73. Cohen-Aubart F, Galanaud D, Grabli D et al (2010) Spinal cord sarcoidosis. Clinical and laboratory profile and outcome of 31 patients in a case-control study. Medicine 89:133–140
74. Mennel HD, Solcher HFK (1984) Infektionen des Nervensystems. Schattauer Verlag, Stuttgart/New York

Metabolic-Toxic Diseases and Atrophic Changes of the Spinal Cord

16

Michael Nichtweiß, Elke Hattingen, and Stefan Weidauer

Contents

16.1	Introduction	370
16.2	Subacute Combined Degeneration of the Spinal Cord (SCDSC)	370
	16.2.1 Pathogenesis	370
	16.2.2 Pattern	370
	16.2.3 Neurological Signs and Symptoms	371
	16.2.4 Vitamin B12 Deficiency	371
	16.2.5 Copper Deficiency	373
16.3	Paraneoplastic Tractopathy	376
16.4	Vitamin E Deficiency	376
	16.4.1 Pathogenesis	376
	16.4.2 Pattern	376
	16.4.3 Neurological Signs and Symptoms	376
16.5	Vacuolar Myelopathy	377
	16.5.1 Pathogenesis	377
	16.5.2 Pattern	377
	16.5.3 Neurological Signs and Symptoms	377
16.6	Spinal Cord Atrophy and Signs of Syndromal Diseases	379
References		387

M. Nichtweiß (✉)
Department of Neurology, Hanse Klinikum Wismar; Wellengang 21,
D-23968 Wismar, Germany
e-mail: michael.nichtweiss@gmail.com

E. Hattingen
Institute for Neuroradiology, Goethe-University,
Schleusenweg 2-16, D-60528 Frankfurt, Germany
e-mail: elke.hattingen@kgu.de

S. Weidauer
Department of Neurology, Sankt Katharinen Hospital,
Seckbacher Landstr. 65, D-60389 Frankfurt, Germany
e-mail: stefan.weidauer@sankt-katharinen-ffm.de

Abbreviations

ADAV	Alexander's disease adult variant
Gd	Gadolinium
LBSL	Leukodystrophy with brainstem and spinal cord involvement and lactate elevation
PGBD	Adult polyglucosan body disease
SCDSC	Subacute combined degeneration of the spinal cord
VM	Vacuolar myelopathy

16.1 Introduction

This chapter is concerned with the depiction of lesions which are confined to individual columns of the spinal cord. They have lengthwise extension, lack of enhancement and swelling in common. Atrophy of the spinal cord should be described, but, for a variety of reasons, radiology does not contribute to the differential diagnosis.

In the case of metabolic toxic and degenerative spinal cord disease there are only a few findings to be expected in gross pathological examination, including possible subtle discolouration of tracts when cut in the transverse plane and possibly some shrinkage of the spinal cord and roots.

Of course, the main contribution to the diagnosis of such diseases is a clinical one, especially since detectable lesions occur neither early nor constantly. However, sometimes radiologists and clinicians may be surprised by certain radiological findings. To offer a rationale for differential diagnosis, some conditions are depicted in the following text. A comprehensive and systematic overview covering not imaging results but most clinical aspects and even geographical predilection is given by Kumar [1]. The approach of this contribution is different: selected entities are displayed, focussing on radiological appearance and differential diagnosis. To elucidate commonalties, some biochemical and immunological findings are detailed.

16.2 Subacute Combined Degeneration of the Spinal Cord (SCDSC)

16.2.1 Pathogenesis

Primarily affection of the myelin sheets: Vitamin B12 deficiency, Copper deficiency.

16.2.2 Pattern

Lesions arise in the centre of the dorsal and on the surface of the lateral columns, and occasionally in the anterior columns.

16.2.3 Neurological Signs and Symptoms

Symmetrical, often heralding dysaesthesia, disturbance of position sense, spastic signs, sometimes arising within weeks.

The first full clinical and pathological description of neurological sequels following vitamin B12 deficiency was given by Russell, Batten and Collier, who coined the term subacute combined degeneration of the spinal cord (SCDSC) more than a century ago (cited by Harper and Butterworth [2]). This term reflects neither the frequent involvement of peripheral nerves nor the occasional effects on the white matter of the brain, but describes the lesion pattern of the spinal cord as it can sometimes be displayed very well radiologically and is therefore preferred. Microscopically these lesions emerge as small foci of perivenular myelin swellings which merge later on. The fibres of greatest diameter are predominantly involved. Yet, the impression of involvement restricted to certain tracts as suggested sometimes by MR images seems to be erroneous [2] (Fig. 16.4). These lesions can be found in any part of the spinal cord and are, as a rule, extended over several segments, up to the whole length of the spinal cord.

Imaging. Signal alterations are depicted consistently in the dorsal columns (Figs. 16.1, 16.2, 16.3 and 16.4), and are sometimes even suspected to be an artifact. However, the reason for the predilection for parts of the spinal cord while sparing the reminder remained unexplained up to now [3].

16.2.4 Vitamin B12 Deficiency

Absorption of vitamin B12 requires a glycoprotein (intrinsic factor) produced by the parietal cells in the gastric fundus. Atrophic gastritis, the autoimmune destruction of parietal cells and inactivation of intrinsic factor, is the most common cause of deficiency, leading to pernicious anaemia and SCDSC. Neuropathy, encephalopathy and white matter lesions, and less often optic nerve atrophy, may be associated. Clinically, SCDSC is characterized by symmetric dysaesthesia, disturbance of the position sense and spastic signs, sometimes arising within weeks. In principle, there seem to be two different enzymes of major importance to discuss regarding the pathogenesis of the nervous system disease, both requiring vitamin B12 as a coenzyme [3]: methylmalonic-coenzyme A (CoA) mutase and methionine synthase. Methylmalonyl-CoA mutase catalyses the isomerization of methylmalonyl-CoA to succinyl-CoA, with methylmalonyl-CoA formed from beta oxidation of fatty acids and catabolism of some amino acids. Methionine synthase helps to catalyse the conversion of homocysteine to methionine. Methionine is then converted to *S*-adenosylmethionine (SAM) which is important in the methylation of myelin basic protein and myelin lipids. Since folate is also integrally involved in the latter pathway, and folate deficiency causes megaloblastic anaemia but not SCDSC, it was assumed that a dysfunction of the first pathway mentioned is causative in vitamin B12 deficiency. However, findings from an animal model provided evidence of the relevance of methionine synthase: N_2O irreversibly oxidizes the active cobalt in

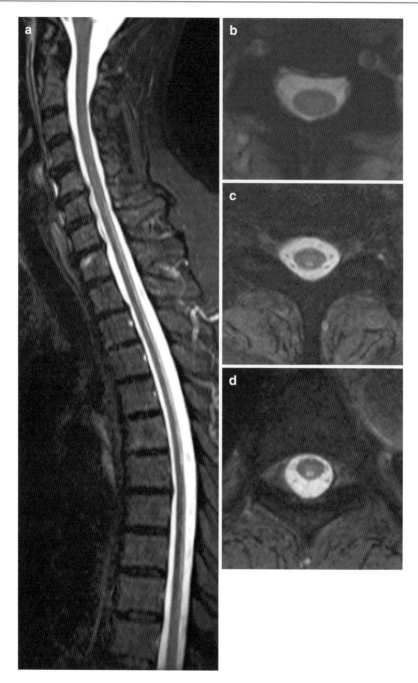

Fig. 16.1 Subacute combined degeneration of the spinal cord (SCDSC) caused by vitamin B12-deficiency with a clinical history of numbness after 6 months, abdominal sensory level, whereas sense for pain and temperature were normal, no paresis. T2 WI sag. (**a**) and axial (**b**–**d**) showing a hyperintense signal conversion through the entire thoracal part of the dorsal columns, but not cervically

16 Metabolic-Toxic Diseases and Atrophic Changes of the Spinal Cord

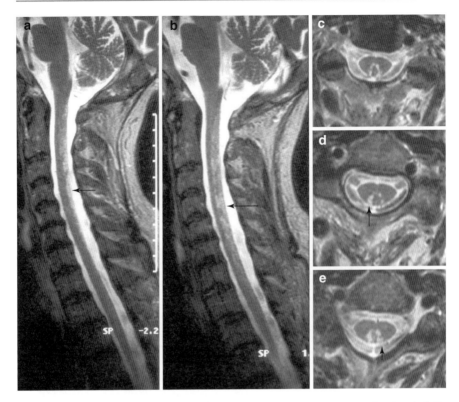

Fig. 16.2 Subacute combined degeneration of the spinal cord (SCDSC) caused by vitamin B12-deficiency in the early course. Sagittal (**a, b**) and axial (**c–e**) T2 WI showing patchy hyperintense signal changes in the dorsal part of the spinal cord, most closely in between gracile and cuneate tract, which were shown to be reversible. *Arrows*, for comarison: Fig. 14.2

methionine synthase, rendering the enzyme inactive. In several species, as well as in humans, this may cause SCDSC [3]. Low or unrecognized vitamin B12 deficiency may become evident with N_2O anaesthesia or the abuse of the agent. Moreover, prolonged N_2O exposure lowers vitamin B12 serum levels for as yet unclear reasons. An entirely new model, independent of vitamin B12 coenzyme functions, considers the pathogenetic role of cytokines and growth factors to explain vitamin B12 deficiency myelopathy [3] (see Sect. 16.5).

16.2.5 Copper Deficiency

Several reports in recent years have revealed that copper deficiency can cause a myelopathy which is clinically and radiologically indistinguishable from SCDSC [4] (Fig. 16.4). Copper is a component of numerous metalloenzymes and proteins which have a key role in maintaining the structure and function of the nervous system.

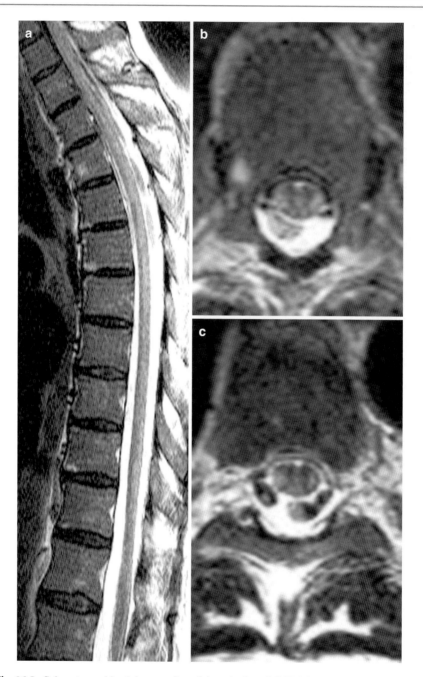

Fig. 16.3 Subacute combined degeneration of the spinal cord (SCDSC) caused by vitamin B12-deficiency in a 63-year-old woman suffering from severe atacic paraparesis with positive pyramidal signs over 9 months; gastrectomy 25 years ago. Sagittal (**a**) and axial (**b–e**) T2 WI disclosing hyperintense signal changes in the thoracic lateral and in addition in the lumbar posterior columns (see difference to Figs. 16.1 and 16.2)

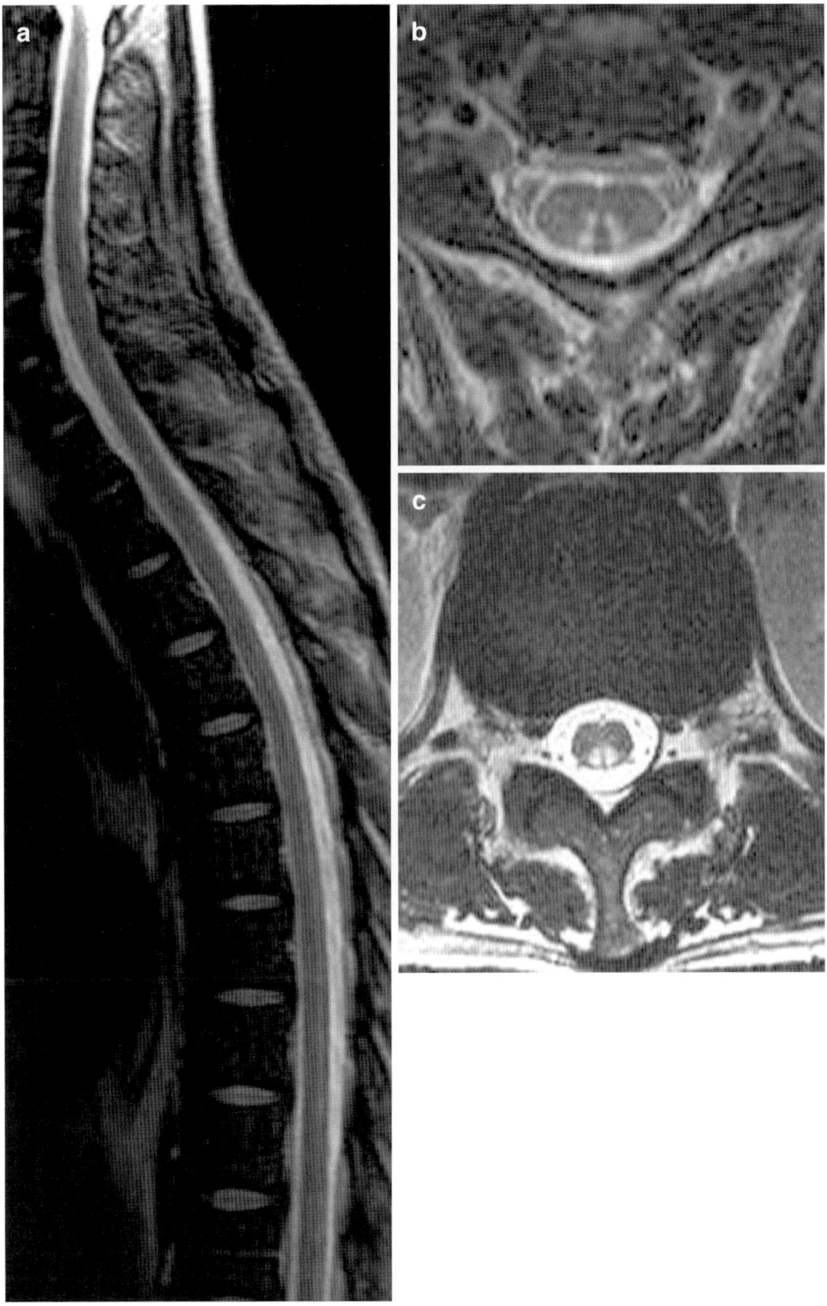

Fig. 16.4 Subacute combined degeneration of the spinal cord (SCDSC) caused by copper deficiency. Extension of hyperintense signal changes on T2 WI in the posterior columns through the whole length of the spinal cord (**a**, sag.), cervically (**b**, ax.) not in the course of lumbar fibres (**c**, ax.); compare with Fig. 16.7

Some of the risk factors for vitamin B12 deficiency, such as malabsorption and previous upper gastrointestinal surgery, are similar. Moreover, an important risk factor for copper deficiency is zinc overload. Zinc interferes with intestinal copper absorption by up-regulating intestinal synthesis of metallothionein, which has a greater affinity for copper. Therefore, the copper bound by the enterocytes is eliminated by their sloughing off into the intestinal lumen. In their review, Jaiser and Winston [4] argued that the phenotypic parallels between vitamin B12 and copper deficiency could be explained by dysfunction of the methylation cycle. The above-mentioned methionine synthase and S-adenosylhomocysteine hydrolase may depend on copper.

16.3 Paraneoplastic Tractopathy

As pointed out by Jacob and Weinshenker [5], the investigation of patients with subacute, evolving and possibly ambiguous symptoms may lead to images which bear a similarity to SCDSC.

Imaging. Symmetric T2 signal abnormalities throughout the thoracic spinal cord seem to be restricted to the corticospinal tract. To our knowledge, there are case reports replicating this finding, but none with neuropathological confirmation. Other than in SCDSC, the tracts showed contrast medium enhancement.

This finding should prompt the search for paraneoplastic antibodies and related cancer (see this review).

16.4 Vitamin E Deficiency

16.4.1 Pathogenesis

Primarily degeneration of axons

16.4.2 Pattern

Posterior columns, most marked in the fasciculus gracilis
 Thoracic course of the tract, sparing the lumbar intumescence

16.4.3 Neurological Signs and Symptoms

A combination of spinocerebellar syndrome and polyneuropathy, possibly with pyramidal signs.

Neuropathologic findings of vitamin E deficiency differ substantially when compared to SCDSC. Irrespective of the kind of primary metabolic events in pathogenesis (which probably concern cellular membranes and subcellular organelles), vitamin E deficiency results first in the degeneration of axons, not in a lesion of the myelin sheath as do the above-mentioned disorders [2].

16 Metabolic-Toxic Diseases and Atrophic Changes of the Spinal Cord

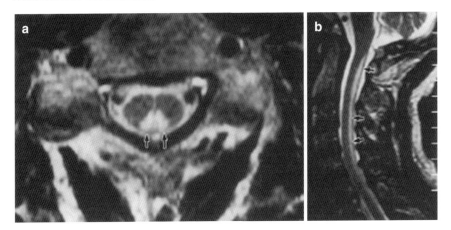

Fig. 16.5 Acquired vitamin E deficiency with axonal degeneration. Axial (**a**) and sag. (**b**) T2 WI showing increased signal intensity in the posterior cervical columns (*arrows*) (From: Vorgerd et al. [6], Springer, Berlin, with kind permission)

Imaging. Vitamin E deficiency results in an axonal neuropathy involving the centrally directed fibres of the "pseudounipolar" sensory neurons located in the spinal ganglia. The large-calibre fibres are predominantly affected, leading to changes in the posterior columns, most marked in the fasciculus gracilis (Fig. 16.5), extending from the gracile nucleus to the thoracic course of the tract, sparing the lumbar intumescence [6].

Despite several acquired circumstances and hereditary conditions leading to vitamin E deficiency, the case report cited is the only one publishing imaging results.

16.5 Vacuolar Myelopathy

16.5.1 Pathogenesis

HIV-infection, non-AIDS immuno-compromised patients

16.5.2 Pattern

SCDSC-like
  Spinal cord atrophy, mainly thoracal

16.5.3 Neurological Signs and Symptoms

Subacutely evolving, painless myelopathy occurring late, mostly in the setting of known infection; see SCDSC.

Vacuolar myelopathy (VM) best known from HIV-infection is mostly looked at as an inflammatory disease. However, from the very beginning there have been discussions on the relationship of vacuolar myelopathy and SCDSC based on a similar lesion pattern and histopathology [7]. Rarely, but repeatedly, VM is observed in non-AIDS immuno-compromised patients, e.g. after steroid medication [7, 8]. The course of the disorders may differ: VM in the case of HIV-infection occurs late and may remain asymptomatic [8], myelopathy as the presenting syndrome of HIV-infection is exceptional [9]. SCDSC with vitamin B12 deficiency, on the other hand, is often heralded by paraesthesia. As supposed by Stacpoole et al. [8], suppression and dysregulation of the immune system may be causative, leading to an impaired repair involving the vitamin B12-dependent transmethylation pathway. S-Adenosylmethionine (SAM; see Sect. 16.1.1), a central component of that pathway, is found to be decreased in AIDS-associated myelopathy. Alternatively, an unidentified infective agent still remains under discussion [8].

In treating the pathogenesis of SCDSC, Hathout and El-Saden [3] commented on the work of Scalabrino and his colleagues [10], which could also be of importance for the development of VM. In the gastrectomized rat, they found sound evidence that vitamin B12 deficiency leads to an imbalance between myelinotoxic and myelinotrophic cytokines and growth factors. Thus, one can speculate that it is dysregulation of the immune system which represents the crucial common part of pathogenesis for VM and SCDSC. A marked macrophage activation and cytokine release was shown in VM as well, and with highly active antiretroviral therapy a decline in incidence has been observed [11].

Imaging. The MRI finding most often observed in patients with the clinical diagnosis of AIDS-associated myelopathy is spinal cord atrophy.

In the series of Chong et al. [12], which was not neuropathologically correlated, 15 of 21 patients showed atrophy, typically involving the thoracic part, with or without association of the cervical segment [12], while 3 of 21 showed no abnormality. Neuropathological studies revealed that the dorsal and lateral white matter columns are mainly affected. The isolated cervical lesion in a rare case of VM with neuropathological confirmation [7], representing a non-enhancing, abnormality without mass effect and moderate T2 hyperintensity, corresponds exactly to SCDSC, restricted to the posterior columns. Enhancement strongly supports HIV-myelitis (Goh et al. [13]; see also Sect. 15.2.6) if lymphoma and the numerous opportunistic infections are ruled out [7]. VM is a diagnosis of exclusion and, as detailed, a categorization as an "immune-mediated" disease one could be justified as well. If any lesion seems to be confined to tracts, brain imaging should be considered in order not to overlook concomitant cerebral pathologies. T2-signal prolongation is caused by every alteration of tissue texture leading to increased water content, or by gliosis, and, thus, vacuolation, axonal loss and Wallerian degeneration all look the same. Nevertheless, knowledge of those underlying pathologies may be of some help for interpretation (Table 16.1).

16 Metabolic-Toxic Diseases and Atrophic Changes of the Spinal Cord

Table 16.1 Lesions of individual columns – hints for differential diagnosis

Pathological definition	Diseases, syndromes	Distribution
Subacute combined degeneration of the spinal cord (SCDSC)	Vitamin B12 deficiency, N$_2$O, copper deficiency	Parts of a tract affected, possibly patchy Length variable, several segments (Figs. 16.1, 16.2, 16.3 and 16.4)
Vacuolar myelopathy		Mostly thoracic
Axonal degeneration		Tracts as a whole affected
	Vitamin E deficiency (Fig. 16.5)	More pronounced distally
	Friedreich's ataxia (Figs. 16.8 and 16.9)	Cervical ascending tracts, descending tracts
	Adrenomyeloneuropathy	Lumbal (compare graphs in Chap. 14)
	Cerebrotendinous xantomatosis	
	Tabes dorsalis (Sect. 15.2.6, Fig. 15.8)	
	Primary lateral sclerosis (Fig. 16.10)	Corticospinal tract
	Polyglucosan body disease (Figs. 16.11, 16.12, 16.13 and 16.14), LBSL, Alexander's disease, adult variant	The entire length may be affected: dorsal column and corticospinal tracts, probably ascending spinocerebellar tracts
Wallerian degeneration Fig. 16.7	Axonal lesions below	Somatotopical (graphs in Sect. 14.1)

LBSL leukoencephalopathy with brainstem and spinal cord involvement and high lactate

16.6 Spinal Cord Atrophy and Signs of Syndromal Diseases

Atrophic changes resulting from circumscribed damage of the spinal cord are easily detected, simply by comparison with the neighbouring, well-preserved parenchyma (Fig. 16.6). A comment on the initial lesion of this case ensuing under therapy with a TNF-alpha-blocker is given in Sect. 15.3.2. Quite similarly, another post-lesional phenomenon, Wallerian degeneration (Fig. 16.7), may be detectable with prolongation of the T2–signal, since the abnormality is confined to an individual tract. Notably, exclusively the fibres from the caudal part of the spinal cord are altered. It is worth mentioning that less conspicuous, subtle shrinkage of the spinal cord and roots may occur in several degenerative disorders such as motor neuron disease or spinocerebellar ataxia affecting the spinal cord [14]. Furthermore, it may be the case in certain minimal volume losses in the course of chronic inflammatory disease. Such changes can be overlooked, in particular when the spinal cord as a whole is affected.

Measurements are appreciated, but their importance is more questionable, apart from probably in multiple sclerosis (see Sect. 15.2.1.). There is considerable interindividual variation of diameters and cross sectional areas seen in healthy individuals

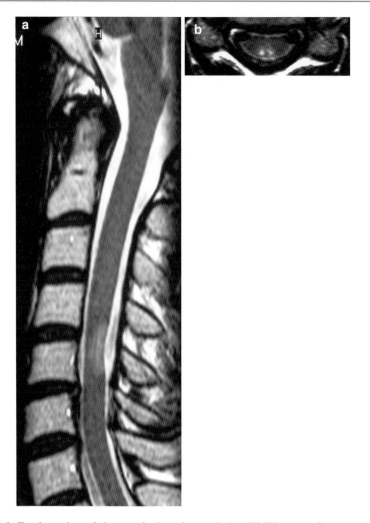

Fig. 16.6 Focal atrophy and circumscript hyperintense lesion (T2 WI; **a**: sag.; **b**: ax.) at the level C5 on follow-up MRI in a 32-year-old female with Crohn's disease (same patient as in Fig. 15.18; Sect. 15.3.2) following anti tumour necrosis factor (TNF; infliximab) therapy

[15, 16] Nevertheless, a description is feasible when the cross sectional area is clearly out of the normal range. Table 16.2 depicts data derived from Thorpe et al. [15]. Anatomical measurements from cadavers give the impression of even lower area values and greater variance, e.g. C5 mean 75 mm^2, ranging from about 56 to 98 mm^2. Considering the widely used lower threshold value for a normal sagittal cervical diameter (atrophy below 6 mm), it is important to know (Thorpe et al. [15]) that atrophic appearance from sagittal scans had cross sectional areas within normal limits. The case presented in Fig. 16.8 is an example of Friedreich's ataxia. The most prevalent (up to 4/100,000) and well described disease among the still growing group of

16 Metabolic-Toxic Diseases and Atrophic Changes of the Spinal Cord

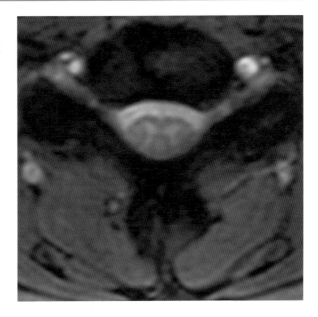

Fig. 16.7 Wallerian degeneration of the lumbar portion in the gracile tract at level C5 11 years after lumbar myeloradiculitis (tick-borne; same patient as in Fig. 15.3, Sect. 15.2.1)

Table 16.2 Spinal cord atrophy

Level	Cross sectional area suggesting atrophy (mm^2)
C5 (cervical intumescence)	<88
T2 (upper thoracic spinal cord)	<52
T7 (lower thoracic spinal cord)	<42
T11 (lumbal intumescence)	<21

From Thorpe et al. [15]

inherited ataxias [17]. In Friedreich's ataxia spinal atrophy is a constant feature, other than cerebellar atrophy, and this is in contrast to common belief. The latter is more prevalent only in late onset cases after age 25 years [18]. Often, spinal cord imaging from degenerative disease is said to show atrophy. This outdated image was coined to demonstrate that, possibly, it may simply be an insufficient resolution which hampers differentiation as opposed to the image from a neuropathology course, accessible via "neuropathology-web.org." (Fig. 16.9). The radiological findings in cases of sporadic, longstanding primary lateral sclerosis (Fig. 16.10) may appear similar. However, on neuropathological examination of the spinal cord there is found degeneration of the corticospinal tract only, which is not discernible from axial images. Again, in some of these cases, brain imaging may give additional information.

Table 16.1 encompasses diseases which come into consideration when a spinal examination performed to elucidate spasticity, ataxia and symptoms from the posterior columns exhibit a hyperintense T2-signal seemingly confined to tracts.

In such cases, nerve conduction and electromyographic studies often reveal peripheral neuropathy as well. More surprisingly, the most common and initial clinical finding of adult polyglucosan body disease (PGBD) in a recent multicenter

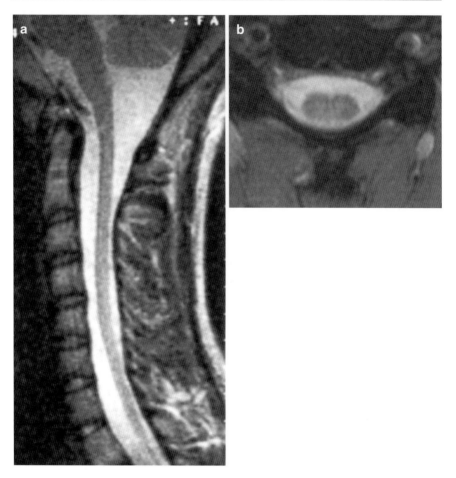

Fig. 16.8 Atrophy of the spinal cord in Friedreich's ataxia. Cross sectional area at the level C5: 40 mm^2; T2 WI sag. (**a**) and ax. (**b**)

study was neurogenic bladder, starting one or two decades before any other deficit [19]. The median age of onset in that study encompassing 50 patients, most of Ashkenazi Jewish background, was 51 years.

With regard to the findings of conventional MR imaging PGBD (Figs. 16.11, 16.12, 16.13 and 16.14), "Leukodystrophy with brainstem and spinal cord involvement and lactate elevation" (LBSL) and the adult variant of Alexander's disease (ADAV) are very similar. LBSL was described as an imaging pattern in 2003, affecting children and younger adults [20]. The patients showed the leading symptoms mentioned above with slow progression and mild cognitive decline. Worth noting is that "lactate elevation" describes a finding of MR spectroscopy, whereas elevated lactate in the spinal fluid is observed in mitochondriopathies only. Imaging of the brain provides additional information in some cases, and some further hints for radiologic differential diagnoses can be can be found in the review by Weidauer et al. [21].

Fig. 16.9 Axonal degeneration: Friedreich's ataxia, myelin stain. Caused by loss of sensory ganglion cells and degeneration of their axons in peripheral nerve (not shown), dorsal roots (pale dyed), posterior columns, spinocerebellar tracts and, to a lesser degree, degeneration of corticospinal tracts (From D.P. Agamanolis: http://neuropathology-web.org with kind permission)

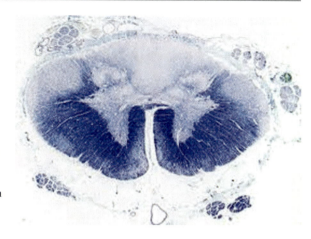

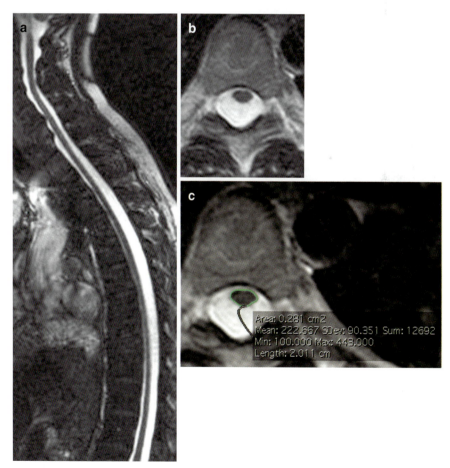

Fig. 16.10 Primary lateral sclerosis, 25 years duration of the disease. Atrophy of the spinal cord in a 44-year-old woman. Transsectional area at T7: 28.1 mm^2; at C5: 65 mm^2 (not shown); T2 WI sag. (**a**) and axial (**b, c**)

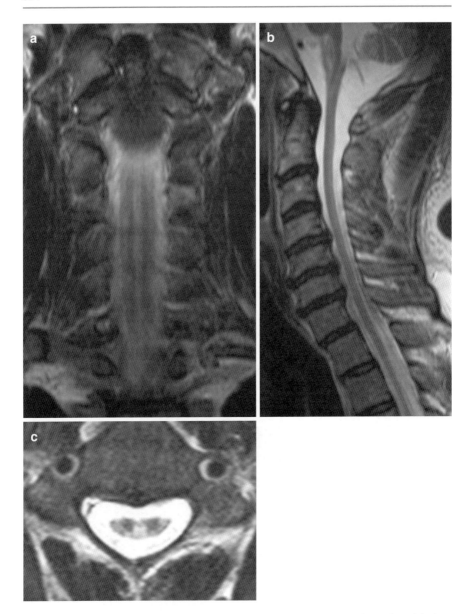

Fig. 16.11 Prominent affection of the posterior column and less pronounced in the lateral funiculus (note brainstem) with hyperintense signal changes on T2 WI (**a–c**: sag., cor., ax.) in a 65year-old male with progressive ataxia, spastic gait and polyneuropathy for several years in adult polyglucosan body disease (PGBD). Same patient as Figs. 16.12, 16.13 and 16.14

16 Metabolic-Toxic Diseases and Atrophic Changes of the Spinal Cord

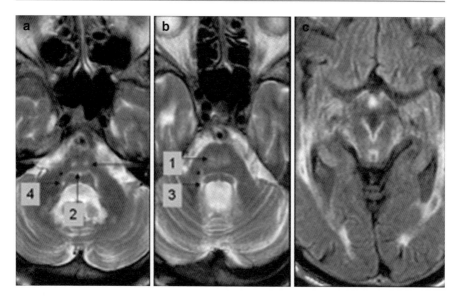

Fig. 16.12 Axial T2 WI (**a–b**) showing hyperintense signal changes of the corticospinal tract (*1*), the medial lemniscus (*2*), the superior peduncle (*3*), the mesencephalic trigeminal tract (*4*) and the intraparenchymal course of the trigeminal nerve (***) in adult polyglucosan body disease (PGBD). Axial FLAIR (**c**) showing a hyperintense rim of the mid brain (From: Weidauer et al. [21], Springer, Berlin, with kind permission)

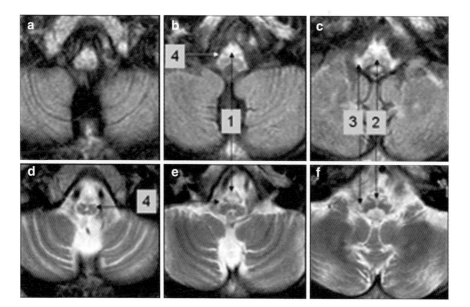

Fig. 16.13 (**a–f**) Fluid attenuated inversion recovery (FLAIR) images (**a–c**) and T2 WI (**e–f**) of the lower brainstem: (*1*) pyramids, (*2*) medial lemniscus, (*3*) inferior cerebellar peduncle and (*4*) spinal trigeminal tract (From: Weidauer et al. [21], Springer, Berlin, with kind permission)

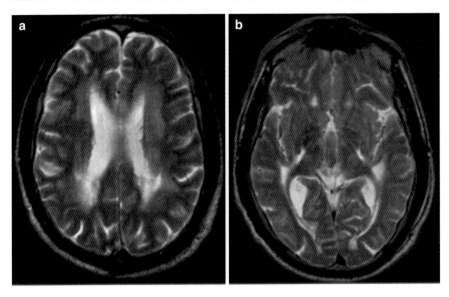

Fig. 16.14 Axial T2 WI (**a, b**; same patient as in Figs. 16.11, 16.12 and 16.13) showing extensive white matter changes (WMC) involving the posterior limb of the internal capsule (**b**) (From: Weidauer et al. [21], Springer, Berlin, with kind permission)

References

1. Kumar N (2012) Metabolic and toxic myelopathies. Semin Neurol 32:123–136
2. Harper C, Butterworth R (1997) Nutritional metabolic disorders. In: Graham DI, Lantos PL (eds) Greenfield's neuropathology, vol 1, 6th edn. Oxford University Press, Arnold/London/Sydney/Auckland, pp 601–655
3. Hathout L, El-Saden S (2011) Nitrous oxide-induced B12 deficiency myelopathy: perspectives on the clinical biochemistry of vitamin B 12. J Neurol Sci 301:1–8
4. Jaiser SR, Winston GP (2010) Copper deficiency myelopathy. J Neurol 257:869–881
5. Jacob A, Weinshenker BG (2008) An approach to the diagnosis of acute transverse myelitis. Semin Neurol 28:105–120
6. Vorgerd M, Tegenthoff M, Kühne D et al (1996) Spinal MRI in progressive myeloneuropathy associated with vitamin E deficiency. Neuroradiology 38(Suppl):S 111–S 113
7. Sartoretti-Schäfer S, Blättler T, Wichmann W (1997) Spinal MRI in vacuolar myelopathy, and correlation with histopathological findings. Neuroradiology 39:865–869
8. Stacpoole SRJ, Phadke R, Jacques TS, Revesz T, Plant GT (2009) Vacuolar myelopathy associated with optic neuropathy in an HIV-negative, immunosuppressed liver transplant recipient. J Neurol Neurosurg Psychiatry 80:581–583
9. Shimojima Y, Yazaki M, Kaneko K et al (2005) Characteristic spinal MRI findings of HIV-associated myelopathy in an AIDS patient. Intern Med 44:763–764
10. Weber D, Mutti E, Galmozzi E et al (2006) Increased levels of the CD40:CD40 ligand dyad in the cerebrospinal fluid of rats with vitamin B 12 (cobalamin)-deficient central neuropathy. J Neuroimmunol 176:24–33
11. Ho EL (2012) Infectious etiologies of myelopathy. Semin Neurol 32:154–160
12. Chong J, Di Rocco A, Tagliati M, Danisi F et al (1999) MR findings in AIDS-associated myelopathy. AJNR Am J Neuroradiol 20:1412–1416
13. Goh C, Phal PM, Desmond PM (2011) Neuroimaging in acute transverse myelitis. Neuroimaging Clin N Am 21:951–973
14. Palau F, Espinos C (2006) Autosomal recessive cerebellar ataxias. Orphanet J Rare Dis 1:47–65
15. Thorpe JW, Kidd D, Kendall BE et al (1993) Spinal cord MRI using multi-array coils and fast spi echo. 1. Technical aspects and findings in healthy adults. Neurology 43:2625–2631
16. Losseff NA, Webb SL, O'Riordan JI et al (1996) Spinal cord atrophy and disability in multiple sclerosis. A new reproducible and sensitive MRI method with potential to monitor disease progression. Brain 119:701–708
17. Finsterer J (2009) Ataxias with autosomal, X-chromosomal or maternal inheritance. Can J Neurol Sci 36:409–428
18. Bhidayasiri R, Perlman SL, Pulst S-M, Geschwind DH (2005) Late-onset Friedreich ataxia. Phenotypic analysis, magnetic resonance imaging findings and review of the literature. Arch Neurol 62:1865–1869
19. Mochel F, Schiffmann R, Steenweg ME et al (2012) Adult polygucosan body disease: natural history and key magnetic resonance imaging findings. Ann Neurol 72:433–441
20. Van der Knaap M, van der Voorn P, Barkhof F et al (2003) A new leukoence-phalopathy with brainstem and spinal cord involvement and high lactate. Ann Neurol 53:252–258
21. Weidauer S, Nichtweiß M, Hattingen E (2014) Differential diagnosis of white matter lesions: nonvascular causes – part II. Clin Neuroradiol 24:93–110

Gray Matter Diseases of the Spinal Cord

17

Johannes C. Klein

Contents

17.1 Introduction 389
17.2 Spinal and Bulbar Muscular Atrophy (SBMA, Kennedy Disease) 390
17.3 Spinal Muscle Atrophy 390
17.4 Poliomyelitis 392
17.5 Progressive Muscular Atrophy (PMA) 393
17.6 Monomelic Amyotrophy (MMA, Hirayama Disease) 393
Further Reading 394

Abbreviations

ALS   Amyotrophic lateral sclerosis
CSF   Cerebrospinal fluid
MMA   Monomelic amyotrophy
MND   Motor neuron diseases
PMA   Progressive muscular atrophy
SBMA   Spinal and bulbar muscular atrophy
SMA   Spinal muscular atrophy

17.1 Introduction

Gray matter diseases of the spinal cord cover a heterogenous group of inherited disorders, infectious and sporadic diseases. Typical examples include the spinal muscular atrophies, poliomyelitis, and motor neuron diseases. Clinical symptoms,

---

J.C. Klein
Brain Imaging Center (BIC), Department of Neurology, Goethe-University,
Schleusenweg 2-16, D-60528 Frankfurt, Germany
e-mail: klein@med.uni-frankfurt.de

age at onset, rate of progression, family history, and electrophysiological findings will help make the diagnosis.

MRI is usually performed to rule out secondary causes of spinal cord involvement, such as compressive myelopathy. Due to the small volume of the spinal cord and the even smaller volume of its gray matter, the diagnostic sensitivity of MRI is low in many of these disorders and rarely helps differentiate between entities.

Gray matter diseases of the spinal cord are not limited to gray matter only, as they will always entail involvement of white matter structures with degeneration of efferents. Consequentially, volume reduction of the whole spinal cord can be seen.

17.2 Spinal and Bulbar Muscular Atrophy (SBMA, Kennedy Disease)

- Rare inherited motor neuron disease affecting motor neurons in the pons, medulla oblongata, and cord, caused by mutation of the androgen receptor gene on the X chromosome.
- Almost exclusively affects males, motor symptoms occur late in life and are slowly progressive.
- Endocrinological symptoms of androgen receptor deficiency usually present before motor symptoms.

SBMA is an inherited motor neuron disease caused by polyglutamine expansion in the androgen receptor gene AR1 on the X chromosome. Because of its X-chromosomal inheritance, SBMA almost exclusively affects males with the very rare exception of women homozygous for the mutation.

Clinically, SBMA presents with progressive muscular atrophy and weakness of the facial, pharyngeal, and tongue muscles, as well as affectation of the proximal shoulder and hip girdle muscles. Patients will show slowly progressive dysphagia, dysarthria, and weakness of proximal muscles of the extremities. Symptoms often begin in one of these regions only and spread to the other regions after years or even decades.

Motor symptom onset is usually late in life. However, patients usually show signs of the underlying androgen receptor mutation before motor symptoms become apparent, such as gynecomastia, testicular atrophy, and fertility problems. Genetic testing is available.

Imaging: On MRI, patients can present with atrophy of the medulla oblongata and pons (Fig. 17.1), while atrophy of the clinically affected anterior horn of the lower spinal cord is usually not visible.

17.3 Spinal Muscle Atrophy

- Group of rare autosomal recessively inherited diseases linked to the same gene.
- Age of onset and progression is determined by specific mutation.
- Spinal MRI typically normal.

17 Gray Matter Diseases of the Spinal Cord

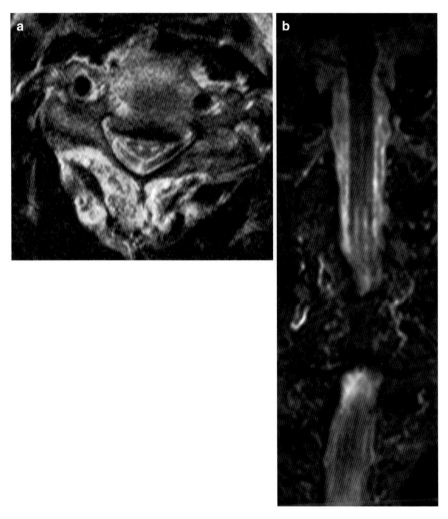

Fig. 17.1 T2-weighted transaxial (**a**) and coronal (**b**) imaging of the upper cervical spine shows marked atrophy, and there is extensive hyperintense gray matter signal. Note CSF flow artifact surrounding the spinal cord

Spinal muscular atrophy (SMA) presents with progressive signs of lower motor neuron disease due to degeneration of the anterior horn of the spinal gray matter. Symptoms include symmetric muscular weakness with loss of deep tendon reflexes and muscular atrophy. Clinically and genetically, SMA is divided into four subtypes, all of which are autosomal recessive disorders caused by specific mutations of the SMN-1 gene. The type and location of mutation determine the age of onset, progression rate, and severity of symptoms. Disease onset can occur at any point in life, and life expectancy can be very limited with SMA type 1, where symptoms present within the first 6 months of life.

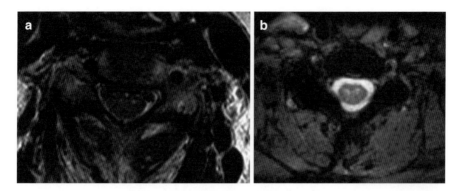

Fig. 17.2 High-resolution transaxial T2-weighted images show hyperintense signal in the anterior horn of the cervical (**a**) and thoracic (**b**) spinal gray matter

Imaging: Typically, MRI is normal in these patients, since the degeneration of the anterior horn of spinal gray matter is beyond the resolution of standard clinical scanning. With high-resolution imaging, however, degeneration can be detected (Fig. 17.2).

17.4 Poliomyelitis

Poliomyelitis, or polio, is caused by the poliovirus. Infection occurs via the fecal-oral route, and effective vaccines are available. Most patients with fresh infections will be asymptomatic or experience gastrointestinal symptoms only. In around 1–3 % of cases, however, the poliovirus enters the central nervous system. It targets spinal and bulbar motor neurons, leading to progressive weakness and muscular atrophy with loss of deep tendon reflexes. Clinically, motor symptoms are preceded by meningeal symptoms or even encephalitis. Diagnosis is made with stool cultures and serology.

The location of motor symptoms depends on the site of viral manifestation within the CNS, leading to spinal, bulbar, and bulbospinal forms of poliomyelitis. Bulbar involvement is particularly dangerous, leading to respiratory deficiency or palsy of pharyngeal muscles with subsequent dysphagia, or even fatal inflammation of the entire brain stem. Most symptomatic infections occur in children, and spinal polio can lead to deformities of the extremities due to insufficient musculature during the growth phase. The virus also targets neurons in the spinal ganglia and the deep cerebellar nuclei. Despite paresthesia during the initial phase, loss of sensation in the extremities is typically absent.

Note that some patients will experience progression of motor symptoms or progressive fatigue decades after the infection, a condition called post-polio syndrome that can be severely disabling.

Imaging: On T2-w, polio can present with hyperintensity of the anterior horn of the spinal gray matter. In cases of bulbar polio, inflammatory disease of the entire medulla oblongata may be seen with T2-w hyperintensity, swelling, and diffuse contrast enhancement.

17.5 Progressive Muscular Atrophy (PMA)

PMA is a variant in the spectrum of sporadic motor neuron diseases (MND), which also includes the more common amyotrophic lateral sclerosis (ALS). PMA refers to exclusive degeneration of the lower motor neuron, leading to muscular weakness, atrophy, and fasciculations. The onset of motor symptoms is usually unilateral (as opposed to SMA or SBMA) and focal. Symptoms spread from one region of the body (upper, lower extremity muscles, thoracic and bulbar muscles) to the contralateral side and to the other regions.

Unlike ALS, where both the lower and upper motor neurons are affected, PMA patients present with decrease or loss of deep tendon reflexes, and not spasticity. PMA accounts for around 5–7 % of MND. Evolution toward full-blown ALS with affectation of the upper motor neuron occurs in around one quarter of cases.

Age of onset is usually between 50 and 70 years of age, and PMA is more common in men than in women (3:1–4:1). Median survival after symptom onset is longer than in ALS and reported at around 2–5 years in studies, with survival beyond 10 years seen in around 10 % of cases.

Imaging: Spinal MRI is typically normal in PMA patients. Unlike ALS, cranial MRI is also normal in PMA.

17.6 Monomelic Amyotrophy (MMA, Hirayama Disease)

MMA presents with unilateral weakness, muscle atrophy, and fasciculations in an extremity, usually in distal muscles innervated by the segments C7–Th1. While the term Hirayama disease is reserved for cases with upper limb involvement, MMA can very rarely present in a lower limb. Upper motor neuron signs are absent. Typically but not exclusively, young males of Asian origin are affected (Japanese and Indian patients in particular). The age of onset is between 10 and 25 years of age. The disease is self-limiting after a progressive phase of 1–5 years. It does not extend beyond the spinal segments controlling one limb, rarely resulting in clinically significant disability.

While the etiology of MMA is not conclusively established, dynamic compression of the spinal cord on the anterior aspect of the spinal canal during neck flexion has been demonstrated with MRI in patients with upper limb involvement.

Imaging: Patients suspected of MMA should receive MRI either of the cervical or the lower thoracic spine including conus, depending on whether an upper or lower limb is affected. On axial T2-w, increased signal in the anterior horn of the affected and neighboring segments may be seen. Segmental atrophy of the spinal cord can occur. MRI also serves to rule out other compressive diseases (Fig. 17.3).

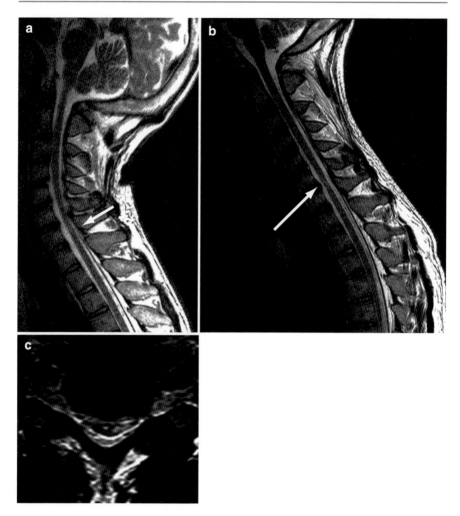

Fig. 17.3 T2-weighted sagittal MRI in retroflexion (**a**) and anteflexion (**b**) shows hypermobility of the cervical spinal cord, as well as hyperintense signal suggestive of myelopathy (*arrows*), presumably caused by dynamic compression. On transaxial imaging (**c**), a flattened appearance of the cord can be seen, and there is marked asymmetry corresponding to unilateral clinical involvement

Further Reading

1. Chahin N, Klein C, Mandrekar J, Sorenson E (2008) Natural history of spinal-bulbar muscular atrophy. Neurology 70(21):1967–1971
2. Choudhary A, Sharma S, Sankhyan N, Gulati S, Kalra V, Banerjee B, Kumar A (2010) Midbrain and spinal cord magnetic resonance imaging (MRI) changes in poliomyelitis. J Child Neurol 25(4):497–499
3. Dejobert M, Geffray A, Delpierre C, Chassande B, Larrieu E, Magni C (2013) Hirayama disease: three cases. Diagn Interv Imaging 94(3):319–323
4. Finsterer J (2009) Bulbar and spinal muscular atrophy (Kennedy's disease): a review. Eur J Neurol 16(5):556–561
5. Lunn MR, Wang CH (2008) Spinal muscular atrophy. Lancet 371(9630):2120–2133
6. Markowitz JA, Singh P, Darras BT (2012) Spinal muscular atrophy: a clinical and research update. Pediatr Neurol 46(1):1–12

Intramedullary Spinal Cord Tumors

18

Kamran Aghayev and Frank Vrionis

Contents

18.1	Introduction	395
18.2	Ependymoma	399
18.3	Astrocytoma	402
18.4	Hemangioblastoma	405
18.5	Intramedullary Spinal Cord Metastasis (ISCM)	406
18.6	Miscellaneous	407
Further Reading		408

Abbreviations

VHL   von Hippel Lindau
VEGF Vascular endothelial growth factor
ISCM Intramedullary spinal cord metastasis

18.1 Introduction

Intramedullary spinal cord tumors are comprised predominantly of intrinsic gliomas such as astrocytomas and ependymomas. In the majority of cases, they are benign (WHO grade 1 or 2) and the primary treatment option is microsurgical

---

K. Aghayev, MD (✉) • F. Vrionis, MD, PhD
Departments of Neurosurgery and Orthopedics, H. Lee Moffitt Cancer Center & Research Institute, Neuro-Oncology Program, 12902 Magnolia Drive, Tampa, FL 33612, USA

Departments of Neurosurgery and Orthopedics, Morsani College of Medicine, University of South Florida, 12902 Magnolia Drive, Tampa, FL 33612, USA
e-mail: kamran.aghayev@moffitt.org

Table 18.1 Intramedullary spinal cord tumor location

Cervical	30 %
Cervicothoracic	25 %
Thoracic	29 %
Conus	15 %

resection. Surgery is usually curative with ependymomas, hemangioblastomas, subependymomas, lipomas, dermoid, and epidermoid tumors due to good cleavage plane from the spinal cord, and when removal is complete, no further therapy is required. Astrocytomas demonstrate infiltrative behavior, and therefore residual and recurrent tumors are frequent. Radiotherapy is indicated for primary malignant tumors (WHO grade 3 and higher), radiosensitive tumors such as lymphoma, germinoma, and for patients in whom surgery is contraindicated. For grade 1–2 tumors, the role of radiotherapy is controversial. Chemotherapy is reserved for recurrent intramedullary spinal cord tumors without other options.

Primary spinal cord tumors account for 5–10 % of all adult spinal tumors and 4.5 % of primary CNS tumors. Unlike intracranial tumors intramedullary spinal cord tumors do not show an association between grade and age at diagnosis.

Because tumor origin varies by anatomic site in the spinal cord, spinal cord tumors are classified by anatomic sublocation as follows: intradural intramedullary, intradural extramedullary, and extradural. Intradural intramedullary spinal cord tumors constitute 20–30 % of all primary spinal cord tumors; the remaining 70–80 % are intradural extramedullary. The distinction between intra- and extramedullary tumor may not be obvious in some cases. For example, astrocytomas may show exophytic growth pattern. The majority (90 %) of intradural intramedullary tumors are either ependymomas (60–70 %) or astrocytomas (30–40 %). For the remaining 10 %, hemangioblastomas account for 3–8 %, of which 15–25 % is associated with von Hippel Lindau syndrome. Another 2 % of intradural intramedullary spinal cord tumors are metastatic.

The clinical presentation of intramedullary spinal cord tumors is determined partially by the location (Table 18.1) and the tumor type (Table 18.2). Regardless of the location, pain is the most common presenting symptom. It manifests as back pain (27 %), radicular pain (25 %), or central pain (20 %), although it is usually not as severe as pain associated with metastatic tumors involving the vertebrae. Neurological deficit is the second most common symptom and usually presents as a combination of motor (72 %), sensory (39 %), or sphincter disturbance (15 %). Intramedullary tumors usually affect the central gray matter and cause a syringomyelitic type syndrome characterized by disassociation between pain/temperature (loss) and tactile sensation (preservation), lower motor neuron dysfunction at the affected level, and upper motor neuron dysfunction caudal to it. No symptoms are pathognomic for spinal cord tumors yet "sacral sparing," i.e., maintenance of sensation in the sacral dermatomes and proximal motor deficits, gradual progressing of symptoms and "ascending" nature of deficits are common in intramedullary tumors.

MRI (with and without contrast) plays an essential role in the diagnosis of primary spinal cord tumors. Currently, no other imaging modality can be utilized alone to establish a diagnosis. Plain X-rays may show scalloping in rare cases of long-standing intramedullary tumors, and CT myelography may show spinal cord

Table 18.2 Intramedullary tumors' major characteristics

Tumor type	Incidence	Presentation	MRI appearance	Treatment	Outcome
Ependymoma	Most common intramedullary spinal cord tumor	Mixed sensorimotor syndrome is most common. Syringomyelic syndrome may be present	Hyperintense on T2 and hypo- or isointense on T1 with heterogeneous contrast enhancement	Surgery is the most effective treatment. Radiotherapy is reserved for recurrent or malignant tumors	Local control rate 90–100 % after complete resection
Astrocytoma	Second most common intramedullary spinal cord tumor	Mixed sensorimotor syndrome is most common. Syringomyelic syndrome may be present	Fusiform expansion with irregular margins. Often with a cystic component, associated edema, or syrinx. Hypo- to isointense on T1, hyperintense on T2, with variable contrast enhancement	Maximal safe surgical resection followed by observation or radiotherapy. Total resection is accomplished infrequently. Radiotherapy only indicated for clinical or radiographic progression, not for pilocytic astrocytoma	Grade is the most important prognostic factor. Five-year survival exceeds 70 %
Hemangioblastoma	Rare, although common in patients with VHL	Usually sensory, especially slowly worsening proprioception. Rarely, patients present with acute hemorrhage	Homogenously enhancing, hypervascular nodule with associated cyst or syrinx. Angiography shows enlarged feeding arteries, intense nodular stains, and early draining veins	Maximal safe surgical resection followed by observation or external beam radiotherapy. There is no role for radiotherapy and experience with VEGF antagonists is limited, although promising. Stereotactic radiosurgery is an option for recurrent or unresectable tumors	Local control rate is almost 100 % after complete resection

Table 18.3 Spinal cord tumors: 5-year survival

Astrocytoma	
Pilocytic	>90 %
Low grade	>70 %
High grade	30 %
Ependymoma	
Low grade	85 %
Anaplastic	30 %

enlargement in cases of intramedullary tumors. However, the internal structure of the spinal cord and tumor as well as the tumor/cord interface cannot be visualized with those modalities.

The presence of mass effect in the form of spinal cord segmental enlargement, cyst formation, contrast enhancement, and peritumoral edema favors the diagnosis of a neoplastic process. Tumor mimicking diseases are multiple sclerosis, transverse myelitis, spinal cord ischemia, cavernous malformation, sarcoid, and CNS angiitis [1] and should be considered as part of the differential diagnosis. Acute demyelination, for example, in multiple sclerosis and transverse myelitis, may be associated with spinal cord edema and segmental enlargement resembling tumor. Additional studies such as brain MRI, CSF analysis, and angiography should be performed in suspected cases to establish the correct diagnosis. In rare cases when diagnosis cannot be established on the basis of clinico-radiological data, patient observation with follow-up imaging in 2–3 months is a reasonable option. The absence of lesion progression, diminished enhancement, and edema on interval MRI favor nonneoplastic process.

Microsurgery is the cornerstone of spinal cord tumor treatment. It has been shown that tumor type and grade are the most important factors affecting outcome (Table 18.3). Surgery provides tissue sampling and consequently, a pathological diagnosis with corresponding prognosis as well as cytoreduction. In the majority of well-defined (circumscribed) low-grade tumors, resective surgery can be curative. In instances of infiltrative tumors, maximal safe resection or biopsy contributes to management by providing diagnosis and defining further treatment. In addition to standard contrast MRI, diffusion tension tractography is a useful tool that can show the passage of fibers around or though the tumor and therefore can be used as part of the preoperative planning [8]. Functional MRI (fMRI), widely used for preoperative planning in eloquent brain areas, has not been utilized for spinal cord tumors, though application for other pathologies such as traumatic injury or multiple sclerosis has yielded encouraging results [4].

Extent of resection has a positive correlation with patient outcome. However, this strategy is counterbalanced with the risk of neurologic injury from aggressive surgery. Most postsurgery deficits are transient and improve with time and rehabilitation. McCormick proposed a grading system of spinal cord tumors and showed that the patient's functional status and limited longitudinal extent of the tumor are the most favorable preoperative functional outcome factors. Delayed postoperative neurological deterioration may occur due to tumor growth (most frequent) or from operative complications such as spinal cord tethering to the dura, spinal instability, and resulting kyphotic deformity. Spinal instability may be present pre- or postoperatively and results from neurologic deficits causing an axial deformity, postlaminectomy kyphosis, radiation injury, syringomyelia, or combination of these factors. Some studies showed an advantage of laminoplasty over laminectomy for prevention of future deformity at least in the pediatric population. This effect seems to be less prevalent in the adult group, though laminoplasty facilitates surgical exposure in recurrent cases. Yasargil et al. reported his series with intraspinal AVMs and tumors approached via hemilaminectomy [10]. Though technically challenging, this approach ultimately eliminates the risk of surgery-induced instability, especially in junctional regions of the spine. Postoperative spinal cord tethering to durotomy site is not infrequent and may be the cause of significant neuropathic pain and deficit. Midline myelotomy, pial suturing after tumor resection, may decrease the likelihood of tethering and should be performed whenever feasible. Reoperation with allo- or autografts usually fails to treat the condition since the granulation tissue inevitably grows into the graft and spinal cord itself. Artificial inert materials, such as Goretex, are an excellent alternative, and in our experience prophylactic grafting at the time of first surgery reduces the risk of tethering (Fig. 18.2).

Radiotherapy is an important adjuvant therapy for the treatment of spinal tumors. Radiotherapy is primarily administered for high-grade gliomas and for recurrent or residual tumors with confirmed progression when surgical resection is deemed not possible. Radiotherapy-associated side effects are characterized as acute, early delayed, and late delayed. Acute reactions usually reflect secondary inflammatory and transient effects on nearby tissues (in-field effects) especially skin and gastrointestinal. Early delayed side effects most often manifest as transient demyelination and commonly posterior column dysfunction (i.e., Lhermitte's sign) that can be seen on T_2-weighted images. Delayed late injuries include secondary malignancies particularly in the pediatric population and patients with genetic tumor predisposition disorders.

18.2 Ependymoma

Ependymoma is the most common intradural intramedullary tumor type in adults. Myxopapillary ependymoma (WHO grade 1) is a distinct type, usually located in the lumbar cistern, and is considered as the intradural extramedullary type. Cellular ependymomas arise from the ependymal lining of the central canal and are classified as WHO grade II tumors. Anaplastic ependymomas are rare and considered as WHO grade III. The most common presentation is pain, followed by neurological deficit. Rare cases of acute neurological compromise due to tumor hemorrhage have been reported.

Histologically, ependymoma cells are characterized by round to oval nuclei containing finely dispersed chromatin with perivascular and ependymal rosettes. The association between neurofibromatosis type 2 (NF-2) and spinal ependymoma is well known. This is an autosomal dominant disease caused by mutation of merlin or schwannomin gene on chromosome 22, which is a member of the protein 4.1 family. Several studies have shown that spontaneous ependymomas also have a high rate of loss of heterozygosity (LOH) on chromosome 22 and/or merlin gene mutation [2]. Furthermore, spinal ependymomas have higher rate of merlin mutation than their cranial counterparts. Therefore, spinal cellular ependymomas (WHO grade II) are considered a distinct type of tumor mostly caused by merlin/schwannomin gene alterations. Nevertheless, the exact pathophysiological mechanism linking the gene function loss and neoplastic transformation is yet to be discovered.

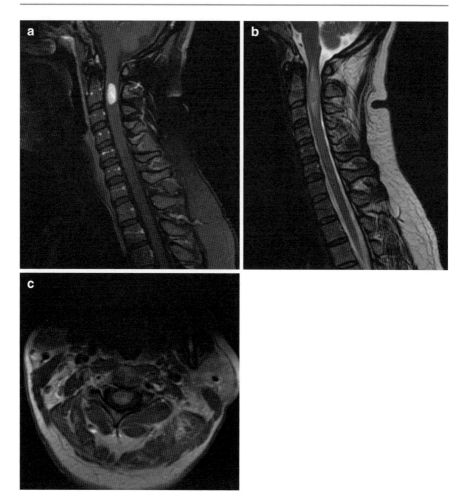

Fig. 18.1 Radiologic appearance of ependymoma. (**a**) Contrast-enhanced T1W image. Note well demarcation from surrounding spinal cord tissue. (**b**) T2W image shows spinal cord edema cranial and caudal to the lesion. (**c**) Axial contrast-enhanced T1W demonstrates central location of the tumor

The most common location of ependymomas is cervical, followed by cervicothoracic and thoracic. Ependymomas are hypointense on T_1 and hyperintense on T_2-weighted MR images (Figs. 18.1 and 18.2). Contrast enhancement is usually present but not in all cases. Ependymomas mostly reside centrally in the spinal cord attributed to the origin of these tumors from the ependymal cells lining the central canal. Reactive

Fig. 18.2 Spinal cord tethering after removal of ependymoma shown in Fig. 18.1. Patient developed intractable neurogenic pain 1 year after surgery. (**a**) T2W images demonstrate site of spinal cord attachment to the dura. Note residual myelomalacia and ongoing cord edema due to tethering. (**b**) T1W contrast-enhanced sagittal image; granulation tissue is growing inside the spinal cord (*arrow*). (**c**) Sagittal T2W image demonstrates status-post detethering with artificial material (Goretex). Note reappearance of CSF posterior to the spinal cord (*arrow*)

18 Intramedullary Spinal Cord Tumors

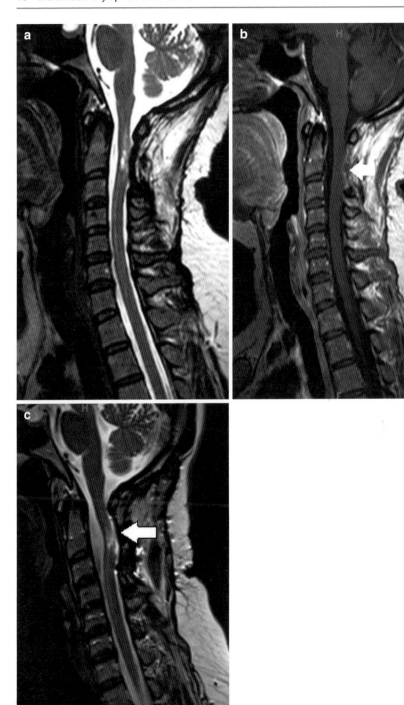

syrinx usually occurs at the superior and/or inferior poles of the tumor and does not require surgical removal. Cyst presence does not appear to have an effect on overall prognosis [7]. The main factor affecting postoperative morbidity is tumor width in relation to spinal cord [7] and preoperative neurological status [7]; tumor length does not have an effect per se, but longer tumors are associated with a higher rate of postoperative dysesthesias [7], possibly due to longer myelotomy. Ependymomas mostly follow a benign course, except for malignant histological subtypes (anaplastic ependymoma; WHO grade 3). Surgery is the most effective treatment for all grades, and the same rate of complete resections can be achieved even for recurrent tumors. With total surgical resection local control rates of 90–100 % have been reported, although in a minority of cases, complete surgical resection is not achieved [5]. There is an inverse relation between preoperative symptom duration and tumor resectability. The possible explanation of this effect is development of microadhesions between tumor and normal tissue in long-standing cases. Overall survival increases with complete resection.

Chemotherapy plays a limited role in the management of ependymomas. Data regarding the effect of chemotherapy for patients with recurrent spinal cord ependymoma is extremely sparse. Etoposide and platinoids are generally considered the agents of choice as commonly used for recurrent intracranial ependymomas. Recently, epidermal growth factor inhibitors (particularly lapatinib) and anti-angiogenic inhibitors (i.e., bevacizumab) have been shown to be useful in recurrent intracranial ependymoma; however, given the different molecular biology, they may not be as effective in spinal ependymomas.

The indications for RT are incomplete resection and malignant grade. In subtotally resected tumors and those with malignant pathology, external beam radiotherapy at a dose of 45–54 Gy is indicated. Several studies have shown that for incompletely resected low-grade ependymoma, no benefit is seen with regard to survival or time to recurrence. Therefore, because of the slow growth of low-grade ependymomas, observation with sequential MRI can be performed and radiotherapy may be reserved for progression. Cases with total resection should also be followed by serial neurological examinations and MRI. If no recurrence is observed, time span between MRI can be increased and patient can be followed neurologically.

> **Take Home Message**
> Spinal ependymomas are distinct type of tumors linked to LOH on chromosome 22q and merlin/schwannomin gene mutation. The main treatment modality is microsurgery.

18.3 Astrocytoma

Astrocytomas are a diverse group of gliomas with differing biological behavior. Histologically, they are classified as pilocytic (WHO grade 1), fibrillary (WHO grade 2), anaplastic (WHO grade 3), and glioblastoma (WHO grade 4). The grade of the tumor is the most important prognostic factor with regard to outcome [3], yet the distinction between anaplastic astrocytomas and glioblastomas is not of prognostic significance. Astrocytomas are associated with neurofibromatosis type 1 (NF1), though the most common spinal tumor encountered with NF1 is neurofibroma.

Radiologically astrocytomas are characterized by heterogeneous contrast enhancement, T_1 iso- or hypointensity, and T_2 hyperintensity on MRI and are sometimes hard to differentiate from ependymomas. Astrocytomas typically occupy eccentric position in the spinal cord and may be associated with cysts that may or may not contrast enhance much as in ependymomas (Fig. 18.3). WHO grade 2–4 astrocytomas lack distinct borders with normal tissue.

Microsurgery is an important part of the treatment of astrocytomas. Total excision rates are lower than in ependymoma, and in most, a partial resection or biopsy is performed. Complete resection significantly reduces the risk of disease progression according to some authors, while others suggest no benefit to extensive resection [3]. Pilocytic astrocytomas have relatively benign course and total resection can be attempted. However, if intraoperative frozen biopsy confirms the diagnosis of astrocytoma grade 2 or higher, and there is obvious infiltration by the tumor, aggressive resection is not recommended.

As with other intramedullary spinal cord tumors, there is limited data addressing the role of chemotherapy. Temozolomide has been used with some success in the recurrent setting, but there are no trials that establish a role for adjuvant (i.e., upfront)

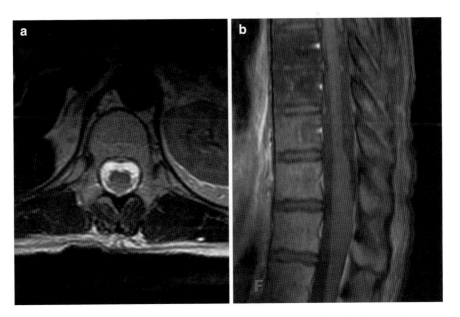

Fig. 18.3 Astrocytoma. Note the diffuse spinal cord thickening (**a**) and absence of contrast enhancement in pilocytic astrocytoma (**b**). Astocytoma WHO grade II, cyst formation (**c**), and nodular enhancement (**d**)

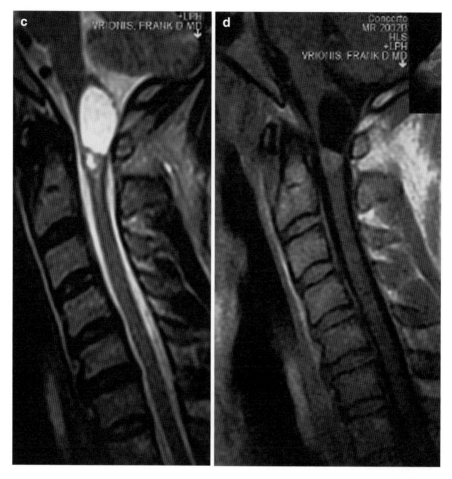

Fig. 18.3 (continued)

chemotherapy. Like intracranial gliomas, spinal cord high-grade tumors are commonly treated with concomitant (chemoradiation) and post-radiotherapy temozolomide. Bevacizumab is of palliative benefit for recurrent spinal cord glioblastoma and may be used as a salvage therapy. Adjuvant radiotherapy plays an important role in the management of spinal cord astrocytomas, since biopsy or partial resection is the surgical result in the majority of cases. Radiotherapy does not confer a benefit on survival in WHO grade 2 tumors [3], but it reduces the risk of disease progression. In high-grade gliomas, the survival benefit of RT is established and commonly applied. In addition, RT is the preferred treatment at recurrence of gliomas if not already irradiated. Serial neurological status assessment and MRI comprise the usual follow-up strategy to monitor tumor recurrence. Pilocytic astrocytomas differ by manifesting a low potential for malignant transformation, and consequently RT is usually deferred notwithstanding incomplete resection. Close follow-up with serial MRI and repeat surgery for recurrence are the usual approaches.

18 Intramedullary Spinal Cord Tumors

> **Take Home Message**
> Astrocytomas are diverse group of tumors with grade ranging from I to IV, although malignant ones are uncommon in the spinal cord. Surgical resection is usually incomplete and RT is an important adjuvant therapy, except for pilocytic astrocytoma.

18.4 Hemangioblastoma

Hemangioblastomas (WHO grade I) are the third most common intramedullary spinal cord tumor in adults, representing 3–8 % of all intramedullary tumors. Males predominate and presentation is usually in the fourth decade [6]. It is estimated that 10–30 % of patients with hemangioblastoma of the spinal cord have von Hippel Lindau (VHL) syndrome, an autosomal dominant disorder caused by deletion of chromosome 3p25. A decreased VHL protein level induces cell proliferation and increases expression of vascular endothelial growth factor (VEGF), platelet-derived growth factor, and erythropoietin. Therefore, chemotherapeutic agents targeting VEGF have been shown to be effective in hemangioblastoma.

The origin of hemangioblastomas is unknown. Anatomically most of them arise from the dorsal portion of the cervical spinal cord, close to the dorsal root entry zone [6], and can be intramedullary (30 %), intra- and extramedullary (50 %), or extramedullary (20 %).

Radiographically, the tumor appearance is as a homogenously enhancing hypervascular nodule with associated cyst or syrinx and peritumoral edema on MRI. Spinal angiography shows enlarged feeding arteries, intense nodular stains, and early draining veins. These tumors are highly vascular and can present with intramedullary or subarachnoid bleeding. Endovascular embolization can be performed to decrease vascularity of tumor and facilitate resection. However, in the majority of cases, neither diagnostic angiography nor endovascular embolization is required for the management of these tumors.

Understanding the natural history of hemangioblastomas in the setting of VHL is an essential part of treatment, and it is typically held that resection of hemangioblastomas should be reserved until the onset of symptoms [9].

Surgical resection is the main treatment modality. Usually there are well-defined margins allowing for total resection and cure. Excessive intraoperative bleeding, obscuring the operative field, can be the limiting factor for total resection. Such complication can be avoided by adherence to the technique of circumferential dissection, much like arteriole-venous malformations, sequential feeder coagulation, preservation of draining vein up to the end of the operation, and en bloc tumor removal.

There is limited role for radiotherapy and experience with chemotherapy is also restricted. Stereotactic radiosurgery is an option for patients with recurrent or unresectable tumors. Since these tumors heavily depend on VEGF, SU5416 (semaxanib, a VEGF receptor inhibitor) and bevacizumab (monoclonal antibody against

VEGF-A) have been tried and demonstrated clinical and radiographic response in individual patients or small case series. Follow-up for sporadic tumors usually includes serial MRI with increasing time span and clinical observation. However, patients with VHL syndrome should be followed by lifelong MRI.

> **Take Home Message**
> Spinal hemangioblastomas are benign tumors occasionally associated with VHL. Radiologically they appear as small highly enhancing nodule within a cyst. Treatment is surgical resection. Anti-angiogenic factors suppressing VEGF may be effective in cases not amenable to surgical resection.

18.5 Intramedullary Spinal Cord Metastasis (ISCM)

With current treatment modalities cancer patients have longer survival time, and thus the incidence of central nervous system metastasis is increasing. However, ISCM are rare tumors representing less than 2 % of primary intramedullary spinal cord tumors. Although any malignant tumor can spread into the spinal cord, the most common types are lung cancer, breast cancer, and melanoma. The presence of ISCM should be suspected in cases of an intramedullary mass in a patient with known malignancy. Clinically, these tumors demonstrate more rapid growth in comparison with intramedullary spinal cord tumors. Therefore, progression of neurologic symptoms is also rapid with higher incidence of complete or near complete deficits [1]. Consequently these tumors have worse outcomes in comparison with intrinsic spinal cord tumors [1]. Radiologically, ISCM may be indistinguishable from intramedullary spinal cord tumors demonstrating contrast enhancement and peritumoral edema formation on T_2-weighted images (Fig. 18.4).

Treatment for ISCM should be individualized on the basis of tumor localization and size, neurological deficit, cancer type, extension of metastatic disease, and other medical conditions. There is a high rate of CSF dissemination with widespread leptomeningeal disease. Therefore, complete brain and whole spine MRI should be obtained prior to treatment. In the majority of cases, there is no need for surgery as these tumors are managed with RT and steroids, especially in cases of radiosensitive tumors. However, given the aggressive behavior of these tumors, with 70–75 % of patients developing complete neurological deficit in 1 month [1], surgical intervention may be warranted in non-radiosensitive tumors and/or rapidly progressing cases. Additionally, in select cases, surgery is necessary as in cancer of unknown origin. Some studies showed that surgically treated patients may have a better prognosis than RT only, though the results are at least partially due to selection bias. Nonetheless, in cases when ISCM is amenable to total removal, vascularity and adhesiveness can impede complete resection [1], making cytoreduction an alternative approach. Additionally, aggressive surgical treatment does not affect overall survival and often is associated with a poor functional outcome. Intraoperative

18 Intramedullary Spinal Cord Tumors

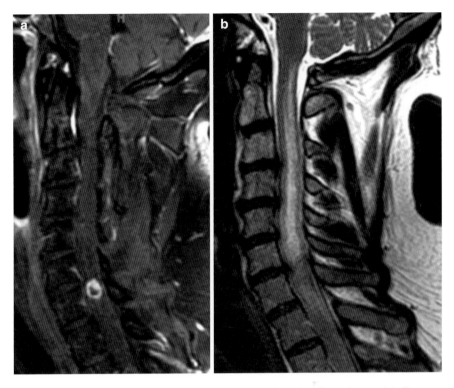

Fig. 18.4 MRI features of intramedullary metastasis of renal cell carcinoma. (**a**) Contrast-enhanced T1W images. Note necrotic core that is not typical for intrinsic spinal cord tumors. (**b**) T2W images; spinal cord edema, much larger than it can be assumed from the tumor size

biopsy is important in selected patients, especially if there is no known history of cancer. Systemic chemotherapy has a very limited role as these tumors are in a relative sanctuary site behind a pharmacological barrier, similar to brain metastasis. Consequently, RT is the primary palliative therapy for the overwhelming majority of patients. Intrathecal chemotherapy has no role in the treatment of ISCM as there is limited diffusion of CSF chemotherapy into the spine parenchyma.

18.6 Miscellaneous

Other rare intramedullary spinal cord tumors include subependymoma, ganglioglioma, lymphoma, germinoma, primitive neuroectodermal tumor, teratoma, dermoid cyst, epidermoid cyst, lipoma, and hamartoma. Except for dermoid/epidermoid cyst and lipoma that have characteristic appearance on MRI (Fig. 18.5), preoperative differential diagnosis is not straightforward, and usually diagnosis is made during or after the surgery. Surgical resection is the main treatment option for lipoma, hamartoma, and dermoid/epidermoid cyst, and repeat surgery should be performed in

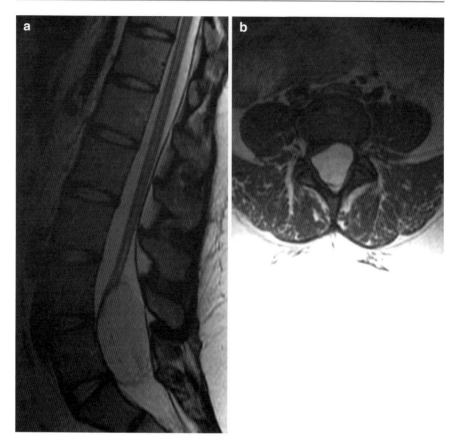

Fig. 18.5 Conus medullaris and filum terminale lipoma associated with tethered cord syndrome. Note the hyperintense nature of the lipoma on both T2W (**a**) and T1W (**b**) images

recurrent/residual cases. Lymphoma and germinoma are radiosensitive tumors, and therefore RT is the primary treatment. Ganglioglioma and subependymoma are rare intramedullary tumors usually diagnosed after the surgery for presumed ependymoma or astrocytoma. Total surgical resection is feasible, and by the time of pathological diagnosis, no further treatment is necessary. Adjuvant RT is not necessary in ganglioglioma due to slow growing nature of these lesions. There is no literature about radiation treatment of subependymomas.

References

1. Dickman CA, Fehlings M, Gokaslan ZL (2006) Spinal cord and spinal column tumors: principles and practice. Thieme, New York
2. Gutmann DH, Giordano MJ, Fishback AS, Guha A (1997) Loss of merlin expression in sporadic meningiomas, ependymomas and schwannomas. Neurology 49:267–270

3. Kim MS, Chung CK, Choe G, Kim IH, Kim HJ (2001) Intramedullary spinal cord astrocytoma in adults: postoperative outcome. J Neurooncol 52:85–94
4. Leitch JK, Figley CR, Stroman PW (2010) Applying functional MRI to the spinal cord and brainstem. Magn Reson Imaging 28:1225–1233
5. McCormick PC, Torres R, Post KD, Stein BM (1990) Intramedullary ependymoma of the spinal cord. J Neurosurg 72:523–532
6. Murota T, Symon L (1989) Surgical management of hemangioblastoma of the spinal cord: a report of 18 cases. Neurosurgery 25:699–707, discussion 708
7. Peker S, Ozgen S, Ozek MM, Pamir MN (2004) Surgical treatment of intramedullary spinal cord ependymomas: can outcome be predicted by tumor parameters? J Spinal Disord Tech 17:516–521
8. Setzer M, Murtagh RD, Murtagh FR, Eleraky M, Jain S, Marquardt G et al (2010) Diffusion tensor imaging tractography in patients with intramedullary tumors: comparison with intraoperative findings and value for prediction of tumor resectability. J Neurosurg Spine 13:371–380
9. Wanebo JE, Lonser RR, Glenn GM, Oldfield EH (2003) The natural history of hemangioblastomas of the central nervous system in patients with von Hippel-Lindau disease. J Neurosurg 98:82–94
10. Yasargil MG, Tranmer BI, Adamson TE, Roth P (1991) Unilateral partial hemi-laminectomy for the removal of extra- and intramedullary tumours and AVMs. Adv Tech Stand Neurosurg 18:113–132

Vascular Diseases of the Spine and Spinal Cord and Basics of Spinal Angiography and Vascular Interventions

19

Joachim Berkefeld, Stefan Weidauer, and Elke Hattingen

Contents

19.1	Introduction	412
19.2	Vascular Anatomy	412
	19.2.1 Arteries	412
	19.2.2 Veins	414
19.3	Basics of Spinal Angiography	414
	19.3.1 DSA	414
	19.3.2 MRI, MRA, and CTA of the Spinal Vasculature	416
19.4	Common Vascular Diseases of the Spine and Spinal Cord	418
	19.4.1 Spinal Cord AVM and Perimedullary AV Fistula	418
	19.4.2 Dural AVF	421
19.5	Vascular Tumors	426
	19.5.1 Tumors of the Spine	426
	19.5.2 Intradural Vascular Tumors	428
19.6	Cavernomas	429
19.7	Variants and Range of Normal Findings	429
Further Reading		432

J. Berkefeld
Institute for Neuroradiology, Goethe-University,
Schleusenweg 2-16, D-60528 Frankfurt, Germany

S. Weidauer
Department of Neurology, Sankt Katharinen Hospital,
Seckbacher Landstr. 65, D-60389 Frankfurt, Germany
e-mail: stefan.weidauer@sankt-katharinen-ffm.de

E. Hattingen (✉)
Institute for Neuroradiology, Goethe-University,
Schleusenweg 2-16, D-60528 Frankfurt, Germany
e-mail: elke.hattingen@kgu.de

Abbreviations

AVF	Arteriovenous fistula
AVM	Arteriovenous malformation
DSA	Digital subtraction angiography
MRA	Magnetic resonance angiography
CTA	Computer tomogram arteriography
WI	Weighted images

19.1 Introduction

The aim of this chapter is a very basic and practical approach to the most common vascular diseases of the spine and spinal cord, and it is beyond the scope of this text to compete with more detailed textbooks ([1]; Lasjaunias 2001).

19.2 Vascular Anatomy

19.2.1 Arteries

The spine is supplied by segmental arteries. From the thoracic level of T5 down to the lumbar levels of L4, normally a pair of arteries originates from the dorsal or dorsolateral aorta and continues as intercostal or lumbar arteries (Fig. 19.1). The upper thoracic levels above the lower aortic arch are supplied by segmental arteries originating in the region of T5 (Fig. 19.1).

In the lower lumbar region, the level of the aortic bifurcation is variable. The median sacral artery originates at the junction between both common iliac arteries (Fig. 19.2). The sacrum and sometimes the lower lumbar spine are supplied by the iliolumbar trunk originating from the internal iliac arteries (Fig. 19.2).

At the level of the intervertebral foramen, small branches to the dura and the nerve roots (radicular arteries) take off from the segmental arteries. The spinal cord arterial supply is provided by the anterior spinal artery running longitudinally at the ventral surface of the spinal cord. In the posterior fossa, the anterior spinal artery arises from the junction of two arteries originating from the V4 segments of the vertebral arteries (Fig. 19.3). The anterior spinal artery is fed by radiculomedullary arteries arising at different levels, but not in every segment. Radiculomedullary arteries can be identified due to the ascending course following a nerve root and a hairpin-shaped curve at the junction with the anterior spinal artery (Fig. 19.4). A larger radiculomedullary artery is frequently located at the thoracolumbar junction between T11 and L2. This artery of the lumbar enlargement (Adamkiewicz) is an important but not the only supply to the lower part of the anterior spinal cord with some variation in the number and location of radiculomedullary arteries. The posterolateral portions of the spinal cord are supplied by two posterior spinal arteries

19 Vascular Diseases of the Spine and Spinal Cord

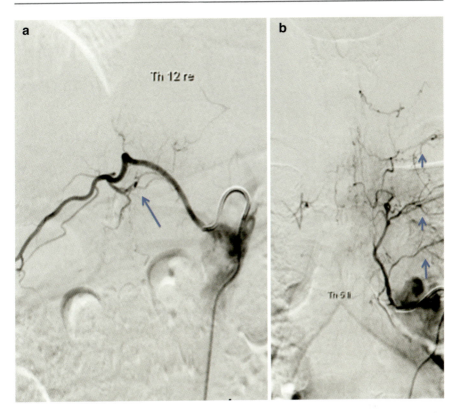

Fig. 19.1 Selective intra-arterial DSA images of the segmental artery at the level of T12 on the right side (**a**). The vessel originates from the thoracic aorta. After giving off branches for the supply of the vertebral body, nerve root, and dura (*arrow*), it continues as an intercostal artery. Above the level of T5, the upper thoracic segmental arteries (*arrowheads*) are supplied from a common trunk (**b**)

and a pair of posterolateral spinal arteries which are part of a pial arterial network. Feeders come from radiculopial arteries, which show also a hairpin shape, but are located lateral to the midline (Fig. 19.4). In the upper cervical spine, the posterior spinal artery equivalent is called lateral spinal artery.

Radial perforators are originating from this pial network (vasa corona) for the supply of the parenchyma. From the anterior spinal artery sulcocommissural branches are arising in the ventral sulcus of the spinal cord penetrating alternate into the left or right parenchyma and supplying the central gray matter and surrounding structures. This is the intrinsic system of the spinal cord supply, whereas the extrinsic system is supplied by the vasa corona. Therefore, in the case of an occlusion of the anterior spinal artery, infarcts may occur in the territory of these sulcocommissural branches (intrinsic system), whereas the periphery is still supplied via the pial network (extrinsic system; see also Chap. 20) (Fig. 19.5).

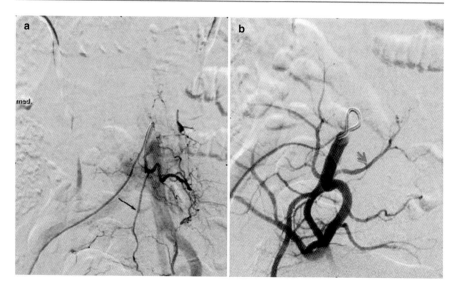

Fig. 19.2 Median sacral artery (*arrow*) originating together with the left L5 segmental artery from the aortic bifurcation (**a**). Selective injection of the internal iliac artery on the right side with iliolumbar truncus (*arrowhead*, **b**)

19.2.2 Veins

The spinal cord is surrounded by a venous network with dominating longitudinal veins at the ventral and dorsal surface of the spinal cord. These venous anastomoses are connected with radicular veins connecting the spinal cord drainage to epidural veins. Normally, a valve-like mechanism prevents reflux from epidural veins into intradural veins.

The epidural venous plexus is draining through the intervertebral foramina into longitudinal venous channels which are connected with the azygos and hemiazygos venous system. Spinal cord veins are visible in the late phase of selective spinal angiograms, especially if varicose enlargement occurs in the presence of AV (arteriovenous) shunts due to vascular malformations (Fig. 19.6).

19.3 Basics of Spinal Angiography

19.3.1 DSA

In former times, spinal angiography was regarded as a difficult, time-consuming, and dangerous examination for imaging of the spinal cord vessels. Adequate catheter techniques, modern nonionic contrast material, and additional use of MRI for targeted examinations have improved feasibility and safety of spinal angiograms.

19 Vascular Diseases of the Spine and Spinal Cord

Fig. 19.3 Segmental arteries arising from the left vertebral artery. Note the weak opacification of the anterior spinal artery fed by radiculomedullary branches at single levels (*arrow*)

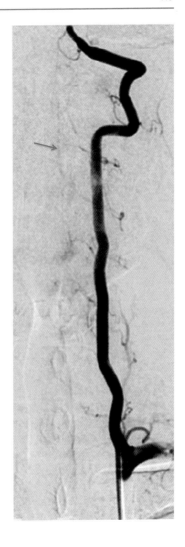

MRI together with contrast-enhanced and time-resolved MR angiography (MRA) may help a lot to localize, e.g., dural AV fistulas (AVF) and other vascular spinal lesions and may abandon catheterization of all segmental arteries; of the external carotid, vertebral, and cervical arteries; and of the iliac arteries.

Spinal angiograms are performed via the transfemoral route with the use of selective catheters with a shape adapted to the course of the initial segments of the segmental arteries. In our experience, the "Michaelsen-type" catheter or renal shape for the lumbar arteries covers most of the anatomic situations. For catheterization of the internal iliac artery, "Sidewinder I" configurations are favorable as well as "vertebral configured" catheters for the cervical vessels, especially the vertebral arteries.

A systematic approach with exact localization of the catheterized segments is mandatory to be sure that the spinal angiogram is complete and that all radicular feeders can be analyzed especially when spinal arteriovenous malformations (AVM) are assumed.

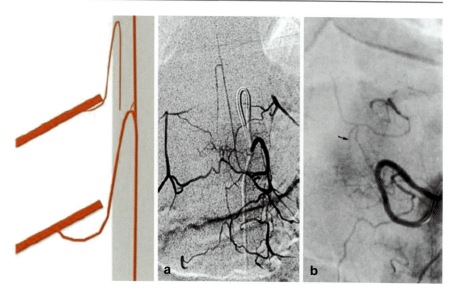

Fig. 19.4 Typical hairpin shape of a radiculomedullary artery supplying the anterior spinal artery in the midline (**a**). Note the paramedian course of the smaller radiculopial artery (schematic representation and **b**) showing also a hairpin shape which is sometimes difficult to distinguish from anastomotic arteries dorsal to the vertebral arch and spinal process (*arrows*)

During catheterization, the catheter tip must be turned away from the ventrally located visceral arteries or the lateral renal arteries. In elderly patients suffering from arteriosclerosis, it is sometimes not easy to find and differentiate a narrowed ostium of a segmental artery from adjacent plaques. Catheterization must be performed gently and dissections have to be strictly avoided. The extent of spinal angiography varied for different indications and is explained in the pathology section.

After catheterization of a segmental artery, we manually inject a few milliliters of nonionic contrast material and perform a DSA series with 2 f/s during breath holding. In the lumbar region, temporary arrest of bowel movements by intravenous injection of butylscopolamine or glucagon is mandatory for good image quality.

19.3.2 MRI, MRA, and CTA of the Spinal Vasculature

On contrast-enhanced T1W MR images, frequently normal spinal veins can be detected. With modern MR equipment, there is a wide range of normal findings (Fig. 19.7).

MRI and MRA are frequently used to localize a vascular lesion at the spine and to guide selective angiography and to avoid injection of all potential spinal arteries. Contrast-enhanced MRA techniques like contrast-enhanced TOF or time-resolved MRA as well as multiplanar reconstructions of contrast-enhanced GRE images allow for reliable visualization of pathological vessels (see Chap. 5). Frequently, the localization of AV shunts can be estimated correctly but should be confirmed by selective angiography (Fig. 19.7). Multidetector or flat panel CTA is also used for imaging of spinal vessels and vascular pathologies (see Fig. 19.5).

19 Vascular Diseases of the Spine and Spinal Cord

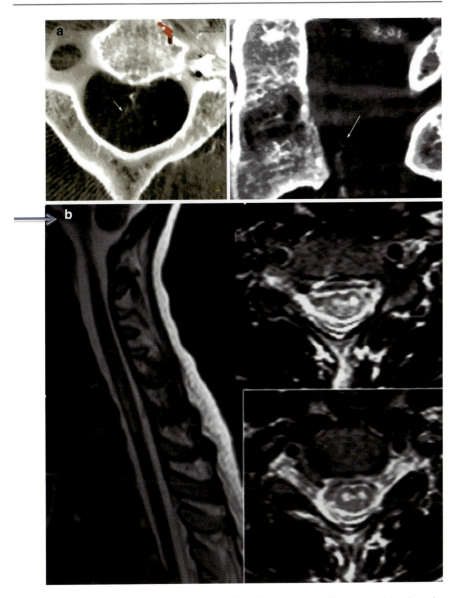

Fig. 19.5 Flat panel CT angiography (CTA) showing sulcocommissural branches arising from the anterior spinal artery at the level of C2 (**a**). MRI shows a patient with a spinal infarction after occlusion of the anterior spinal artery (**b**) Note that the periphery of the spinal cord is preserved due to supply via the pial network (extrinsic system)

Fig. 19.6 Varicose enlargement of an ascending and descending spinal cord vein in a case with dural AV fistula (AVF)

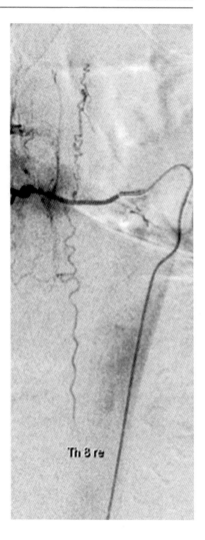

19.4 Common Vascular Diseases of the Spine and Spinal Cord

19.4.1 Spinal Cord AVM and Perimedullary AV Fistula

Vascular malformations involving the spinal cord or the surrounding pial vessels are rare diseases and uncommon. They may become symptomatic with subarachnoid or parenchymal hemorrhage or with ischemic neurological deficits related with AV shunting. MRI and MRA are the methods of choice if spinal AVMs are suspected, and angiography is often not needed for screening or even for making the diagnosis (Fig. 19.8).

19 Vascular Diseases of the Spine and Spinal Cord

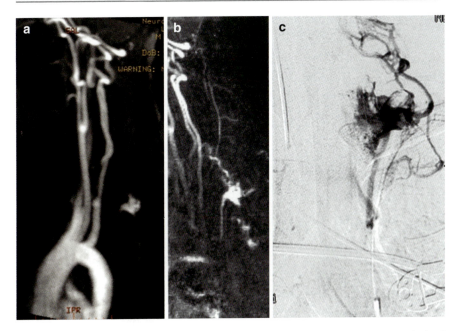

Fig. 19.7 Contrast-enhanced and time-resolved MRA in a patient with radicular pain at the level of T1. MRA shows pathological veins in projection on the upper thoracic spine (**a**, **b**). Selective angiography of the left upper thoracic segmental artery shows the opacification of a mainly venous vascular malformation

Spinal cord vascular malformations are supplied by the anterior or posterior spinal arteries fed by radiculomedullary or radiculopial branches as mentioned above. The AVM nidus or AVF as zones of AV shunting are supplied by branches of these arteries. Draining veins fill early and show frequently varicose enlargement (Fig. 19.9).

Endovascular and surgical treatment of spinal cord AVM and AVF are risky procedures with the aim of selective obliteration of the nidus without compromise of the anterior spinal artery and the spinal cord parenchyma due to reduced arterial perfusion. Treatment should be confined to few specialized centers with sufficient expertise. It does not make sense to embolize one case per year which is the average case load in a region of around one million people.

Spinal angiograms showing the anterior spinal artery and other possible feeders in the region of the AVM may be helpful for the referral in a specialized center. However, embolizations outside of such institutions are not recommendable. Even after spinal subarachnoid or parenchymal hemorrhage, there is hardly an indication for immediate interventional or surgical treatment, and thus referral to a specialized neurovascular center is recommended.

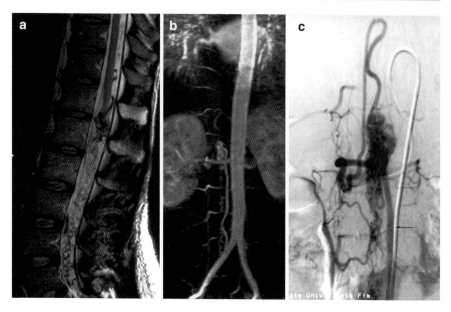

Fig. 19.8 Spinal AVM at the level T12/L1 with pathological flow void and dilated vessels on sagittal T2WI (**a**). CE MRA disclosed in addition a part of vascular structures (**b**), and selective spinal DSA showed angioarchitecture in detail with dilated arteria radicularis magna (**c**)

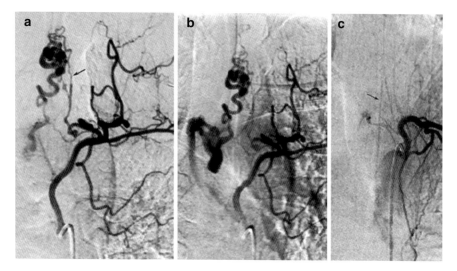

Fig. 19.9 Spinal cord AVM (**a**) with a small nidus fed by a thoracic radiculopial artery (*arrow*). Venous drainage into descending spinal cord veins, a radicual vein which exits the intradural space and is connected with epidural and paraspinal veins (**b**). The anterior spinal artery is not involved (**c**)

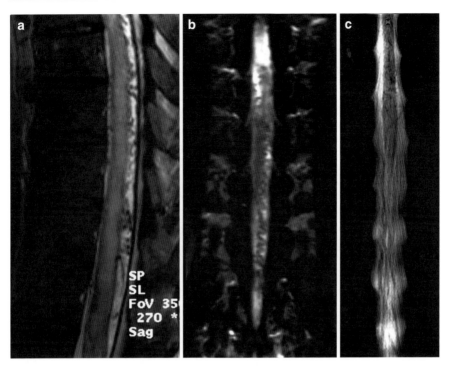

Fig. 19.10 Venous congestion of the spinal cord with edema and hyperintense signal changes on sag. T2WI (**a**) and in addition pathological juxtamedullary pathological flow voids (**a, b**: coronal T2WI; **c**: MR myelography) due to dural AVF

19.4.2 Dural AVF

Although spinal dural AVF are rare diseases of the spinal cord, they are much more common than spinal AVM. Most frequently elderly male patients are involved. Clinically, the patients suffer from progressive gait disturbance, pain, bowel, and bladder disturbances up to incomplete paraplegia symptoms. MRI shows characteristic intramedullary edema with centrally accentuated bright signal on T2WI. These hyperintense signal changes are most likely caused by venous congestion of the spinal cord in consequence of overcharged veins due to arteriovenous shunting. Varicose enlargement and increased visibility of ascending or descending spinal cord veins are also characteristic (Figs. 19.6 and 19.10). In the former literature, before dural AVF could be diagnosed by spinal angiography, this disease perhaps might be misdiagnosed as the so-called necrotizing myelopathy Foix-Alajouanine with varicose enlargement of spinal veins. In many instances, localization of pathological vessels and edema on MRI and recent techniques of spinal MRI and in addition MRA can provide major contributions to the localization of the fistula.

The fistula is fed from a network of dural artery branches at the level of the foramen with retrograde filling of the radicular vein which ascends to longitudinal spinal cord veins (Fig. 19.11). Therefore, edema of the spinal cord is caused by venous congestion due to retrograde venous inflow of the AV shunt.

The aim of spinal angiography is to identify the level of the fistulous point. A targeted approach guided by MRI findings is recommendable. Most of the dural

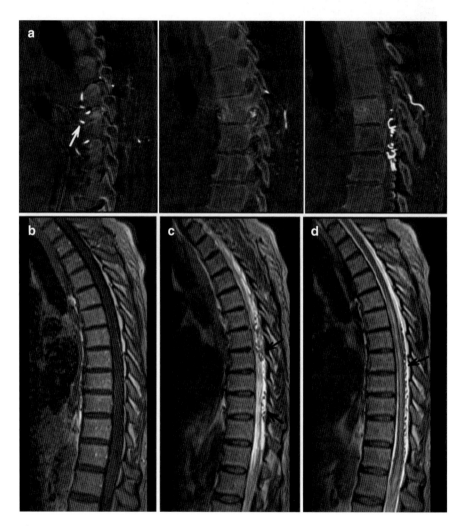

Fig. 19.11 (a–d) Typical spinal AVF supplied from level TH6 on the left side of a patient with incontinence, sensible deficits of the legs, and gait ataxia. The MIP reconstruction of rotational selective angiography (**a**) from intercostal artery level TH6 (*arrow*) reveals the nidus in the intervertebral foramen and the corkscrew-like perimedullary veins. The conventional MRI shows pronounced enhancement around the spinal cord on contrast-enhanced T1WI. The T2WI clearly depicts the dilated perimedullary veins (**c**) and the extensive centromedullary edema of the spinal cord (**d**). (**e**) The selective angiography with VRT reconstructions of the rotational angiography shows the nidus (*arrow*) which is best seen on the oblique VRT reconstruction. Note angiographically proven anastomoses from adjacent levels above (*dashed arrow*)

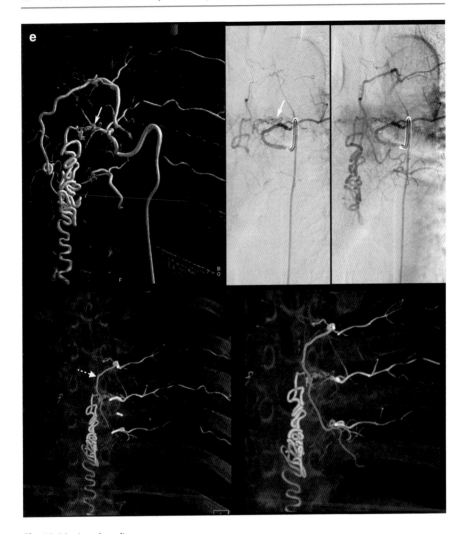

Fig. 19.11 (continued)

AVF are located in the thoracolumbar region. Currently, there is a debate on whether complete spinal angiography is necessary to rule out single cases with a second fistula. Especially in severely atherosclerotic patients with increased angiographical risks, we tend to avoid complete spinal angiography and confine the examination to the level of the fistula and the adjacent levels above or below.

It is important to know whether a radiculomedullary or radiculopial artery arises from the level of the dural AVF and how these vessels can be preserved during treatment.

If the fistula is identified, indication for treatment is clearly given. One has to decide whether interventional embolization or surgical therapy is preferable. The

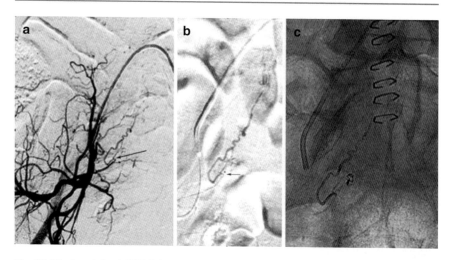

Fig. 19.12 Sacral dural AVF fed by branches of the right iliolumbar trunk (**a**, *arrow*). Selective catheterization after unsuccessful surgery shows the fistulous point (*small arrow*) open (**b**). Glue cast of the draining radicular vein with occlusion of the fistula after superselective embolization (**c**)

aim of endovascular or surgical therapy is obliteration of the fistulous point and the initial segment of the draining radicular vein. Incomplete treatment will result in recanalization of the fistula and recurrence of symptoms.

Interventional embolization with liquid embolic agents is possible if a microcatheter can be placed close to the fistulous point. Diluted glue or Onyx® has to be pushed from the arterial to the venous side without compromising longitudinal spinal cord veins (Fig. 19.12).

Surgical treatment is done by clipping or coagulation of the initial segment of the draining vein at the level of the entrance into the intradural space. For surgical purposes, exact localization of level and side of the fistula is mandatory. The use of endovascular coils as fluoroscopically visible markers is useful especially in the thoracic spine.

3D reconstructions of rotational angiography may also be helpful for treatment planning and surgical guidance (Figs. 19.11, 19.13, and 19.14).

Postoperative or postinterventional angiograms are strongly recommendable to be sure that the fistula is completely occluded and not supplied by collateral vessels (Fig. 19.15). Postoperative angiograms can be done early after surgery. After interventional treatment, we have a completion angiogram, and controls should be done after 3–6 months to exclude revascularization of the fistulous point.

Clinical and MRI controls should be performed to watch regression of symptoms, intramedullary edema, or pathologically enlarged juxtamedullary vessels. A regression of symptoms can be expected in many but not all cases. Long duration of symptoms and edema of the whole cross section of the spinal cord are unlikely to be associated with a good clinical outcome.

Complications of endovascular or surgical treatment are rare. The highest risk of interventional embolization is insufficient penetration of the liquid embolic agent

19 Vascular Diseases of the Spine and Spinal Cord

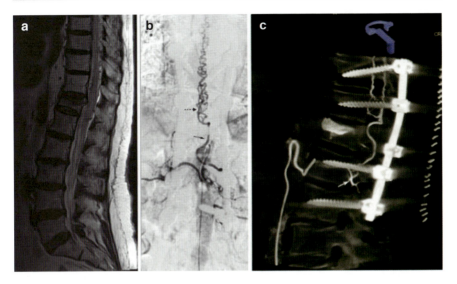

Fig. 19.13 MRI of a patient with compression fracture of the 12th thoracic vertebra. In addition to the fracture, spinal cord edema and pathologically enlarged veins are visible on T2-weighted images (**a**). Spinal angiography confirmed dural AVF with fistulous point at the foramen T11–T12 on the left side and venous drainage into an ascending vein which becomes connected to the longitudinal anterior and posterior spinal cord veins (**b**). Flat panel CTA shows the fistulous point as well as the connection of the draining vein to ascending spinal cord veins after surgical stabilization of the fracture (**c**)

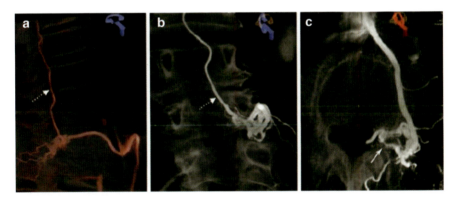

Fig. 19.14 Typical pathoanatomy of a spinal dural AVF shown on reconstructions of a flat panel CT angiogram after selective injection of contrast agent (**a**). Dural arteries arising from a segmental artery are divided into an arterial network which is connected to the ascending draining vein (*arrow*) which enters the intradural space at the level of the foramen just below the vertebral pedicle (**b**, **c**)

into the first segment of the draining radicular vein with incomplete occlusion of the fistula. In experienced hands, dislodgement of embolic material into spinal cord veins and damage of radicular arteries with segmental deficits are rare complications in single cases.

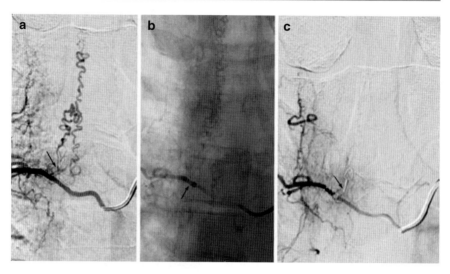

Fig. 19.15 Dural AVF with fistulous point at the level of TH 6 on the right side. (**a**) Placement of an embolization coil into the segmental artery for guidance of surgery (**b**, *arrow*). Successful clipping of the initial segment of the draining vein with complete occlusion of the AV shunt (**c**)

19.5 Vascular Tumors

19.5.1 Tumors of the Spine

The most frequent hypervascular tumors of the spine are bone metastases from renal or thyroid carcinoma. Aneurysmal bone cysts or vertebral hemangiomas may also show increased vascularity.

Tumor vascularity is frequently detected on MR images showing intensive contrast enhancement as well as hypertrophy of feeding arteries and draining veins. Spinal angiography is indicated for planning of surgery or preoperative embolization. Spinal angiograms have to cover the involved levels as well as the adjacent segments above and below. The tumor blush on angiography indicates increased vascularity compared with the normal bone structures. A careful analysis whether radiculomedullary or radiculopial arteries arise from segmental arteries involved in surgical or embolization procedures is absolutely mandatory (Fig. 19.16). Feeding branches from the segmental arteries to the tumor frequently show increased calibers. Early venous draining into enlarged epidural veins may occur in highly vascular metastases.

In hypervascular tumors, vertebral body replacement and other surgical procedures are associated with high amounts of intraoperative blood loss. Therefore, preoperative embolization is strongly recommended. Most frequently, transarterial embolization with midsize PVA particles (150–350 μ) is used after superselective catheterization of the segmental arteries or feeding branches with a microcatheter.

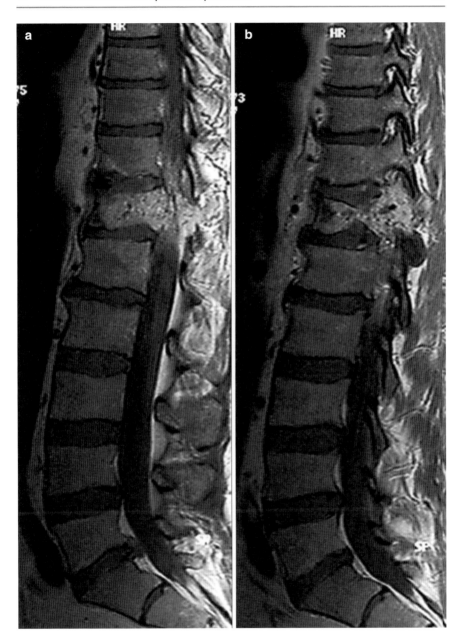

Fig. 19.16 (**a**, **b**) Hypervascular metastasis of a renal cell carcinoma at T12. Sagittal MRI postcontrast T1WI showing partial destruction of vertebra T12, ventral and dorsolateral compression of the spinal canal, and intense contrast enhancement. In addition, note flow voids intratumoral. (**c–h**) Selective angiography reveals hypertrophy of feeding arteries, intensive tumor blush, and early venous drainage. After embolization of the right side with 150–250 μ PVA particles, the tumor is devascularized in large part for preparation of surgery. Note the radiculomedullary artery arising from the contralateral segmental artery, which was not embolized

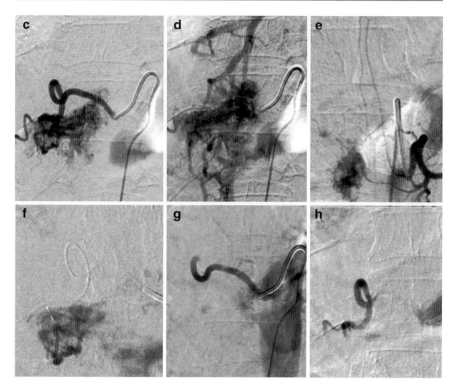

Fig. 19.16 (continued)

Careful analysis of the spinal angiogram regarding the opacification of radiculomedullary or radiculopial arteries avoids inadvertent embolization of the spinal cord supply. Suspensions of particles are injected until the tumor blush disappears. Due to the risk of revascularization, surgery should follow early during the next few days after embolization. With the above-mentioned precautions, complications of preoperative embolization with particles are extremely rare. With medium particle size, we avoid skin necrosis or permanent nerve root damage is unlikely to occur.

19.5.2 Intradural Vascular Tumors

In single cases, hemangioblastomas or paragangliomas are located in the parenchyma of the spinal cord or at the filum terminale (Fig. 19.17). Tumors in connection with the spinal cord may use spinal cord vessels for arterial supply or venous drainage, and intense tumor blush is visible on angiograms.

The most intrinsic tumors of the spinal cord are not highly vascularized and spinal angiography is not indicated. Neurinomas may show increased vascularity on MR images, and in some instances, neurosurgeons request an angiogram for surgical planning.

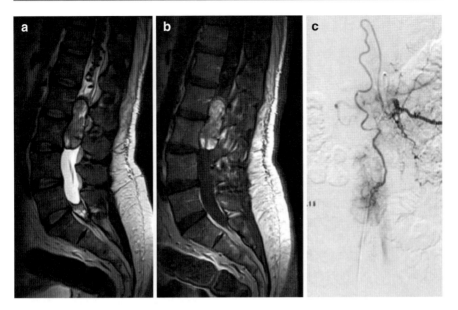

Fig. 19.17 Hypervascular intradural tumor in the lumbar spinal canal fed by the anterior spinal artery. Histology proved a paraganglioma of the filum terminale. Note also the large flow void signals around the conus medullaris on T2WI (**a**). Enhancement of the tumor on contrast enhanced T1WI (**b**). Spinal angiography shows the enlarged anterior spinal artery, tumor vessels and an intense blush (**c**)

19.6 Cavernomas

Cavernomas of the spinal cord may cause acute neurological symptoms due to hemorrhage into the malformation. MRI shows circumscribed lesions with signal loss in the periphery and high signal on T2WI in the center in line with imaging findings of intracerebral cavernoma (Fig. 19.18). In the case of recent hemorrhage, the cavernoma may be surrounded by edema. Post-contrast T1WI may show contrast enhancement in the center of the lesion. Cavernomas are angiographically negative due to very slow uptake of contrast material. Spinal angiography may only be indicated in single cases to rule out other sources of hemorrhage.

19.7 Variants and Range of Normal Findings

With increasing use of spinal MRI, there are borderline findings concerning the spinal cord vasculature. Sometimes, it is difficult to distinguish between normal veins and draining veins of a dural fistula with low shunt volume (Fig. 19.19). With modern MR equipment, some veins are always visible on contrast-enhanced T1WI. Absence of neurological symptoms and lack of spinal cord edema on T2WI are arguments against the presence of a dural AV fistula. However, in doubt spinal angiography may be indicated to rule out a vascular malformation.

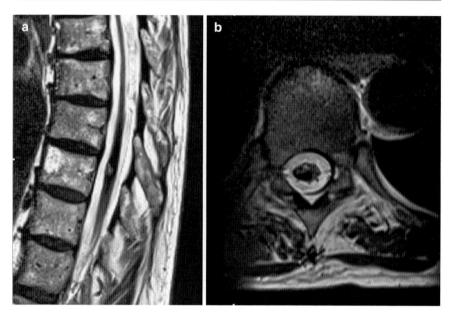

Fig. 19.18 (**a**, **b**) Cavernoma of the lower thoracic spinal cord with central hyperintense signal and hemosiderin deposits in the periphery with lowered signal on T2WI. (**c**) Cavernoma of the cervical spinal cord at level C6 on sag. T2WI with typical inhomogeneous signals ("popcorn pattern")

Fig. 19.18 (continued)

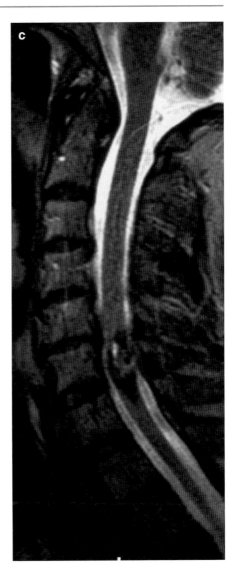

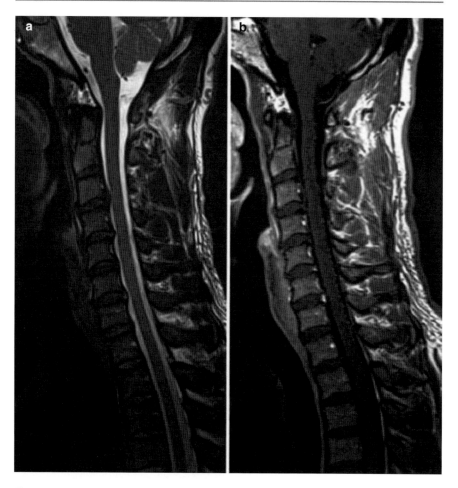

Fig. 19.19 Variant with strongly visible dorsal spinal cord veins on contrast-enhanced T1WI (**b**). Note the absence of clear varicose enlargement. No AVM nidus or intramedullary edema was visible on T2WI (**a**). Spinal angiogram was negative

Further Reading

1. Andres RH Barth A, Guzman R, Remonda L, El-Koussy M, Seiler RW, Widmer HR, Schroth G (2008) Endovascular and surgical treatment of spinal dural arteriovenous fistulas. Neuroradiology 50:869–76
2. Krings T (2010) Vascular malformations of the spine and spinal cord. Clin Neuroradiol 20:5–24
3. Krings T, Lasjaunias PL, Hans FJ, Mull M, Nijenhuis RJ, Alvarez H, Backes WH, Reinges MH, Rodesch G, Gilsbach JM, Thron A (2007) Imaging in spinal vascular disease. Neuroimaging Clin N Am 17:57–72
4. Lasjaunias P, Berenstein A, Ter Brugge KG Surgical Neuroangiography 2nd Edition. Springer Berlin, Heidelberg, New York 2001

5. Mull M, Nijenhuis RJ, Backes WH, Krings T, Wilmink JT, Thron A (2007) Value and limitations of contrast – enhanced MR angiography in spinal arteriovenous malformations and dural arteriovenous fistulas. AJNR Am J Neuroradiol 28:1249-58.
6. Rodesch G, Hurth M, Alvarez H, David P, Tadie M, Lasjaunias PL (2003) Embolization of spinal cord arteriovenous shunts: morphological and clinical follow-up and results – review of 69 consecutive cases. Neurosurgery 53: 40–9
7. Rodesch G, Hurth M, Alvarez H, Ducot B, Tadie M, Lasjaunias PL (2004) Angio-architecture of spinal cord arteriovenous shunts at presentation. Clinical correlations in adults and children. The Bicêtre experience on 155 consecutive patients seen between 1981-1999. Acta Neurochir (Wien) 146:217–26
8. Thron A (ed) (1988) Vascularisation of the spinal cord. Springer, Wien/New York
9. Weidauer S, Nichtweiß M, Lanfermann H, Zanella FE (2002) Spinal cord infarction: MR imaging and clinical features in 16 cases. Neuroradiology 44:851–857

Spinal Cord Infarction

20

Stefan Weidauer, Michael Nichtweiß, and Joachim Berkefeld

Contents

20.1	Vascular Anatomy	435
	20.1.1 Extrinsic Spinal Cord Arteries	436
	20.1.2 Extrinsic and Intrinsic System	438
	20.1.3 Sulcal Arteries (Syn.: Central or Sulcocommissural Arteries)	439
20.2	Aetiology of Spinal Ischemia	439
20.3	Clinical Symptoms	440
	20.3.1 Syndrome of the Anterior Spinal Artery (ASA)	440
	20.3.2 Syndrome of the Posterior Spinal Artery (PSA)	441
	20.3.3 Syndrome of the Artery of Adamkiewicz	441
	20.3.4 Syndrome of the Sulcal (Syn.: Central, Sulcocommissural) Artery	443
	20.3.5 "Man-in-the-Barrel" Syndrome	445
20.4	MR Imaging Features	447
References		451

20.1 Vascular Anatomy

The spinal cord is supplied by the radiculomedullary artery (synonyma: nervomedullary arteries or spinal branches) originating in the thoracic region from the

S. Weidauer (✉)
Department of Neurology, Sankt Katharinen Hospital,
Seckbacher Landstr. 65, D-60389 Frankfurt, Germany
e-mail: stefan.weidauer@sankt-katharinen-ffm.de

M. Nichtweiß
Department of Neurology, Hanse Klinikum Wismar; Wellengang 21, D-23968 Wismar, Germany
e-mail: michael.nichtweiss@googlemail.com

J. Berkefeld
Institute for Neuroradiology, Goethe-University,
Schleusenweg 2-16, D-60528 Frankfurt, Germany
e-mail: joachim.berkefeld@kgu.de

E. Hattingen et al. (eds.), *Diseases of the Spinal Cord*,
DOI 10.1007/978-3-642-54209-1_20, © Springer-Verlag Berlin Heidelberg 2015

posterior intercostal artery, which arises from the aorta (Fig. 20.1a) [1–4]. In the cervical section of the spinal cord the feeders originate from the vertebral artery (VA) and also from deep cervical arteries arising from the thyreocervical trunk via ascending cervical artery and the costocervical trunk. In the lumbar region pelvic arteries and the lateral sacral arteries arising from the internal iliac artery also supply the lumbar section with the conus medullaris [1–4].

The radiculomedullary artery may divide into an anterior and a posterior radicular artery, but most often in man there is only one branch running with the dorsal or ventral nerve root [2, 4]. Three types of radicular arteries could be defined: (1) some radicular arteries (RA) end with the nerve root at the level of the dura mater without reaching or supplying the spinal cord, (2) other RA do not enter the surrounding arterial system of the spinal cord (vasocorona) and (3) another type of RA feeds the spinal vascular system. In total, there are 31 pairs of RA and the distribution of the 10–23 (mean: 12–16) posterior RA over the spine is homogeneous without lateral preference. The posterior RA supply the pial arterial plexus (vasocorona) of the lateral and dorsal spinal cord, the dorsal nerve roots and the sensoric spinal ganglia. As mentioned above, the number and locations of posterior RA are different to the anterior RA. Only in a few segments is the common extradural trunk, i.e. the radiculomedullary artery, branching into an anterior and posterior RA (Fig. 20.1a) [2, 4].

In contrast to the posterior RA, the number of the anterior RA is related to segments of the spinal cord [1–4]. The mean number in the cervical part is 0–6, at the thoracic part 1–4 and at the thoracolumbar level 1–2 [4].

In the lower thoracic and thoracolumbar region there is one dominant anterior RA, the arteria radicularis magna or artery of Adamkiewicz, with a diameter of 1.0–1.3 mm, in comparison with the other anterior RA with a mean diameter of 0.2 mm. About 75 % of arteries of Adamkiewicz originate from the aorta at levels Th 9–12, 10 % at levels L1–L2 and often the artery is left sided (80 %). The artery of Adamkiewicz has two branches, the smaller ascending and the larger descending branch, the latter supplying the lower thoracic and the lumbar part of the spinal cord including the conus medullaris. Therefore there is a greater flow of blood in the downward branch of the artery of Adamkiewicz [4].

20.1.1 Extrinsic Spinal Cord Arteries

20.1.1.1 Anterior Spinal Artery (ASA)
At the craniocervical level, the confluence of two intradural feeders arising from the distal VA, i.e. the V4-segment forms the ASA, which runs downwards in the anterior spinal fissure (see Fig. 20.2). However, the two vertebral branches may not fuse with the consequence of a double ASA. In this case, each of the two ASA supplies one inner half of the spinal cord via sulcal arteries (syn.: central artery or sulcommisural artery) (see Fig. 20.1a). The size of the ASA is variable because of the different number and calibres of the anterior RA, especially at the level of the artery of

20 Spinal Cord Infarction

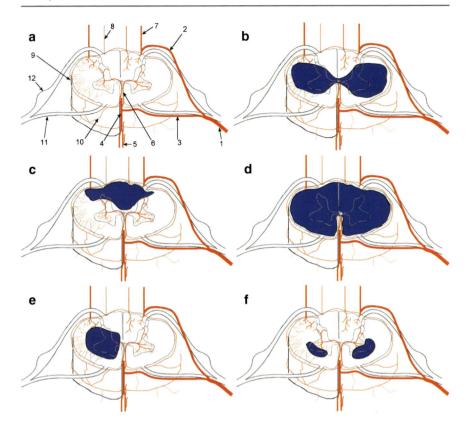

Fig. 20.1 (**a**) Vascularization of the spinal cord. *1* Radiculomedullar artery (syn.: nervomedullar artery); *2* posterior radicular artery; *3* anterior radicular artery; *4* anterior spinal artery (ASA); *5* duplication of the anterior spinal artery, *6* sulcal artery (syn.: central artery, sulcocommissural artery); *7* posterolateral spinal artery (PLSA); *8* posterior spinal artery (PSA); *9* vasocorona; *10* transverse and longitudinal interconnections; *11* anterior nerve root; *12* dorsal nerve root with sensoric spinal ganglion. (**b–f**) Different infarct types and presumed vascular territories. (**b**) Anterior spinal artery (ASA) territory infarct (syn.: centromedullar infarct; ASA syndrome). (**c**) Posterior spinal artery (PSA)/posterolateral spinal artery territory infarct. (**d**) Artery of Adamkiewicz territory infarct. (**e**) Infarct in the sulcal artery territory (spinal sulcal artery syndrome). (**f**) Watershed infarcts between intrinsic and extrinsic system at the level of the anterior horns ("man-in-the-barrel" syndrome)

Adamkiewicz. Beside missed fusion of the cranial VA feeders, segmental duplication of the ASA for a short distance is frequent (50 %) (see Fig. 20.1a) [2, 4].

20.1.1.2 Posterior Spinal Artery (PSA)

The dual posterior spinal artery (PSA) also arises from the distal intradural V4 segments and may have additional feeders originating from the posterior inferior cerebellar artery (PICA) or from the rope ladder-like collateral vascular system of the medulla oblongata. With variable calibre there are, in addition, dual posterior lateral spinal arteries (PLSA) and these four arteries supply the dorsal and dorsolateral transverse section of the spinal cord (see Fig. 20.1a) [2, 4].

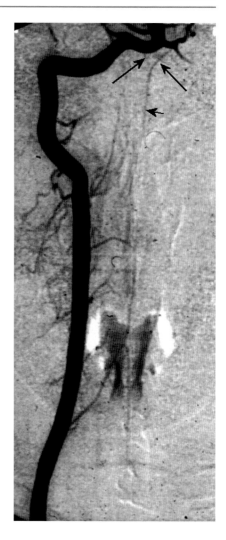

Fig. 20.2 Digital subtraction angiography (DSA, posterior anterior projection) of the right VA showing bilateral feeders from the V4 segment (*arrow*) fusing to the ASA (*short arrow*)

20.1.2 Extrinsic and Intrinsic System

The vasocorona is a circumference transverse and longitudinal collateral network on the surface around the spinal cord connecting the ASA, the PSA and the PLSA. Beside the ASA and PSA/PLSA territories, vascular supply of the spinal cord could be separated into extrinsic and intrinsic systems. The circumference of the spinal cord is supplied by numerous small penetrating arteries originating from the vasocorona, running directly perpendicular to the surface into the spinal cord representing the extrinsic or peripheral vascular system (see Fig. 20.1a) [1–4].

20.1.3 Sulcal Arteries (Syn.: Central or Sulcocommissural Arteries)

The sulcal arteries (SA) originate from the ASA and enter the spinal cord in the anterior fissure and represent the intrinsic central vascular system. Within the spinal cord they run alternating to the left or right side. However, when there is a duplication of the ASA, the SA supply only the side of the ASA from which they originate. There may be a common trunk of the SA with bifurcation in the sagittal plane in 7–9 % but never in the transverse sections. The number and size of SA depend upon the extent of the grey matter, especially at the level of the cervical and thoracolumbar intumescences of the spinal cord (Fig. 20.1a) [2].

Therefore, in the cervical section there are 5–8 SA and in the thoracolumbar region 5–12 SA per centimetre in the sagittal direction, whereas at the thoracic level with a smaller amount of grey matter the number of SA at 2–6 per centimetre is lower. In consequence, in the thoracic region the intramedullary course of the SA in sagittal plane is much more longitudinal, resulting in traversing branches up to 3 cm in length in comparison to the cervical and thoracolumbar section, whereas the SA has a more horizontal intramedullary course [2, 4].

A watershed region is also described at the level of the anterior and posterior horns, and there is no fixed border between the extrinsic or peripheral system and the intrinsic, i.e. central vascular system [2]. Consecutively there is an overlap and intermediate region nearby the anterolateral horns and the central part of the dorsal horns which is variably supplied by one system or the other. Regarding the perfusion of the spinal cord, the vasocorona with the penetrating perforators exhibit a centripetal bloodflow and the SA represent a centrifugal vascular system [4].

However, there is no fixed watershed region and the so-called "dead point" between neighbouring radicular arteries or the intrinsic and extrinsic system with blood flow in neither direction changes constantly over time [4, 5].

The capillary bed in the grey matter of the spinal cord is up to a five times densely because of the higher oxygen uptake. Especially the anterior horns with numerous motorneurons and the base of the posterior horns including the substantia gelantinosa need a thick capillary bed [4, 6]. The course of the capillaries in the white matter is be geared to the orientation of the fibre tracts. Whereas circumscribed loss of grey matter may be tolerated without neurological deficits, segmental loss of white matter may cause functional diachisis of fibre tracts, resulting in distinct clinical disorders.

However, in contrast to cerebral ischemia, spinal cord infarcts are rare because of the good collateral vascular supply.

20.2 Aetiology of Spinal Ischemia

Aetiology of spinal cord infarction is heterogeneous, including spontaneous or traumatic uni- or bilateral vertebral artery (VA) dissection [7–9], hypotension, e.g. caused by cardiac failure [7], fibrocartilaginous embolism [10–12], cocaine misuse

Table 20.1 Aetiologies of spinal cord infarcts

Aortal surgery
Systemic arteriosclerosis (risk factors, e.g. hypertension, diabetes)
Dissection (aorta, VA dissection – uni/bilateral)
Hypotension (cardiac failure)
Cocaine
Vasculitis
Fibrocartilaginous embolism
Embolic occlusion of the VA
Diagnostic blockade of cervical nerve roots
Spinal decompression sickness
Scoliosis operation
Compression of a lumbar artery
Spinal AVM, dural fistula
Spinal tumour
Idiopathic

[13, 14], arteriosclerosis of the VA and cardioembolic occlusion of the VA (see Table 20.1) [7, 9]. In the elderly, arteriosclerosis of the aorta and infrarenal aneurysm repair with potential occlusion of the artery of Adamkiewiecz are considerable risk factors for medullar ischemia. Further etiologies are vasculitis, e.g. panarteriitis nodosa or antiphospholipid antibody syndrome, neurosyphilis, spinal decompression sickness after diving, scoliosis operation with erection of the spine, diagnostic blockade of cervical nerve roots, spinal tumours and spinal arteriovenous malformation AVM (see Table 20.1). However, in about one third of spinal cord infarcts, aetiology remains unclear (idiopathic) [9].

20.3 Clinical Symptoms

20.3.1 Syndrome of the Anterior Spinal Artery (ASA)

Ischemia in the ASA territory, including the SA with bilaterally and sometimes asymmetric lesions of the anterior horns, the lateral corticospinal tract, the thalamic pathways and the area around the central canal (commissural pathways), causes the "centromedullar syndrome" or syndrome of the ASA (see Fig. 20.1b and 20.3). This dramatic clinical feature is characterized by spastic para- or tetraparesis, dissociated sensation deficits with loss of pain and temperature sense below the lesion level of the spinal cord. In addition, there are bladder and bowel dysfunction, and when the vasoconstrictor tract in the lateral medullary part is affected, neurological syndrome including different temperature of the limbs and ipsilateral Horner's syndrome in the case of cervical infarction. As a consequence of direct lower motor neuron damage, floppy paresis at the level of infarct occurs (Figs. 20.3) [3].

However, in contrast to cerebral infarction with acute onset, the clinical deficits caused by spinal cord ischemia manifest over 30–45 min, accompanied by a radicular belt-like pain representing the start of this severe neurological disease.

20.3.2 Syndrome of the Posterior Spinal Artery (PSA)

Due to dual posterior (PSA) and posterolateral (PLSA) spinal arteries in combination with a pial collateral network, infarcts are more often located in the ASA territory than in the PSA/PLSA territories (see Fig. 20.4 and 20.1c) [15]. Disturbance of proprioception reflecting light touch and vibration sense due to damage of the dorsal columns causes atactic gait disturbances.

20.3.3 Syndrome of the Artery of Adamkiewicz

In lower thoracic levels, especially with occlusion of the artery of Adamkiewicz, both ASA and PSA/PLSA territories are affected. Neurological examinations often show complete transverse spinal cord syndrome (Fig. 20.1d and 20.5) [3, 7, 9, 16].

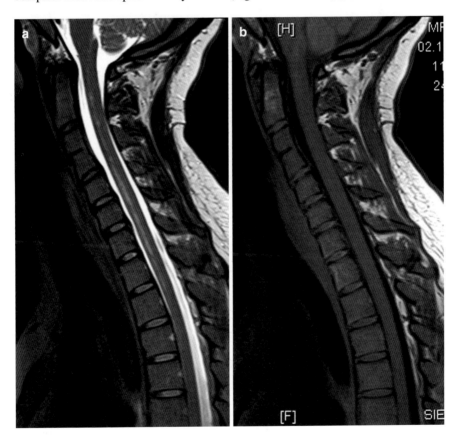

Fig. 20.3 (a–f) A 24-year-old woman suffering from ASA syndrome and rapid progressive tetraparesis within 3 h. Sagittal T2 WI (a) showing a "pencil-like" longitudinal hyperintense medullary lesion ventrally accentuated. Axial T2 WI (d–f) disclosing at the level C2/3 bilateral nearly symmetrical hyperintense signal changes probably in the anterior horns (d; "snake eyes"), which increase at level C4 (e) and lastly affect large parts of the transverse section sparing the PSA territories. T1 WI sag. before (b) and after contrast medium application (c) revealing slight inhomogeneous enhancement

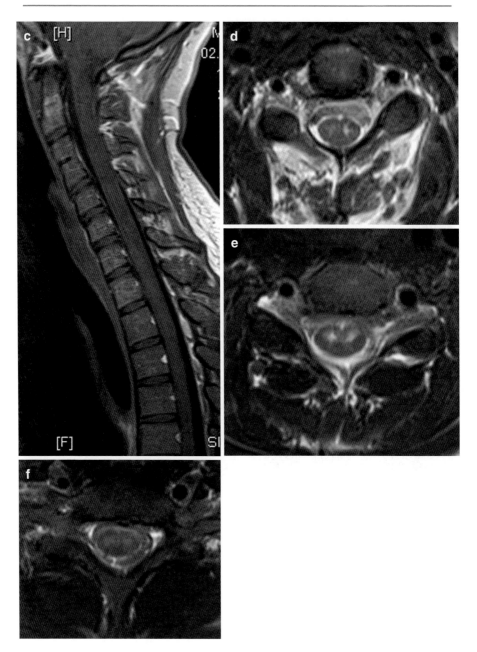

Fig. 20.3 (continued)

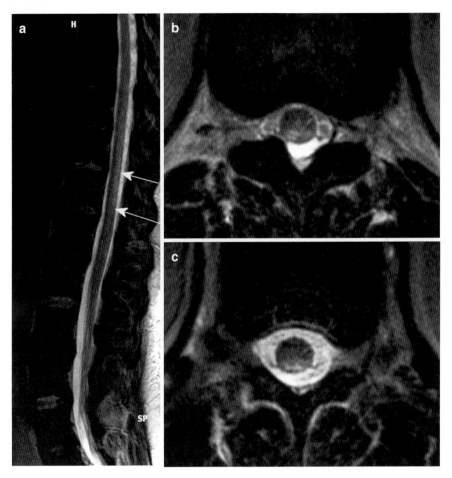

Fig. 20.4 (**a–c**) A 42-year-old man with sudden onset of mild paraparesis and severe gait ataxia caused by ischemia in the PSA territory of unknown aetiology. Sagittal (**a**, *arrows*) and axial T2 WI (**b, c**) showing a hyperintense lesion at the level Th 9–12 preferentially in the dorsal medullar circumference (From: Weidauer et al. [7])

20.3.4 Syndrome of the Sulcal (Syn.: Central, Sulcocommissural) Artery

Duplication of the ASA is quite likely and, as a probable consequence, ischemia in one of the two ASA may cause ipsilateral infarcts in the sulcal artery (SA) territory. A clinical feature is the spinal "sulcal artery syndrome" and, in contrast to the Brown Séquard's syndrome, (hemi spinal cord syndrome) posterior columns are not affected (Fig. 20.6 and 20.1e) [8, 17–19].

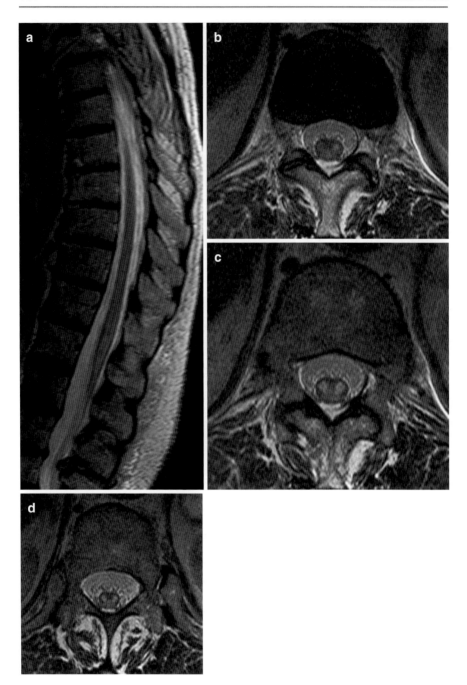

Fig. 20.5 Syndrome of the artery of Adamkiewicz. Sag. T2 WI (**a**) showing inhomogeneous signal conversion of the lower thoracic and thoracolumbar spinal cord; axial T2 WI (**b–d**; downwards) revealing increasingly hyperintense intramedullary signal changes, which encompass finally nearly the whole transverse section

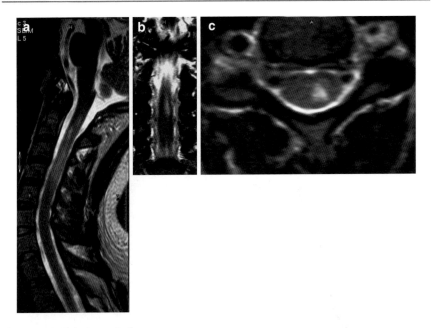

Fig. 20.6 Spinal sulcal artery (SA) syndrome. Sag. T2 WI (**a**) showing inhomogeneous hyperintense lesion of the cervical spinal cord. Coronal (**b**) and axial (**c**) T2 WI disclosing left sided centromedullar lesion in the spinal sulcal artery territory as a likely consequence of anterior spinal artery duplication and occlusion of the left branch. Note dissection of the left VA (**c**).

20.3.5 "Man-in-the-Barrel" Syndrome

Comparable to cerebral ischemia, watershed infarcts may also occur, especially in the border zones between the central and peripheral system (see Fig. 20.1f and 20.7). In the case of spinal hypoperfusion, hemodynamic infarcts often occur in the anterior horns, because the grey matter and particular the motor neurons exhibit a much higher vulnerability to anoxia as shown by Gelfan and Tarlov [6]. A typical clinical feature of watershed infarcts in the spinal cord is the "man-in-the-barrel" syndrome with bilateral atonic paresis of the upper limbs without motor deficits in the legs [20]. MR imaging shows bilateral hyperintense lesions on axial T2 WI in the region of the anterior horns ("snake-eye" configuration) (see Fig. 20.7) [21–23]. Also in lower motor

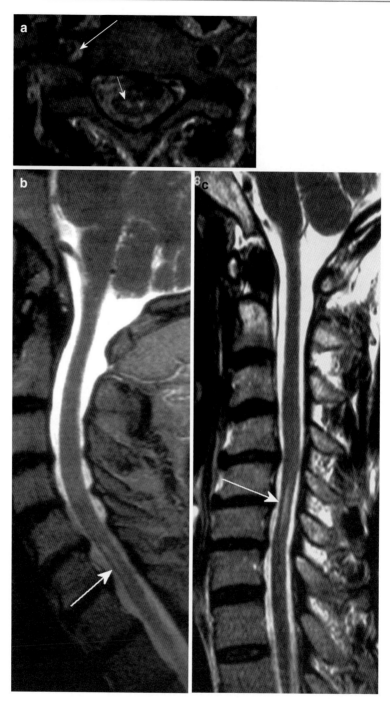

Fig. 20.7 (a–c) "Man-in-the-barrel" syndrome in a 61-year-old male caused by right VA dissection (**a**, T2 WI, ax., *arrow*) with small hyperintense intramedullary lesions at the level of the anterior horns (**a**, *short arrow*). T2 WI sag. (**b**) showing hyperintense pencil-shaped signal conversion (*arrow*) at the level C6/7 and follow-up imaging 1 year later circumscribed medullar atrophy (**c**, *arrow*)

neuron disease, e.g. spinal muscle atrophy bilateral hyperintense lesions at the level of the anterior horns and possible additional cord atrophy may be visible (see Fig. 20.8).

However, there are three types of "man-in-the-barrel" syndrome. The initial type was described as a consequence of bilateral watershed infarctions between the anterior cerebral artery (ACA) and middle cerebral artery (MCA) territories caused by global hypoperfusion or occlusive bilateral diseases of internal carotid artery (ACI) with isolated lesions of the corticospinal tract to the upper limbs with sparing of the fibres to the legs, resulting in a pure motor syndrome with proximally accentuated central paresis of the upper limbs. In addition, bilateral pontine infarcts may also cause a "man-in-the-barrel" syndrome [20].

Hemodynamically appearing lesion patterns with bilateral hyperintense signal changes on axial T2 WI are also seen in the upper part of thoracolumbar medullary infarcts caused by occlusion of the artery of Adamkiewicz (see Fig. 20.5b) [7]. A likely cause is a watershed zone between the territory of this artery and upper thoracic feeders or between the central and peripheral system (Fig. 20.7).

Review of the literature yielded no definite spinal watershed zone in the upper thoracic cord as supposed in some publications [5]. Numerous spinal infarcts are located in the cervical cord, especially at the C2–C4 level [7]. Therefore the reasons might be insufficient anastomoses for the higher perfused segments of the cervical intumescence, e.g. absence of direct communications between the proximal ASA and the intradural (V4) vertebral artery segments or unilateral existence of radiculomedullary branches at the cervical level in up to 20 % [7]. The corpus vertebra and the dura mater are also supplied by the segmental arteries. Whereas the anterior and lateral parts of the corpus vertebra are fed by proximal originating branches of the segmental arteries, the dorsal part of the corpus vertebra is supplied by branches originating from the RA [9, 24]. Therefore additional vertebral body infarcts may be a hint of the location of vessel occlusion and are best seen on MRI one or two weeks after onset [24].

Table 20.2 Differential diagnosis of acute spinal cord symptoms

Extradural	Tumour
	Medial disc herniation
	Spinal stenosis ± perfusion impairment
	Spinal trauma (contusio/compressio spinalis)
	Epidural abscess, empyema
Intradural	Myelitis (meningomyeloradiculitis; immune associated, viral, bacterial)
	Vascular malformation (intra-/perimedullar angioma, dural av fistula; bleeding – hemorrhagic myelopathy, ischemia, venous congestion)
	Cavernoma
	Infarct
	Metabolic/toxic
	Post radiation

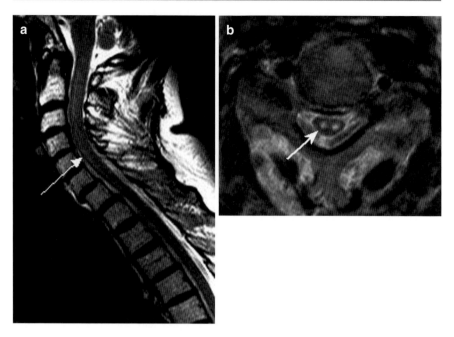

Fig. 20.8 (**a**, **b**) Lower motor neuron disease (spinal muscle atrophy); 73-year-old man suffering from spinobulbar muscle atrophy (Kennedy type) for 8 years. T2 WI (**a**: sag.; **b**: ax.) exhibit bilateral lesions accentuated in the anterior horns (*arrow*), comparable to those in spinal watershed infarcts (see Fig. 20.7)

20.4 MR Imaging Features

In an emergency setting with acute spinal-cord symptoms, MRI is the method of choice for differential diagnosis. Especially space-occupying lesions with consecutive cord compression have to be excluded, such as epidural hematoma, epidural inflammatory disturbances, i.e. abscess or empyema, intra- or extradural tumours and medial disc herniation. Furthermore, possible treatable intramedullary pathologies should be excluded, such as intramedullary tumours, vascular malformations and bleedings as well as myelitis (see Table 20.2) [7].

Medullary lesions caused by spinal cord infarcts are best demonstrated on sagittal T2 WI showing longitudinal extended "pencil-like" hyperintense signal changes, accompanied by swelling and consecutive cord enlargement in the subacute stage (see Figs. 20.3a, 20.4a, 20.5a, 20.6a, 20.9) [7, 24]. Comparable to cerebral infarcts post contrast (pc) T1 WI disclose variable contrast enhancement from day 3 forward after onset caused by disruption of blood brain barrier (see Fig. 20.3c) [7, 24]. In this stage, especially in cervical infarcts, imaging features may mimic spinal cord tumours and hemorrhagic transformation may also occur. Infarcts are most frequent in the ASA territory showing bilateral symmetric or asymmetric hyperintense signal

20 Spinal Cord Infarction

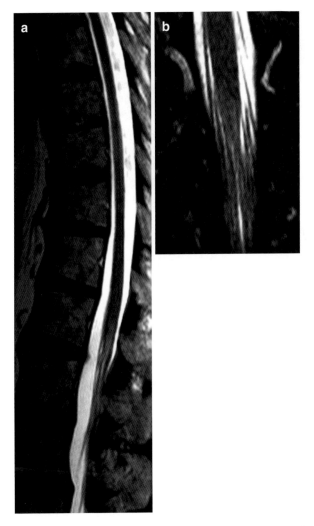

Fig. 20.9 (a–d) Infarct of the conus medullaris caused by infrarenal aortic dissection in a 77-year-old man with sudden onset of breeches-like sensation deficits, urinary retention and bowel incontinence. T2 WI (**a**: sag.; **b**: cor.; **c**: ax.) showing circumscribed hyperintense signal changes of the conus medullaris; (**d**) contrast enhanced axial CT exhibiting aortic dissection (*arrow*: dissection membrane) with "double lumen"

abnormalities in the central part of the spinal cord, sparing the peripheral circumference because of the collateral network of the vasocorona at cervical and upper thoracic location (see Fig. 20.3) [7]. In the lower thoracic and thoracolumbar regions infarcts are often caused by occlusion of the artery of Adamkiewicz and transverse sections often exhibit nearly complete hyperintense signal changes of the cord (see Figs. 20.5 and 20.9). However, as mentioned above, in the upper part of these

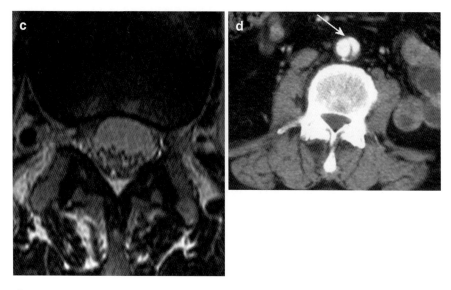

Fig. 20.9 (continued)

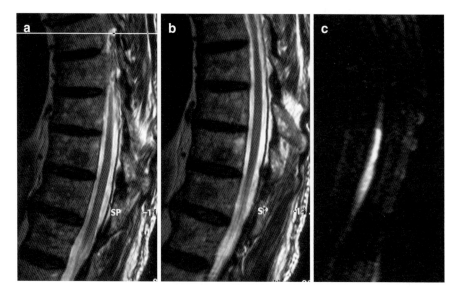

Fig. 20.10 Sag. T2 WI (**a**, **b**) in a 74-year-old woman showing questionable slight signal inhomogeneity 3.5 h after onset of progressive paraparesis. Additional DWI (**c**, sag.; TR 1,500 ms; TE/TE diff.:13/75 ms; **b** – value: 700 s/mm^2; EPI – factor: 11; pulse-triggering; NSA: 4) disclosing distinct signal intensity caused by restricted diffusion in the spinal cord at the level Th 9 downward (From: Weidauer et al. [25])

extended lesions, a hemodynamic lesion pattern with bilateral signal abnormalities at the level of the anterior horn may be visible (see Figs. 20.3d and 20.5b).

Assessment of infarct pattern disclosed that not all lesions fit to an assumed ASA or PSA territory, probably because of variable spinal vascular supply and individual hemodynamic watershed zones [7, 9, 24].

Slight signal conversions on T2 WI may be visible as early as 3 h after onset of ischemia, although they are unspecific at this time (see Fig. 20.10) [25]. Reliable hyperintense signal changes on T2 WI are detectable 12–24 h later, potentially accompanied by subtle cord swelling. Whereas diffusion weighted imaging (DWI) is well implemented in routine cerebral imaging protocols and plays a key role in the diagnostic set-up of acute cerebral stroke and consecutive therapeutic strategies, up to now DWI of the spinal cord is unusual in clinical routine. Although spinal DWI is feasible, there are several problems regarding data acquisition, e.g. cerebrospinal fluid (CSF) motion artefacts, huge susceptibility problems and the small cord size [25–30]. In contrast to normal T2 WI or unspecific slight hyperintense signal changes, DWI shows significant intensity conversion with lowered apparent diffusion coefficient (ADC) in the first hours after symptom onset, comparable to that in acute cerebral ischemic stroke (Fig. 20.10). Therefore, DWI is a useful tool in emergency imaging of acute spinal cord symptoms [29, 30]. However, from the clinical point of view, it is crucial to exclude space-occupying lesions with consecutive spinal cord compression, epidural inflammatory diseases, i.e. abscess or empyema, and myelitis (see Table 20.2). Comparable to cerebral ischemia, signal abnormalities on DWI with restricted diffusion are typical but not pathognomonic for spinal cord infarction [29, 30]. Thus, high signal intensities on DWI may also occur in acute myelopathy caused by severe spinal canal stenosis, in tumours, e.g. epidermoid, in inflammatory diseases and in spinal traumata [27, 29, 30].

References

1. Turnbull IM, Brieg A, Hassler O (1966) Blood supply of cervical spinal cord in man. A microangiographic cadaver study. J Neurosurg 24:951–965
2. Thron A (ed) (1989) Vascularisation of the spinal cord. Springer, Wien, New York
3. Lazorthes G (1972) Pathology, classification and clinical aspects of vascular diseases in spinal cord. In: Vinken PJ, Bruyn GW (eds) Handbook of clinical neurology, vol 12. North Holland, Amsterdam, pp 492–506
4. Martirosyan N, Feuerstein J, Theodore N, Cavalcanti D, Spetzler R, Preul M (2011) Blood supply and vascular reactivity of the spinal cord under normal and pathological conditions. J Neurosurg Spine 15:238–251
5. Jellinger KA (1997) Spinal cord watershed. Neurology 48:1474
6. Gelfan S, Tarlov IM (1955) Differential vulnerability of spinal cord structures to anoxia. J Neurophysiol 18:170–188
7. Weidauer S, Nichtweiss M, Lanfermann H, Zanella FE (2002) Spinal cord infarction: MR imaging and clinical features in 16 cases. Neuroradiology 44:851–857
8. Weidauer S, Gartenschläger M, Claus D (1999) Spinal sulcal artery syndrome due to bilateral vertebral artery dissection. J Neurol Neurosurg Psychiatry 67:550–551
9. Mull M (2005) Acute spinal cord ischemia: diagnosis without therapeutic options? Clin Neuroradiol 15:79–88

10. Masson C, Boukriche Y, Berthelot JL, Colombani JM (2001) Vertebra, rib and spinal cord infarction caused by probable fibrocartilaginous embolism. Cerebrovasc Dis 12:142–143
11. Tosi L, Rigoli G, Beltramello A (1996) Fibrocartilaginous embolism of the spinal cord: a clinical and pathogenetic reconsideration. J Neurol Neurosurg Psychiatry 60:55–60
12. Mikulis DJ, Ogilvy S, McKee A, Davis KR, Ojeman RG (1992) Spinal cord infarction and fibrocartilaginous emboli. AJNR Am J Neuroradiol 13:155–160
13. Di Lazzaro V, Restuccia D, Oliveiro A, Profice P, Nardone R, Valeriani M, Colosimo C, Tartaglione T, Della Corte F, Pennini MA, Tonali P (1997) Ischaemic myelopathy associated with cocaine: clinical, neurophysiological and neuroradiological features. J Neurol Neurosurg Psychiatry 63:531–533
14. Qureshi AI, Akbar MS, Czander E, Safdar K, Janssen RS, Frankel MR (1997) Crack cocaine use and stroke in young patients. Neurology 48:341–345
15. Bergqvist C, Goldberg HI, Thorarensen O, Bird SJ (1997) Posterior cervical spinal cord infarction following vertebral artery dissection. Neurology 48:1112–1115
16. Berg P, Kaufmann D, van Marrewijk CD, Buth J (2001) Spinal cord ischemia after stent – graft treatment for infrarenal abdominal aortic aneurysms. Analysis of the Eurostar data base. Eur J Vasc Endovasc Surg 4:342–347
17. Laufs H, Weidauer S, Heller C, Lorenz M, Neumann-Haefelin T (2004) Hemi-spinal cord infarction due to vertebral artery dissection in congenital afibrinogenemia. Neurology 63:1522–1523
18. Lipper MH, Goldstein JH, Do HM (1998) Brown – Séquard syndrome of the cervical spinal cord after chiropractic manipulation. AJNR Am J Neuroradiol 19:1349–1352
19. Goldsmith P, Rowe D, Jäger R, Kapoor R (1998) Focal vertebral artery dissection causing Brown – Séquard`s syndrome. J Neurol Neurosurg Psychiatry 64:415–416
20. Urban P, Gawehn J, Ringel K (2005) "Man–in–the–barrel" syndrome. Clin Neuroradiol 15:190–194
21. Pullicino P (1994) Bilateral upper limb amyotrophy and watershed infarcts from vertebral artery dissection. Stroke 25:1870–1872
22. Stapf C, Mohr JP, Straschill M, Mast H, Marx P (2000) Acute bilateral arm paresis. Cerebrovasc Dis 10:239–243
23. Berg D, Mullges W, Klotzenburg M, Bendszus M, Reiners K (1998) Man-in-the-barrel syndrome caused by cervical spinal cord infarction. Acta Neurol Scand 97:417–419
24. Yuh W, Marsh EE, Wang AK, Russel JW, Chiang F, Koci TM, Ryals TJ (1992) MR imaging of spinal cord and vertebral body infarction. AJNR Am J Neuroradiol 13:145–154
25. Weidauer S, Dettmann E, Krakow K, Lanfermann H (2002) Diffusion-weighted MRI of spinal cord infarction – description of two cases and review of the literature. Nervenarzt 73:999–1003
26. Bammer R, Fazekas F, Augustin M, Simbrunner J, Strasser-Fuchs S, Seifert T, Stollberger R, Hartung HP (2000) Diffusion weighted MR imaging of the spinal cord. AJR Am J Neuroradiol 21:587–591
27. Lanfermann H, Pilatus U, Weidauer S (2004) Diffusion-weighted MRI of the spinal cord in spinal stroke. Riv Neuroradiol 17:309–313
28. Thurnher MM, Bammer R (2006) Diffusion-weighted MR imaging (DWI) in spinal cord ischemia. Neuroradiology 48:795–801
29. Marcel C, Kremer S, Jeantroux J, Blanc F, Dietemann JL, De Sèze J (2010) Diffusion-weighted imaging in noncompressive myelopathies: a 33-patient prospective study. J Neurol 257:1438–1445
30. Tanenbaum LN (2013) Clinical applications of diffusion imaging in the spine. Magn Reson Imaging Clin N Am 21:299–320

Index

A
Abt–Letterer–Siwe disease, 210
Acceleration techniques, 68–70
Accessory process, 17
Achondroplasia, 133
Acquired lumbal canal stenosis, 182–188
Acute disseminated encephalomyelitis
 (ADEM), 331
 acute transverse myelitis, 357–358
 monophasic disorder, 354
 Mycoplasma pneumonia-associated
  myelitis, 354, 355
 prototypical, 356
Adult polyglucosan body disease
 (PGBD), 381–382, 384, 385
Aliasing, 96
Aneurysmal bone cyst, 206
Ankylosing spondylitis, 160, 161
Anterior longitudinal ligament, 24
Anterior spinal artery (ASA)
 clinical symptoms, 440, 441
 extrinsic spinal cord arteries, 436–437
 hypervascular intradural tumor, 429
 radiculomedullary, 415, 416
 sulcocommissural branches, CTA, 417
AOD. *See* Atlantoccipital dislocation (AOD)
Apparent diffusion coefficient
 (ADC), 88, 89
Arachnopathy, 296–299
Arteriovenous malformations (AVM)
 MRI and MRA, 418, 420
 radiculomedullary artery, 419, 420
 surgical treatment, 419
Artery of Adamkiewicz
 clinical symptoms, 441, 444
 vascular anatomy, 435–437

Astrocytoma
 classification, 402–403
 microsurgery, 403
 radiologic appearance, 403–404
Atlantoaxial dislocations
 axial/cranial, 254
 translatory, 252, 253
 traumatic rotatory, 252–254
Atlantoccipital dislocation
 (AOD), 247–248
Atlantodens interval (ADI), 119, 120
Atlanto-occipital joints, 20
Atlanto-occipital membrane, 24–25
Atlas fractures, 249–252
Atlas malformations, 125–126
Axis malformations, 126–130

B
Back pain
 local pain
  ankylosing spondylitis, 160, 161
  epidural abscess, 160, 162
  spondylodiscitis, 160, 163–165
 muscle spasm, 167
 radicular pain, 161–162, 165, 166
 referred pain, 163, 165, 167
Bacterial spinal meningitis, 272–274
Basilar invagination, 118, 119,
 120, 122, 126
Behcet's disease, 359–361
Benign tumor
 intradural extramedullary
  ependymomas, 238
  ganglioneuromas, 237–238
  meningiomas, 231–235

Benign tumor (*cont.*)
  neurofibromas, 235–236
  paragangliomas, 237
  schwannomas, 235–237
  primary epidural
    diagnosis, 204
    oncological staging system, 205
    origin, 203
    outcome, 204
    prevalence, 203
    surgical staging system, 205
    symptoms, 203–204
    therapy, 204
Bevacizumab, 404
Bladder disturbances, 313–314
Borreliosis. *See* Lyme disease
Brown tumours, 210

C
Cauda equina, 33–35
Caudal regression syndrome (CRS), 154–156
Cavernomas, 429, 430
Centromedullary lesions,
  space-occupying, 306–309, 311–313
Cerebrospinal fluid (CSF) flow
  arachnoid cysts, 97–99
  ECG triggering, 96
  indications, 97
  MRI, 91
  phase contrast MRI, 94–96
  phase-difference images, 94
  physiological principles, 94
  pulsation, 93
  suitable maximum flow value, 96
Cervical disc herniation, 192–197
Cervical meningocele, 141, 144
Cervical rib syndrome, 13
Cervical spine
  alignment, 6, 7
  characteristics, 12–15
  diagnosis, 244–245
  function, 16
  intervertebral foramen, 13, 16, 19, 26–28
  origin, 244
  os odontoideum, 12, 15
  prevalence, 244
  symptoms, 244
  therapy and outcome, 245
  transverse foramen, 12, 16
  upper cervical spine (*see* Upper
    cervical spine)
Cervical spondylosis, 193–194, 198–200
Chamberlain line, 22, 23

Chondrosarcoma, 208
Chordoma, 208, 209
Claudicatio spinalis, 185, 187, 188
Clefts of atlas arches, 126
Clinical isolated syndrome (CIS)
  cervical trauma, 341
  hyperintense lesion, 343
  swollen lesion, 340
  symptoms, 335
  thoracic pain, 342
Closed spinal dysraphisms (CSD)
  dermal sinus, 140–142
  vs. open spinal dysraphisms, 138
  in postnatal phase, 139
  taillike lipoma, 139, 140
Contrast-enhanced magnetic resonance
    angiography (CE-MRA)
  high-resolution, 87
  with spinal arteriovenous
    malformation, 87, 88
  standard and dynamic, 86
Contrast-enhanced MR myelography
  advantages, 102
  CSF leakage, 103–105
  demerits, 103
  MR imaging protocol, 103
  technique, 102
Contrast-to-noise ratio (CNR), 57
Conus medullaris, 34, 35, 108, 112, 118,
    168, 280, 322, 408, 448, 449
Copper deficiency, SCDSC, 373–376
Corticospinal tract, topography of, 304
Costal process, 17
Craniocervical junction (CCJ)
  atlanto-axial joint, 21, 22
  atlantoccipital dislocation, 247–248
  atlanto-occipital joints, 20
  imaging, 22–23
  ligaments
    atlanto-occipital membrane, 24–25
    cruciate ligament, 24
    ligamentum flavum, 26
    odontoid ligaments, 24
    tectorial membrane, 24
  occipital condyle fractures, 245–247
Craniocervical junction (CCJ) anomalies, 118
  atlantodens interval, 119, 120
  atlas malformations, 125–126
  axis malformations, 126–130
  MRI, 119
  occipital bone malformations, 122–125
  odontoid process,
    malformation of, 126–130
  representative inherited syndromes

Index

achondroplasia, 133
Down syndrome, 129–131
juvenile rheumatoid arthritis, 131–132
Larsen syndrome, 133
mucopolysaccharidoses, 132–134
neurofibromatosis, 131
osteogenesis imperfecta, 133
spondyloepiphyseal dysplasia, 133
symptoms, 119
Crohn's disease, TNF, 347
Cruciate ligament, 24
Cuneate fascicles tracts, topography of, 304
Cysticercosis, 328
Cytomegalovirus (CMV), 322–323

D

Degenerative diseases
  back pain, 160–167
  myelon compression syndromes, 188–200
  radicular compression syndromes (*see* Radicular compression syndromes)
  sinuvertebral nerves, 160
Degenerative vertebral endplate, 174, 175
Dermal sinus, 140–142
Devic's disease. *See* Neuromyelitis optica (NMO)
Diffusion tensor imaging (DTI), 89
Diffusion-weighted imaging (DWI), 89
Digital subtraction angiography (DSA), 414–416
Disc extrusion, 176
Disc herniation, 174
  classifications, 176, 178
  disc extrusion, 176
  focal herniation, 176
  intervertebral disc herniation, 176
  lateral foraminal and extraforaminal disc herniation, 179, 180
  medial (central/paracentral), 176–178
  mediolateral/subarticular, 176
  protrusion, 176
  sequestration, 176
Down syndrome, 129–131
Duplex sonography, 96
Dural AVF
  compression fracture, 424–425
  fistulous point, 424, 426
  pathoanatomy, 424, 425
  radiculomedullary artery, 423
  sacral, 424
  venous congestion, 421
  vertebral foramen, retrograde filling, 421–422

E

Echo planar imaging (EPI), 67
Echo time, 46
End-plates, 6
Enneking system, 204, 205
Eosinophilic granuloma, 210–212
Ependymoma
  characteristics, 399
  chemotherapy, 402
  radiologic appearance, 400–401
Ependymomas, 89, 90, 238
Epidural abscess, 160, 162
Epidural empyema
  diagnosis, 226, 227
  neurological symptoms, 225
  origin, 222, 224–225
  outcome, 227–228
  prevalence, 225
  therapy, 226, 228–229
Epidural hemorrhage
  differential diagnosis, 230
  neurological symptoms, 230
  origin, 229–230
  outcome, 231
  prevalence, 230
  therapy, 230–231
Epidural space, 31–32
  anatomy, 202–203
  lymphoma, 217–218
  sacrococcygeal teratoma, 218
  vertebral venous plexus, 202
Epidural tumours
  aneurysmal bone cyst, 206
  brown tumour, 210
  chondrosarcoma, 208
  chordoma, 208, 209
  eosinophilic granuloma, 210–212
  Ewing sarcoma, 216
  fibrosarcoma, 216
  fibrous dysplasia, 210
  giant cell tumour, 208, 209
  langerhans cell histiocytosis, 210–211
  lymphoma, 212, 215, 217–218
  malignant, 203–205
  malignant fibrous histiocytoma, 217
  metastases, 218–222
  multiple myeloma, 211–212, 216
  osteoblastoma, 206, 208
  osteochondroma, 208
  osteoid osteoma, 206, 208
  osteosarcoma, 215
  primary benign
    diagnosis, 204
    oncological staging system, 205

Epidural tumours (cont.)
  origin, 203
  outcome, 204
  prevalence, 203
  surgical staging system, 205
  symptoms, 203–204
  therapy, 204
 sacrococcygeal teratoma, 218
 secondary malignant
  diagnosis, 219, 220, 221
  outcome, 222
  prevalence, 218–219
  symptoms, 219
  therapy, 219, 222, 223
 solitary plasmacytoma, 211–215
 vertebral hemangioma, 206, 207
Epstein–Barr virus (EBV), 323
Ewing sarcoma, 216
Extradural extramedullary pathologies, 202–203
Extradural process, 109–110
Extrinsic spinal cord arteries
 anterior spinal artery, 436–437
 posterior spinal artery, 437

F
Facet joints
 degeneration, 181
 description, 20
Fast spin-echo (FSE) readouts, 67
Fibrosarcoma, 216
Fibrous dysplasia, 210
Filum terminale, 152–154
Flip angle, 46
Flow artefacts
 inflow signal enhancement, 76
 outflow signal loss, 76
 from pulsatile flow, 76
 single dephasing, 74, 75
Focal herniation, 176
Foraminal epidural fat, 180
Foraminal stenosis
 facet joint degeneration, 181
 foraminal epidural fat, classification of, 180
 juxtaarticular cysts, 181–182
 narrowed intervertebral foramen, 179
 spondylolisthesis, 181, 183, 184
 spondylolysis, 181, 185
Fractional anisotropy (FA), 89
Fractures
 atlas, 249–252
 atypical, 258–259
 occipital condyle, 245–247
 odontoid, 255–258
 sacral, 264–267
 types, 254–255
Frequency encoding process, 59–63
Friedreich's ataxia, 380, 382–383

G
Ganglioneuromas, 237–238
GBS. See Guillain–Barré syndrome (GBS)
Giant cell tumour, 208, 209
Gibb's ringing artefacts, 72–73
Glioblastoma, metastases, 288
Gnathostomiasis, 329
Gracile tracts, topography of, 304
Gray matter diseases
 monomelic amyotrophy, 393–394
 MRI, 390
 poliomyelitis, 392–393
 progressive muscular atrophy, 393
 SBMA, 390
 spinal muscle atrophy, 390–392
Guillain–Barré syndrome (GBS), 279–281

H
Hand–Schüller–Christian disease, 210
Hangman fracture, 258–261
Hemangioblastoma, 405–406
Hemangioma, vertebral, 206, 207
Hemangiopericytoma, 240
Herniation, spinal cord, 291–293
Herpes simplex virus (HSV), 321–322
Hirayama disease. See Monomelic amyotrophy (MMA)
HIV myelitis, 332–333
Human T-cell lymphotrophic virus (HTLV), 333
Hydromyelia, 306–307

I
Idiopathic acute transverse myelitis, 330
Idiopathic hypertrophic spinal pachymeningitis, 294–296
Image artefacts/errors
 chemical shift, 71–72
 flow artefacts
  inflow signal enhancement, 76
  outflow signal loss, 76
  from pulsatile flow, 76
  single dephasing, 74, 75

Index

Gibb's ringing, 72–73
magnetic susceptibility and metallic implants, 70–71
patient motion, 73–74
Image contrasts, 47
  proton density weighting, 50–51
  signal and contrast-to-noise ratios, 53–57
  T1 weighting, 48, 49
  T2 weighting, 48, 49
  T2* weighting, 51–53
Image formation, 57
  magnetic field gradients, 58, 59
  slice selection, 58, 60
  spatial localisation
    acceleration techniques, 68–70
    frequency encoding, 59–63
    k-space, 61–68
    phase encoding, 60
    readout methods, 67–68
Image quality, improvement of
  adjacent tissue suppression, 77
  contrast agents, 80–81
  fat suppression, 78–81
  inversion recovery, 78, 79
  physiological fluctuations, reduction of, 76–77
  protocols, 82, 83
  short tau inversion recovery, 78–80
  spectrally selective saturation, 78
Immune-mediated myelopathies
  acute disseminated encephalomyelitis, postvaccination myelopathies, 351–358
  multiple sclerosis (*see* Multiple sclerosis (MS))
  neuromyelitis optica, 346–351
  SAD and sarcoidosis, 358–362
  tumor necrosis factor, 345–346
Inflammation
  acute myelopathy
    CMV, 322–323
    Epstein–Barr virus, 323
    Herpes simplex virus, 321–322
    HIV, 322
    poliomyelitis, 324
    varicella zoster virus, 320–321
    West Nile virus, 324–325
  acute transverse myelitis, 318–319
  clinically definite multiple sclerosis, 317–318
  idiopathic acute transverse myelitis, 330
  immune-mediated myelopathies
    ADEM, postvaccination myelopathies, 351–358
    multiple sclerosis (*see* Multiple sclerosis (MS))
    neuromyelitis optica (*see* Neuromyelitis optica (NMO))
    SAD and sarcoidosis, 358–362
    tumor necrosis factor, 345–346
  infectious myelopathies agents, 319–320
  parainfectious myelitis, post-infectious myelitis, 330–332
  subacute and chronic infections, 332–334
  subacute myelopathy
    bacteria, 326–328
    fungi and parasites, 328–329
  transverse myelitis, 316–317
Intervertebral discs, 17–18, 20
  degeneration, 172–173
  herniation, 176
Intervertebral (neural) foramen, 11, 13, 16, 19, 26–28
Intradural extramedullary pathologies, 231
  ependymomas, 238
  ganglioneuromas, 237–238
  hemangiopericytoma, 240
  leptomeningeal metastases, 241
  meningiomas
    diagnosis, 232–234
    origin, 231
    outcome, 235
    prevalence, 232
    symptoms, 232
    therapy, 233–235
  MPNST, 238–240
  neurofibromas, 235–236
  paragangliomas, 237
  schwannomas, 235–237
Intradural extramedullary space-occupying lesions, 111
Intradural intramedullary space-occupying lesions, 111, 112
Intramedullary spinal cord metastasis (ISCM)
  MRI features, 406–407
  treatment, 406
Intramedullary spinal cord tumors, 407–408
  astrocytoma, 402–405
  clinical presentation, 396–397
  ependymoma, 399–402
  hemangioblastoma, 405–406
  ISCM, 406–407
  microsurgery, 398
  MRI, 396
  radiotherapy, 399

J

Joints
　craniocervical junction, 21–23
　facet joints, 20
　uncinate process, 20, 21
　uncovertebral joints, 20, 21, 23
Joints of Luschka. *See* Uncovertebral joints
Juvenile rheumatoid arthritis, 131–132
Juxtaarticular cysts, 181–182

K

Kennedy disease. *See* Spinal and bulbar muscular atrophy (SBMA)
k-space, 61–68

L

Langerhans cell histiocytosis, 210–211
Larsen syndrome, 133
Lasègue manoeuvre. *See* Straight leg raising
Lateral foraminal and extraforaminal disc herniation, 179, 180
Lateral recess, 11, 14
Leptomeningeal metastases, 241
Ligamentum flavum, 26
Lipomyelomeningocele, 142, 144–146
Local pain
　ankylosing spondylitis, 160, 161
　epidural abscess, 160, 162
　spondylodiscitis, 160, 163–165
Locked facet, 20
Longitudinally extensive transverse myelitis (LETM), 312, 331–332
Lower motor neuron disease, 445, 448
Lumbar spine, 17, 18
Lung carcinoma, osteolytic metastasis of, 223
Lyme disease, 326, 327
Lymphoma, 212, 215, 217–218

M

Magnetic resonance angiography (MRA), 85
　contrast-enhanced, 86–88
　diffusion imaging, 88–90
　indications, 87
　inflow enhancement effect, 85
Magnetic resonance imaging (MRI), 82, 83
　advantages, 40–41
　arteriovenous malformations, 418, 420
　CCJ anomalies, 119
　challenges, 41
　detection, 44
　excitation, 44
　gray matter diseases, 390
　intramedullary spinal cord tumor, 396, 406–407
　polarisation, 42–44
　precession, 44
　pulse sequence, 46–47
　radicular compression syndromes, 169–172
　relaxation process, 44–45
　scanner components, 42, 43
　spinal cord infarction
　　conus medullaris, 448, 449
　　differential diagnosis, 447
Malignant fibrous histiocytoma, 217
Malignant peripheral nerve sheath tumours (MPNST), 238–240
Malignant tumours
　epidural tumours, 203–205
　secondary epidural tumours
　　diagnosis, 219, 220, 221
　　outcome, 222
　　prevalence, 218–219
　　symptoms, 219
　　therapy, 219, 222, 223
Mamillary process, 17
Man-in-the-barrel syndrome, 445–447
Medial (central/paracentral) disc herniation, 176–178
Median atlanto-axial joints, 21
Mediolateral/subarticular disc herniation, 176
Medulloblastoma, 287
Meningeal disorders, 271–272
　neoplastic meningeosis, 280, 282–286
　pachy-and leptomeningeal diseases
　　arachnopathy, 296–299
　　idiopathic hypertrophic spinal pachymeningitis, 294–296
　　spinal cord herniation, 291–293
　　spinal CSF leakage, 286–291
　　subdural hematoma, 293–294
　spinal meningitis
　　bacterial, 272–274
　　empyema, 275
　　Guillain–Barré syndrome, 279–281
　　neurosarcoidosis, 276, 278–279
　　subdural abscess, 275
　　tuberculous, 276, 277, 278
Meningeosis carcinomatosa
　manifestations, 282
　with scrotal teratocarcinoma, 283–284
Meningeosis leucemica, 284, 285, 286
Meningeosis neoplastica, 280, 282–286
Meninges

Index

dura (pachymeninx) layer, 29
MRI, 30–31
tubular prolongations, of dura, 29, 30
Meningiomas
   diagnosis, 232–234
   origin, 231
   outcome, 235
   prevalence, 232
   symptoms, 232
   therapy, 233–235
Meningocele
   cervical, 141, 144
   Chiari I malformation, 140, 143
   lipomyelomeningocele, 142, 144–146
   split cord malformations, 146–147
   terminal myelocystocele, 148
Monomelic amyotrophy (MMA), 393–394
MPNST. *See* Malignant peripheral nerve sheath tumours (MPNST)
Mucopolysaccharidoses, 132–134
Multi-Echo Data Image Combination (MEDIC), 53, 54
Multiple Echo Recombined Gradient Echo (MERGE), 53, 54
Multiple myeloma, 211–212, 216
Multiple sclerosis (MS)
   clinically isolated syndromes, 335–336
      cervical trauma, 341
      hyperintense lesion, 343
      swollen lesion, 340
      thoracic pain, 342
   diagnosis, 334
   McDonald criteria, 334–335
   MRI criteria, 334–335
   primary progressive, 336
   relapsing-remitting
      acute partial transverse myelitis, 344
      gait disturbance, 337
   secondary progressive, 337, 338
   STIR, 337, 339
Myelitis, 326–327
Myelography, 1–2
   contraindications, 111–113
   description, 107
   procedure and imaging features
      dose limits, 108
      extradural process, 109–110
      intradural extramedullary space-occupying lesions, 111
      intradural intramedullary space-occupying lesions, 111, 112
      standard lumbar examination, 108
Myelomeningocele, 149–151
Myelon compression syndromes
   cervical disc herniation, 192–197
   cervical spondylosis, 193–194, 198–200
   spinal cord compression
      extradural or intradural/extramedullary lesions, 188
      location of, 190–191
      time course of, 189–190
Myelopathy, extramedullary
   cause of, 309–311

N

Narrowed intervertebral foramen, aetiology of, 179
Neoplastic meningeosis, 280, 282–286
Nerve roots, 33–35, 203
Neurofibromas, 235–236
Neurofibromatosis, 131
Neuromyelitis optica (NMO)
   hyperintense lesion, 352
   intense contrast enhancement, 351
   perimetric investigation, 350
   second spinal attack, 353
   spectrum disorders, 346, 350
   spinal lesions, extension and enhancement, 354–355
Neurosarcoidosis, 276, 278–279

O

Occipital assimilation, of atlas, 126
Occipital bone malformations, 122–125
Occipital condyle fractures, 245–247
Odontoid fractures, 255–258
Odontoid ligaments, 24
Odontoid process, malformation of, 126–130
Open spinal dysraphisms (OSD)
   vs. closed spinal dysraphism, 138
   incidence, 148
   myelomeningocele, 149–151
Os odontoideum, 12, 15
Osteoblastoma, 206, 208
Osteochondroma, 208
Osteogenesis imperfecta, 133
Osteoid osteoma, 206, 208
Osteosarcoma, 215

P

Pain
   back pain (*see* Back pain)
   in spinal tumours, 203
Paired lateral atlanto-axial joints, 21
Paragangliomas, 237

Parainfectious myelitis, 330–331
Parallel imaging approach, image acquisition, 69, 70
Paraneoplastic tractopathy, 376
Partial Fourier approach, image acquisition, 69, 70
Patient motion artefacts, 73–74
Pediatric cervical spine, 118
PGDB. *See* Adult polyglucosan body disease (PGBD)
Phase contrast MRI, CSF flow, 94–96
Phase encoding process, 60
Pilocytic astrocytomas, 403, 404
Platybasia, 122
Poliomyelitis, 324, 325, 392–393
Posterior longitudinal ligament, 24
Posterior spinal artery (PSA)
 clinical symptoms, 441, 443
 extrinsic spinal cord arteries, 437
Post-myelographic CT, 110. *See also* Myelography
Primary lateral sclerosis, 381, 383
Primary progressive MS (PPMS), 336
Progressive muscular atrophy (PMA), 393
Proton density weighting, 50–51
Protrusion, 176
Psoriasis arthritis, TNF, 348
Pulse sequence, MRI, 46–47

R
Radial readouts, 68
Radicular compression syndromes
 acquired lumbal canal stenosis, 182–188
 degenerative vertebral endplate changes, 174, 175
 disc herniation, 174, 176–182
 foraminal stenosis
  facet joint degeneration, 181
  foraminal epidural fat, classification of, 180
  juxtaarticular cysts, 181–182
  narrowed intervertebral foramen, 179
  spondylolisthesis, 181, 183, 184
  spondylolysis, 181, 185
 intervertebral disc degeneration, 172–173
 MRI, 169–172
 and neurological deficits, 168, 171
 pathophysiological and clinical aspects, 167–169
Radicular pain, 161–162, 165, 166
Radiculomedullary artery. *See also* Artery of Adamkiewicz
 anterior spinal, 415, 416
 arteriovenous malformations, 419, 420
 dural AVF, 423
 vascular anatomy, 412–413, 416
Radiculopial artery. *See* Radiculomedullary artery
Radiotherapy
 intramedullary spinal cord tumors, 399
 spinal cord astrocytomas, 404
Readout methods, 67–68
Referred pain, 163, 165, 167
Relapsing-remitting MS (RRMS)
 acute partial transverse myelitis, 344
 gait disturbance, 337
Renal cell carcinoma, osteolytic metastasis of, 220–221
Repetition time, 46
Representative inherited syndromes, instability associated with
 achondroplasia, 133
 Down syndrome, 129–131
 juvenile rheumatoid arthritis, 131–132
 Larsen syndrome, 133
 mucopolysaccharidoses, 132–134
 neurofibromatosis, 131
 osteogenesis imperfecta, 133
 spondyloepiphyseal dysplasia, 133
Resonance frequency, 46

S
Sacral fractures
 classification, 264–266
 diagnosis, 266
 origin, 264
 outcome, 267
 prevalence, 266
 symptoms, 266
 therapy, 266
Sacrococcygeal teratoma, 218
Sarcoidosis, 276
 intraparenchymatous cerebral perivascular enhancements, 362, 364
 meningovascular syphilis, 362, 364
 paraparesis, 363
SCDSC. *See* Subacute combined degeneration of the spinal cord (SCDSC)
Schistosomiasis, 313–314, 329
Schwannomas, 235–237
SCI. *See* Spinal cord injury (SCI)
Secondary progressive MS (SPMS), 337, 338
Sequestration, 176
Short tau inversion recovery (STIR), 78–80, 337, 339

Index

Signal-to-noise ratio (SNR)
    definition, 54
    factors affecting, 55
    relative, 56
Solitary plasmacytoma, 211–215
Space available for the cord (SAC), 119
Spina bifida, 134
    caudal regression syndrome, 154–156
    filum terminale, 152–154
    meningocele
        cervical, 141, 144
        Chiari I malformation, 140, 143
        lipomyelomeningocele, 142, 144–146
        split cord malformations, 146–147
        terminal myelocystocele, 148
    spinal dysraphisms (*see* Spinal dysraphisms)
Spinal and bulbar muscular atrophy (SBMA), 390, 391
Spinal angiography
    DSA, 414–416
    MRI, MRA, and CTA, 416, 419
Spinal arachnoid cysts, 97–99
Spinal canal structures
    meninges, 29–31
    nerve roots, 33–35
    spaces, 31–33
Spinal cord, 5
    cervical spine (*see* Cervical spine)
    compression, 203
        extradural or intradural/extramedullary lesions, 188
        location, 190–191
        time course, 189–190
    formation, 118
    intervertebral discs, 17–18, 20
    joints (*see* Joints)
    ligaments, 24–26
    lumbar spine, 17, 18
    thoracic spine, 16–17
    vertebral body
        appearance, 7–11
        epiphysis, 6
        MRI, 8–12
        non-ossified epiphysis, 6, 8
    vertebral column, 6
Spinal cord atrophy
    anatomical measurements, 380, 381
    circumscript hyperintense lesion, 379, 380
    Friedreich's ataxia, 380, 382–383
    hyperintense signal changes, axial T2 WI, 385
    lower brainstem, FLAIR and T2 WI images, 385
    PGBD, 384
    primary lateral sclerosis, 381, 383
    Wallerian degeneration, 379, 381
    WMC, axial T2 WI, 386
Spinal cord infarction
    aetiology, 439–440
    clinical symptoms
        anterior spinal artery, 440, 441
        artery of Adamkiewicz, 441, 444
        lower motor neuron disease, 445, 448
        man-in-the-barrel syndrome, 445–447
        posterior spinal artery, 441, 443
        sulcal artery syndrome, 443, 445
    MR imaging, 450
        conus medullaris, 448, 449
        differential diagnosis, 447
    vascular anatomy
        extrinsic and intrinsic system, 438
        extrinsic spinal cord arteries, 436–437
        radiculomedullary artery, 435–437
        sulcal arteries, 439
Spinal cord injury (SCI)
    diagnosis, 269
    origin, 267
    outcome, 269
    prevalence, 267
    symptoms, 267–268
    therapy, 269
Spinal CSF leakage, 286–291
Spinal dysraphisms, 117. *See also* Closed spinal dysraphisms (CSD); Open spinal dysraphisms (OSD)
    Chiari II malformation, 138
    CT scanning, 137, 138
    description, 135
    MRI, 135
    MR myelography, 137
    neurosonography, 135
Spinal meningitis
    bacterial, 272–274
    empyema, 275
    Guillain–Barré syndrome, 279–281
    neurosarcoidosis, 276, 278–279
    subdural abscess, 275
    tuberculous meningitis , 276, 277, 278
Spinal muscular atrophy (SMA), 390–392
Spinal trauma
    cervical spine
        diagnosis, 244–245
        origin, 244
        prevalence, 244
        symptoms, 244
        therapy and outcome, 245

Spinal trauma (cont.)
craniocervical junction
atlantoccipital dislocation, 247–248
occipital condyle fractures, 245–247
sacral fractures
classification, 264–266
diagnosis, 266
origin, 264
outcome, 267
prevalence, 266
symptoms, 266
therapy, 266
subaxial cervical spine
type A fractures, 259–262
type B fractures, 262–263
type C fractures, 263–264
traumatic spinal cord injury
diagnosis, 269
origin, 267
outcome, 269
prevalence, 267
symptoms, 267–268
therapy, 269
upper cervical spine
atlas fractures, 249–252
atypical fractures of axis, 258–259
fractures of axis, 254–255
odontoid fractures, 255–258
traumatic atlantoaxial
dislocations, 252–255
Spin echo, 52
Spinocerebellar tracts, topography of, 305
Spinothalamic tracts, topography of, 304
Spiral readouts, 68
Split cord malformations, 146–147
Spoiling technique, 48
Spondylodiscitis, 160, 163–165
Spondyloepiphyseal dysplasia, 133
Spondylolisthesis, 181, 183, 184
Spondylolysis, 181, 185
Spontaneous intracranial hypotension
(SIH), 102, 104
Standard lumbar examination, 108
STIR. See Short tau inversion recovery (STIR)
Straight leg raising, 161
Subacute combined degeneration of the
spinal cord (SCDSC)
copper deficiency, 373–376
neurological signs and symptoms, 371
pathogenesis, 370
pattern, 370
vitamin B12 deficiency
atacic paraparesis, 374
numbness, 372
patchy hyperintense signal changes, 373

Subarachnoid space, 33
Subaxial cervical spine
type A fractures, 259–262
type B fractures, 262–263
type C fractures, 263–264
Subdural abscess, 275
Subdural empyema, 275
Subdural hematoma, 293–294
Subdural space, 32
Sulcal artery
clinical symptoms, 443, 445
vascular anatomy, 439
Sulcocommissural artery. See Sulcal artery
Syphilis, 326
Syringomyelia, 308
Systemic lupus erythematosus (SLE)
Behcet's disease, 359, 361
gray matter myelitis, 359
white matter myelitis, 359

T
Tabes dorsalis, 333–334
Tectorial membrane, 24
Temozolomide, 403–404
Terminal myelocystocele, 135–137, 148
Thoracic spine, 16–17
Time-of-flight angiography, 85, 86
Time-resolved angiography with interleaved
stochastic trajectories
(TWIST), 86
Time-resolved imaging of contrast
kinetics (TRICKS), 86
Time-resolved MRA, advantage of, 86
Toxocara infection, 329
Tractography, 89
Traumatic spinal cord injury (SCI)
ASIA Impairment Scale, 269
diagnosis, 269
origin, 267
outcome, 269
prevalence, 267
symptoms, 267–268
therapy, 269
Traumatic spondylolisthesis. See Hangman
fracture
Tuberculous spinal
meningitis, 276, 277, 278
Tumor necrosis factor (TNF)
cranial MRI, 349
Crohn's disease, 347
psoriasis arthritis, 348
Turbo spin echo (TSE) readouts.
See Fast spin-echo (FSE) readouts
T1 weighting, 48

Index

T2 weighting, 48, 49
T2* weighting, 51–53

U
Uncovertebral joints, 23
Upper cervical spine
  atlas fractures, 249–252
  atypical fractures of axis, 258–259
  fractures of axis, 254–255
  odontoid fractures, 255–258
  traumatic atlantoaxial dislocations, 252–255

V
Vacuolar myelopathy (VM), 332
  neurological signs and symptoms
    differential diagnosis, 378–379
    HIV-infection, 377–378
  pathogenesis, 377
  pattern, 377
Variants, 429, 432
Varicella zoster virus (VZV), 320–321
Vascular anatomy
  arteries
    intra-arterial DSA images, 412, 413
    median sacral artery, 412, 414
    radiculomedullary artery, 412–413, 416
    sulcocommissural branches, CTA, 413, 417
    vertebral artery, 412, 415
  spinal cord infarction
    extrinsic and intrinsic system, 438
    extrinsic spinal cord arteries, 436–437
    radiculomedullary artery, 435–437
    sulcal arteries, 439
  veins, 414, 418

Vascular endothelial growth factor (VEGF), 405–406
Vascularization, of spinal cord, 437
Vascular tumors
  hypervascular metastasis, 426–428
  intradural vascular tumors, 428–429
Vertebral canal, 11
Vertebral hemangioma, 206, 207
Vertebral venous plexus, internal, 202
Vitamin B12 deficiency
  atrophic gastritis, 371
  numbness, 372
  patchy hyperintense signal changes, 373
  risk factors, 376
  SCDSC, 372, 374
Vitamin E deficiency
  neurological signs and symptoms, 376–377
  pathogenesis, 376
  pattern, 376
VM. See Vacuolar myelopathy (VM)
von Hippel Lindau (VHL), 405–406

W
Wackenheim line, 22, 23
Wackenheim's clivus baseline, 122
Wallerian degeneration, 379, 381
WBB surgical staging system, 204, 205
West Nile virus, 324–325
White matter tracts, 303–306

Z
Zygapophyses, 10

Printing: Ten Brink, Meppel, The Netherlands
Binding: Ten Brink, Meppel, The Netherlands